ADVANCES IN
CARDIOVASCULAR NURSING

Sr. aloysius

gift 1976

Titles in the *Contemporary Nursing Series*

A compilation of articles selected
and reprinted from the *American Journal of Nursing,
Nursing Research,* and *Nursing Outlook*

Contemporary Nursing Series

ADVANCES IN
CARDIOVASCULAR NURSING

compiled by
Andrea B. O'Connor, R.N.

The American Journal of Nursing Company
New York

FOREWORD

This present publication is the thirteenth book in the CONTEM-PORARY NURSING SERIES. Launched in 1970 by the Educational Services Division of The American Journal of Nursing Company, the series has covered a wide range of subjects, ranging from such areas as nursing in cardiovascular and respiratory conditions to the broader issues of the expanded role of the nurse and the nurse in community mental health.

As readers of the series know, these paperback books are collections of selected articles in a particular subject area, all of the material having originally been published in one of The American Journal of Nursing Company's three periodicals: the *American Journal of Nursing, Nursing Outlook,* and *Nursing Research.* The selection of articles for inclusion is not random. Instead, the three magazines are carefully searched to identify the best and most appropriate material, the articles are subgrouped within each volume for the reader's convenience, and the final product is a compact reference source for the nurse who wishes to broaden or update her knowledge in a given subject area.

The response to the CONTEMPORARY NURSING SERIES has been both enthusiastic and gratifying. This encourages the Journal Company to believe that, through these books, it is continuing to expand its services to the nursing profession. In so doing, the Company is also accomplishing the goal established for it by its founders in 1900: "to present the most useful facts, the most progressive thought, and the latest news the profession has to offer in the most attractive form that can be secured."—PHILIP E. DAY, R.N., Publishing Director, The American Journal of Nursing Company.

PREFACE

Advances in Cardiovascular Nursing is the thirteenth book in the CONTEMPORARY NURSING SERIES and the second volume to be concerned with the nursing care of patients with cardiovascular diseases. Since the early days of the coronary care unit, nurses have assumed and sustained a primary role in the care of such patients. Knowledge and technology have expanded rapidly, and nurses must keep abreast of these developments in order to acquire, perfect, and maintain their skills. Directed toward practicing nurses, nursing students, and their instructors, this book explores aspects of the broad field of cardiovascular nursing, with special emphasis on intervention and therapy.

Drawn from material printed in the Journal Company's three publications, this compilation contains the most up-to-date information about assessment and intervention in cardiac care, the pathophysiologic bases of therapy, the use of drugs in the treatment of cardiovascular disorders, and new developments in cardiac surgery. Attention has also been given to the care of patients with hypertension and special considerations in the nursing management of peripheral vascular disease. While this book is by no means comprehensive, it does represent the latest thinking of experts across the country. As in the previous books in the CONTEMPORARY NURSING SERIES, the biographies accompanying the articles identify each author's background and position at the time the article was originally written and published.

Contents

Section I Cardiac Care: Assessment Techniques

The initial assessment and ongoing monitoring of the cardiac patient's condition are vital elements in therapy, requiring astute nursing observation and the skilled use of increasingly complex technology. The techniques and equipment described in the articles in this section have applicability to the care of patients with acute cardiovascular diseases, as well as to the care of other critically ill patients.

From the *American Journal of Nursing* 72:1242-1246, July 1972.

Auscultation of Heart Sounds

SISTER JANET LEHMANN

Nurses have long been using stethoscopes to listen to the heart. Most often, however, they were listening for the rate and character of the apical pulse. They heard, but seldom identified, heart sounds. Today, the nurse, as the person most consistently at the patient's bedside, can and ought to develop skills in cardiac auscultation so that changes in cardiac sounds, which may indicate a need for therapeutic intervention, can be detected early.

Auscultation of the heart is a skill which involves practice in listening for specific heart sounds and murmurs. It also involves an understanding of the basic facts of heart sound production. The beginning listener must know in what area of the chest wall particular sounds are transmitted and must understand the characteristics of sound that determine which end piece of a stethoscope is needed to pick up each sound.

CHARACTERISTICS OF SOUND

For sound waves to be produced, there must be an object that is in motion, for it is the vibratory movement of the object that initiates the sound wave cycles(1). Four aspects of sound are important to consider: frequency and pitch; intensity and loudness; quality; and duration.

The frequency of a vibration is the number of wave cycles generated per second by the vibrating body(2). This determines the pitch of the sound. The higher the frequency, that is, the greater number of wave cycles per second, the higher is the pitch of a particular sound. Low frequency vibrations produce low-pitched sounds(3).

The intensity of the vibrations and the loudness of the sound are dif-

SR. LEHMANN *is a cardiovascular nursing specialist at St. Joseph's Hospital in Paterson, N.J. She was graduated from All Souls Hospital School of Nursing, Morristown, N.J., received her B.S.N. degree from Seton Hall University, South Orange, N.J., and her M.S.N. degree in cardiovascular nursing from St. Louis University, Mo.*

1

ferent phenomena but, for our purposes, they will be considered synonymous. The intensity of sound is related to the height or amplitude of the sound wave produced by the vibrating object(4). The height of the wave, in turn, depends on the energy with which the object vibrates. Vibrations of great energy produce waves of high amplitude and are heard as loud sounds, for example, the clanging of cymbals. A low energy system produces waves of low amplitude which are heard as soft sounds, such as the light tapping of one's fingertips on a table top.

Two sounds with the same degree of loudness and the same pitch, but coming from different sources are distinguished by their quality. Just as the same note, produced with the same degree of loudness, from a violin and from a piano can be distinguished by their difference in quality, sounds of equal loudness and pitch from different organs, such as the heart and the lungs, can be differentiated(5).

Duration refers to the number of continuous vibrations. As the energy given to the vibrating system is diminished by frictional resistance, the duration of the vibratory movement is reduced. The vibratory motion is then said to have been "damped." Vibrations coming from the internal organs of the body are damped by the soft tissues that cover these organs(4).

There are four major heart sounds, each with diverging theories to explain their cause and production. Two basic mechanisms operate to cause the vibrations in the cardiovascular system: sudden acceleration or deceleration of blood and turbulent blood flow. The opening and closing of the heart valves influence sudden acceleration and deceleration of blood. The vibrations, generated by the sudden acceleration or deceleration of blood, tend to be of a higher intensity and frequency and therefore produce louder sounds than the vibrations caused by turbulent blood flow. In general, the high intensity and high frequency cardiac sounds are called the heart sounds, and the low intensity and low frequency cardiac sounds are called the heart murmurs(4).

The ability to hear these sounds on the chest wall depends both on the intensity and frequency of the vibrations and on the use of the stethoscope. The diaphragm of the stethoscope is used to hear high-pitched sounds, which include both components of the first heart sound, both components of the second heart sound, and the ejection clicks and opening snaps[1] of the heart valves. The bell of the stethoscope is used to hear

---

[1] Ejection clicks are extra sounds which occur early in systole, close to the onset of right or left ventricular systolic ejection. Opening snaps are sounds produced by a thickened or otherwise altered mitral or tricuspid valve as it opens. Normally there is no sound when these valves open.

2

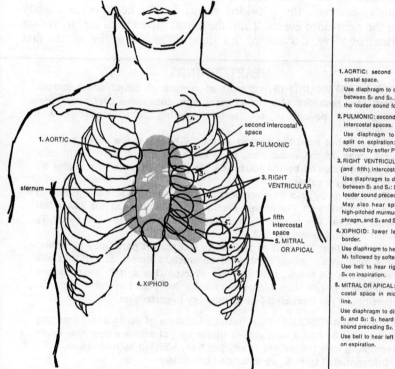

second intercostal space

1. AORTIC

sternum

2. PULMONIC

3. RIGHT VENTRICULAR

fifth intercostal space

5. MITRAL OR APICAL

4. XIPHOID

1. AORTIC: second right intercostal space.
   Use diaphragm to differentiate between S_1 and S_2. S_2 heard as the louder sound following S_1.

2. PULMONIC: second (and third) intercostal spaces.
   Use diaphragm to detect S_2 split on expiration: louder A_2 followed by softer P_2.

3. RIGHT VENTRICULAR: fourth (and fifth) intercostal spaces.
   Use diaphragm to differentiate between S_1 and S_2: S_1 heard as louder sound preceding S_2.
   May also hear split S_2 and high-pitched murmurs with diaphragm, and S_3 and S_4 with bell.

4. XIPHOID: lower left sternal border.
   Use diaphragm to hear S_1 split: M_1 followed by softer T_1.
   Use bell to hear right S_3 and S_4 on inspiration.

5. MITRAL OR APICAL: fifth intercostal space in midclavicular line.
   Use diaphragm to differentiate S_1 and S_2: S_1 heard as louder sound preceding S_2.
   Use bell to hear left S_3 and S_4 on expiration.

A suggested sequence for auscultating heart sounds is to proceed from the aortic area to the mitral or apical area.

3

low-pitched sounds, which include third and fourth heart sounds and most murmurs(6).

FIRST HEART SOUND (s₁) The first heart sound (s₁) is thought to be caused by mitral and tricuspid valve closure. Right ventricular contraction follows tricuspid valve closure; left ventricular contraction follows mitral valve closure. The closure of the two valves occurs *almost* simultaneously; however, the left-sided events in the heart occur slightly before the right-sided events. Thus, the mitral valve closes slightly before the tricuspid valve. Because of this slight difference in timing, the first

---

HEART SOUNDS

FIRST HEART SOUND (S_1): Result of closure of mitral and tricuspid valves. May be heard with closed diaphragm chestpiece over entire precordium with patient in any position during both inspiration and expiration.

Differentiated from the second sound (S_2) best at the aortic and the apical areas. At the aortic area, S_2 is more prominent: S_1 is heard as a soft sound followed by the louder S_2. At the apical area, the louder S_1 is followed by a softer S_2.

The split of S_1 into its components parts—mitral (M_1) and tricuspid (T_1)—is heard with the closed diaphragm chestpiece at the lower left sternal border. The louder M_1 is followed immediately by the softer T_2 (which is then followed by S_2).

Abnormalities: The split of S_1 into its component parts may be abnormally long with such a right-sided conduction defect as right bundle branch block. Or the S_1 split may be reversed (the soft T_1 heard before the louder M_1) with such a left-sided mechanical defect as mitral stenosis. Intensity of T_1 is increased with pulmonary hypertension.

SECOND HEART SOUND (S_2): Result of closure of aortic and pulmonary valves. May be heard with closed diaphragm chestpiece over the entire precordium with the patient in any position. Affected by respiration.

Differentiated from S_1, as described previously.

The split of S_2 into its component parts—aortic (A_2) and pulmonic (P_2)—is wider than the S_1 split and is heard with the closed diaphragm chestpiece at the pulmonic area during inspiration. Here, the louder A_2 is followed by a softer P_2.

Abnormalities: The S_2 split may be abnormally long in right bundle branch block, pulmonic stenosis, atrioseptal defect, mitral insufficiency, and ventricular septal defect. Paradoxical splitting, in which S_2 is split during expiration instead of inspiration, may occur with left bundle branch block, aortic stenosis, patent ductus arteriosis, and, occasionally, coronary insufficiency. Intensity of A_2 may increase with systemic hypertension; intensity of P_2 may increase with pulmonary hypertension.

heart sound can actually be "split" into two components—the mitral (M_1) and the tricuspid (T_1).

The vibrations generated by mitral valve closure are of higher intensity and frequency than those generated by tricuspid valve closure, and the sound produced can be heard over much of the precordium. The mitral component is actually the main component of the first heart sound heard at the apex(7).

Vibrations of the tricuspid valve closure, on the other hand, have a very low intensity. This sound is poorly transmitted over the precordium,

---

Detection of P_2 at the apical area usually occurs only in pathologic conditions.

THIRD HEART SOUND (S_3): Result of vibration produced during ventricular filling. It is a dull, soft sound heard best with the bell chestpiece at the apical area at the beginning of expiration with the patient recumbent on his left side. Occurs 0.12 to 0.20 seconds after A_2 and may be picked up by listening for the word "Ken-tuc-ky."

$$S_1 \quad S_2 \quad S_3$$

Abnormalities: S_3 normally heard only in children and young adults; in older adults, the presence of S_3 may indicate myocardial failure or atrioventricular valve incompetence and is called a ventricular gallop. Also, in pathologic states, the S_3 may continue to be heard instead of disappearing when the patient is sitting or standing.

A left S_3 may be heard at the apical area. In an older adult, a left S_3 may indicate left-sided cardiac failure. A right S_3 may be heard at the xiphoid or lower left sternal border. In an older adult, a right S_3 may indicate right-sided cardiac failure.

FOURTH HEART SOUND (S_4): Result of recoil of vibrations between the atria and ventricles following atrial contraction. It is a very soft sound heard best with the bell chestpiece at the apical area during expiration with the patient recumbent. It is rarely heard in normal patients. When present, it occurs immediately before S_1; since S_1 is not normally split at the apical area, the suggestion of a split S_1 heard with the bell chestpiece at the apical area may indicate S_4. The listener should listen for the word, "Ten-nes-see" to detect S_4.

$$S_4 \quad S_1 \quad S_2$$

Abnormalities: A right S_4 heard at the xiphoid or the lower left sternal border may indicate increased right ventricular resistance to filling, as in pulmonic stenosis, primary pulmonary hypertension, and cor pulmonale. A left S_4 heard at the apical area may indicate left ventricular resistance to filling, as in hypertensive cardiovascular disease, coronary artery disease, cardiomyopathy, and aortic stenosis.

and therefore is not usually heard at the apex, but it is heard at the lower left sternal border. Thus, it is at the lower left sternal border that the two components of the first heart sound can be distinguished. In this area, the mitral component will be heard as a louder sound than the soft tricuspid component(8).

Splitting of the first and second heart sounds is more evident with the diaphragm chestpiece than with the bell chestpiece. In order to hear the two components of the first heart sound, the diaphragm of the stethoscope should be applied firmly to the skin at the lower left sternal border(9).

The first heart sound may be abnormally split as the result of electrical or mechanical causes. With either an electrical or mechanical delay, the two ventricles may contract at different times. For example, in an electrical delay in the conduction pathway to the ventricular muscle, as in right bundle branch block, the time between the two components of the first heart sound increases. Although an abnormally long split may be present with right bundle branch block, it is rarely present with left bundle branch block(10).

If there is a mechanical delay in the closing of the mitral valve, as in mitral stenosis in which the tricuspid valve closes before the mitral valve, there may be a reversal of the splitting sounds. In this situation the soft tricuspid component will be heard before the loud mitral component of the heart sound(11).

The first heart sound is normally louder than the second heart sound at the apex. And, the second heart sound is normally louder than the first heart sound at the second right intercostal space. It is in this latter region that the first two heart sounds (S_1 and S_2) can usually be differentiated most easily.

SECOND HEART SOUND (S_2) The second heart sound (S_2) is the result of vibrations produced by aortic and pulmonic valve closures. Right ventricular ejection time is slightly longer than left ventricular ejection time. Thus, the vibrations set up by the aortic valve closing (left side) will occur before those of the pulmonic valve closing (right side).

The closure sound generated by the aortic valve is generally heard over the entire precordium. The vibrations caused by pulmonic closure are poorly transmitted and are usually heard at the second left intercostal space. It is in this area that the splitting of the second heart sound into its component parts will be heard best; the louder aortic component (A_2) will be followed by the softer pulmonic sound (P_2). However, in pathologic states, the pulmonic closure sounds may be detected at the apex(12).

The components of the second heart sound are normally affected by respiration in a phenomenon called physiologic splitting, in which the difference in sounds is more apparent during inspiration than expiration.

During inspiration, the intrathoracic pressure decreases, which increases the venous return into the intrathoracic veins and the right atrium. Because of this, the right ventricular and end-diastolic volume is increased, and right ventricular contraction takes a little longer, which delays the pulmonic valve closure. However, filling of the left ventricle does not increase and, in fact, may actually decrease during inspiration(13). Therefore, left ventricular contraction is unaltered or slightly shortened during inspiration, aortic valve closure occurs before the pulmonic valve closure, and the split is heard on inspiration.

On the other hand, during expiration, there is increased filling of the left ventricle and contraction of the left ventricle takes a little longer. The aortic closure sound during expiration generally occurs at the same time as the pulmonic closure sounds, so that splitting heard over the pulmonic area during inspiration disappears during expiration(13).

Variations in the normal splitting pattern may occur in some pathologic states. Although there are other deviations from the normal splitting pattern of the second heart sound that might occur, only paradoxical splitting and fixed splitting will be considered here.

Paradoxical splitting of the second heart sound is a reversal of the normal splitting pattern in response to respiration. It occurs when there is a delay in aortic valve closure due to such situations as aortic stenosis, patent ductus arteriosus, and left bundle branch block. Because of this delay, the pulmonic component of the second heart sound may occur first. During inspiration when the pulmonic closure sound normally occurs slightly after the aortic closure sound, these two closure sounds come closer together and may fuse(14). Then during expiration, instead of the two components of the second heart sound fusing, in paradoxical splitting, the sounds are more widely split.

In fixed splitting, the split in the two components of the second heart sound is unaffected by respiration. The two components are heard with equal intensity and duration during both inspiration and expiration. Fixed splitting is commonly present in atrioseptal defects(15).

THIRD HEART SOUND (S_3) Third heart sound is synonymous with such terms as ventricular gallop, early diastolic rapid ventricular filling sound, protodiastolic gallop, early diastolic gallop, and the physiologic third heart sound (S_3). The third heart sound occurs during early diastole, right after the second heart sound, and is thought to be caused by vibrations produced during left ventricular filling. As a person becomes older, apparently there is either a lessening of sound transmission to the surface of the body or a decrease in the actual formation of this sound, for it is normally not heard in older adults, but may be heard in children and young adults(16).

When listening for the low-pitched third heart sound, it is necessary to use the bell endpiece of the stethoscope. This endpiece should be placed lightly against the chest wall. Too much pressure will cause "damping" of those low-pitched sounds and may obliterate them completely(17).

The third heart sound is best heard in the apical area with the patient in a recumbent position or turned on his left side. Sitting up tends to diminish this sound or cause it to disappear. The intensity of a normal third heart sound is related to the respiratory cycle; it is best heard at the beginning of expiration. Exercise also tends to increase the intensity of this sound. Accommodation to this sound apparently occurs very rapidly. Thus the third heart sound is best heard when the examiner initially begins to listen at the apical area(18). Andreoli and her associates suggest listening for the word, "Ken-tuc'-ky" when trying to determine the
$$S_1 \quad S_2 \quad S_3$$
presence of a third heart sound(19).

An abnormal third heart sound may be produced by various pathologic states in either the left or right ventricle. As opposed to a normal physiologic third heart sound which disappears when a patient sits up or stands, a pathologic third heart sound persists regardless of the patient's position. Generally, when the patient's condition improves, the third heart sound disappears. A persistent third heart sound, particularly in an older adult, may indicate an unfavorable prognosis(20).

Mitral regurgitation tends to produce a left-sided third heart sound because blood flow into the ventricle is rapid and under pressure. A left-sided third heart sound may also indicate left ventricular failure due to such conditions as coronary artery disease, hypertension, or aortic valve disease(20). Left-sided third heart sounds are heard at the apical region with the bell endpiece of the stethoscope. They are loudest on expiration.

A right-sided third heart sound may be indicative of right-sided cardiac failure. Since pulmonary hypertension and pulmonary emboli result in right-sided failure, these conditions need to be considered in the presence of a right-sided third heart sound(20).

Right-sided third heart sounds are heard at the lower left sternal border with the bell endpiece of the stethoscope. These sounds are loudest on inspiration.

FOURTH HEART SOUND (S_4) The fourth heart sound (S_4) occurs during the last third of diastole, immediately before the first heart sound, and is believed to be caused by a recoil of vibrations between the atria and ventricles following atrial contraction. These vibrations are of such low intensity and frequency that they often cannot be heard with a stethoscope(21).

The fourth heart sound is an atrial sound and may be referred to as atrial gallop, presystolic gallop, or the physiologic fourth heart sound. Three points are important to remember when considering the significance of an atrial sound: atrial sounds are usually not heard in normal patients; they are the result of increased resistance to filling; and, their presence does not imply cardiac failure(22).

When listening for atrial sounds, it is necessary to apply the bell end piece of the stethoscope lightly to the chest wall in the apical area. Andreoli and others suggest listening for the word "Ten' nes-see" when

$$S_4 \quad S_1 \quad S_2$$

trying to determine the presence of a fourth heart sound(19).

Since the first heart sound is not normally split at the apex, the suggestion of a split first heart sound in this region should lead one to consider the possibility of an atrial sound. However, if the splitting of the first sound is picked up with a stethoscope using the diaphragm, the sound heard is probably not an atrial sound. It is more likely that the sound is a ventricular systolic ejection sound(23).

Left atrial sounds are best heard at the apex with the patient in a recumbent position. Sitting or standing tends to lessen the intensity of this sound so that it can no longer be heard. When the patient is turned on his left side, the left atrial sound will diminish during inspiration. Even when the patient is not on his left side, it frequently happens that a left atrial sound is heard only on expiration(23). Left atrial sounds become audible when there is an increased resistance to filling in the left ventricle, such as occurs in hypertensive cardiac disease, coronary artery disease, and aortic stenosis(22).

Right atrial sounds are best heard just to the left of the lower sternal border. A right atrial sound, in contrast to a left atrial sound, is generally loudest during inspiration. Right atrial sounds can be heard in conditions resulting in increased resistance to filling of the right ventricle, such as severe pulmonic stenosis and cor pulmonale(22).

Each practitioner will develop his own sequence of steps as he listens to the heart sounds and murmurs. It seems advisable to repeat the same sequence with each patient in order to develop the skills and correlated thought patterns that auscultation requires.

Before auscultation of the heart, as much extraneous noise as possible should be eliminated from the environment. Also, the listener must understand the effects of respiration and the patient's position on the heart sounds and consider these factors during auscultation.

Finally, Hurst and Schlant recommend that a problem solving technique be used during cardiac auscultation. One should think and then listen selectively for each sound. When he hears the sound, he should concentrate on listening for a split(24).

If the examiner is unable to distinguish the first from the second heart sound, it is often useful to palpate a carotid artery. The first heart sound coincides with the initial upstroke of the carotid pulse(25).

Learning the art of cardiac auscultation takes much time, practice, and patience on the part of the learner. But, a nurse who can learn to recognize the basic heart sounds and detect changes and abnormalities in them greatly enhances her assessment abilities.

REFERENCES

1. WHITE, H. E. *Modern College Physics.* 4th ed. Princeton, N.J., D. Van Nostrand Co., 1962, p. 250.
2. *Ibid.*, p. 253.
3. *Ibid.*, p. 257.
4. RUSHMER, R. F. *Cardiovascular Dynamics*, 3d ed. Philadelphia, W .B. Saunders Co., 1970, p. 303.
5. SEARS, F. W., AND ZEMANSKY, M. W. *College Physics,* 3d ed. Reading, Mass., Addison-Wesley Publishing Co., 1960, p. 438.
6. HURST, J. W., AND SCHLANT, R. C. Auscultation of the heart. IN *The Heart*, edited by J. Willis Hurst and R. Bruce Logue, 2d ed. New York, McGraw-Hill Book Co., 1970, p. 232.
7. RAVIN, ABE. *Auscultation of the Heart,* 2d ed. Chicago. Year Book Medical Publishers, 1967, p. 41.
8. LEONARD, JAMES, AND KROETZ, F. W. *Examination of the Heart: Part 4. Auscultation.* New York, American Heart Association, 1967, p. 8.
9. HURST AND SCHLANT, *op. cit.*, p. 234.
10. LEATHAM, AUBREY. First and second heart sounds. IN *The Heart,* edited by J. Willis Hurst and R. Bruce Logue, 2d ed. New York, McGraw-Hill Book Co., 1970, pp. 241-242.
11. *Ibid.*, p. 240.
12. LEONARD AND KROETZ, *op. cit.*, p. 12.
13. RAVIN, *op. cit.*, p. 49.
14. LEONARD AND KROETZ, *op. cit.*, pp. 15-16.
15. RAVIN, *op. cit.*, p. 57.
16. *Ibid.*, p. 81.
17. WESTURA, E. Personal communication, 1971.
18. RAVIN, *op. cit.*, p. 60.
19. ANDREOLI, KATHLEEN G., AND OTHERS. *Comprehensive Cardiac Care*, St. Louis, C. V. Mosby Co., 1968, p. 12.
20. RAVIN, *op. cit.*, p. 83.
21. RUSHMER, *op. cit.*, p. 305.
22. LEONARD AND KROETZ, *op. cit.*, pp. 29-30.
23. RAVIN, *op. cit.*, pp. 65-66.
24. HURST AND SCHLANT, *op. cit.*, pp. 230-231.
25. *Ibid.*, p. 236.

From the *American Journal of Nursing* 74:48-53, Jan. 1974.

Intra-Arterial Monitoring
of Blood Pressure

MARY A. NIELSEN

For 90 minutes the surgeons have operated on the patient's quivering heart while his need for oxygenated blood was met by a pump-oxygenator. Now the time has come to restore the heartbeat, to again impose on the weakened myocardium the task of pumping blood. Will it be able to carry the load? The heart is shocked, and the rhythmic contractions return. The aorta feels firmer to the surgeon's fingers. But how strong are the beats? The anesthesiologist scans a manometer dial for the oscillations coming from the blood pressure cuff that might give the answer. But is the pressure really good enough to assure that the patient is getting the circulation he requires?

Another patient has suffered a ruptured viscus and the toxins in his blood are threatening the vascular bed. His nurse must administer intravenous vasopressors at a rate adquate to maintain a systolic pressure over 80 mm. Hg. She wraps a cuff around the brachial artery and listens carefully for the Korotoff sounds. How faint they are. Did she hear them correctly? Does the cuff measurement represent the central arterial pressure, or is she being misled by the peripheral vasodilatation or vasoconstriction that may accompany sepsis?

Uncertainty in cardiovascular crises like these is common enough to warrant employing an alternative technique to evaluate blood pressure —a technique that is continuous and direct. By passing a catheter into the artery and attaching it to an electronic measuring system, one can measure arterial pressure as it is transmitted directly to an electronic pressure sensor called a transducer. The transducer converts the mechan-

MS. NIELSEN *is a nurse computer specialist with the computerized Bio-Physical Monitoring Service at the Minneapolis Veterans Administration Hospital. She earned a B.S.N. and an M.Ed. at the University of Minnesota.*

ical pressure of the pulses to electrical impulses which are transmitted to a bedside monitor. Just as the familiar central venous pressure can be monitored via a catheter in the great veins, a direct arterial pressure measurement comes from within the vessel. The pressure appears as a waveform rising and falling as it sweeps across the oscilloscope. This is a visual and vastly more precise representation of what the nurse is accustomed to feeling under her fingertips on a patient's wrist.

The first blood pressure measurement in recorded history was a direct measurement with a intra-arterial cannula. In the early 1700's, Stephen Hales inserted the end of a nine-foot glass rod into an artery of a horse, and noted that the blood rose 8 feet, 3 inches above the level of the heart(1). For more than 250 years, investigation of blood pressure using the direct (intra-arterial) technique has been carried on, improved, and reported in the technical literature. In many studies, the technique served as a standard by which indirect techniques of pressure measurement could be developed and evaluated.

In 1905 Korotkoff reported how the characteristic sounds of the pulse under an inflated cuff surrounding the artery could be used to approximate the intra-arterial pressure in most circumstances(2). The American Heart Association, cooperating with similar groups in Great Britain, published recommendations for carrying out the now familiar measurement of blood pressure by sphygmomanometer(3,4,5,6). These recommendations were based on reseach comparing measurements obtained directly from intra-arterial catheters with measurements resulting from variations in cuff techniques. However, studies have demonstrated discrepancies between simultaneous direct and indirect measurements of arterial pressure(7).

With the increased dependability and miniaturization of electronic equipment and the development of heparin and plastic catheters that resist clotting, long-term, direct, arterial pressure measurement has become part of the management of critically ill patients. The nurse has gained an accurate, continuous resource for her assessment of the patient, and it may lead her to more appropriate, perhaps lifesaving, intervention.

THE CATHETER-TRANSDUCER-MONITOR SYSTEM

An effective direct pressure monitoring system consists of four major components:

1. A **catheter**, filled with fluids, carries the pressure wave to the manometer. It must be rigid enough to carry the pulse faithfully (unlike a soft catheter of the type used for intravenous infusions, which would

dissipate the pressure in its walls) and nonirritating to the artery.

2. A **transducer** is the manometer. It converts the mechanical signal (pressure) to an electrical signal (voltage). It fits tightly into the hub of the catheter so that pulses traveling down the fluid in the catheter bombard the delicate face of the transducer, distorting its shape, thereby pushing and pulling on the fine wires (strain gauge) attached to the back side of the transducer face. When the transducer is plugged into a bedside monitor, these wires become part of an electrical circuit arising from the monitor. The changes in shape of these fine wires are, in effect, changes in electrical resistance which cause the rising and falling voltage output displayed as a beam on the monitor.

3. A beside **monitor** amplifies the signal coming from the transducer and displays it on an oscilloscope so that the patient's pressure can be observed. This display is continuous, although monitoring can be interrupted, if necessary, by unplugging the transducer from the monitor.

4. A **fluid source** for flushing the catheter is made an integral part of the monitoring system for patient safety. If the catheter can be flushed without opening the system to air, there is no chance of introducing air through the catheter, whose tip may lie close to the base of a carotid artery. The hazard comes not from oxygen or carbon dioxide, which are soluble in body fluids, but rather from nitrogen, which is not. Constituting 78 percent of air, nitrogen occupies space which should be occupied by blood.

A plastic bag (*Fenwall Transfer Pack or Travenol Vioflex*) is used to hold the flush solution, usually heparinized saline, so that pressure can be applied to it without introducing air. Pressure is applied by placing an inflatable sleeve around the plastic bag of solution and pumping enough pressure against the solution to force it to flow against the systolic pressure in the artery.

BEGINNING MONITORING

With the catheter-transducer assembly filled with fluid and attached to the bedside monitor, and the transducer balanced to establish the zero point, the equipment is ready. The catheter is introduced through a 17- or 18-gauge needle into a radial or brachial artery. There is no backing of blood into the catheter when the needle enters the artery because the catheter is already filled with fluid and sealed off at the hub by the transducer or stopcock. Observation of the monitor confirms the catheter's entry into the artery at the moment the languid beam on the scope leaps into the conformation of the arterial pulse. Repeated trauma to the arterial wall is avoided.

The catheter is advanced up the arterial channel into the chest, so that the measurement is free of peripheral variations due to position, vasoconstriction, vasodilatation, and obstruction in the vessel. A central measurement also allows the calculation of cardiac output by the pulse contour method when a computer is available for this purpose(8).

With the catheter in place, the needle is withdrawn and pressure applied to the puncture site. The catheter is secured with tape, and a loop of catheter is left protruding from the dressing so that it can be retracted easily if it later becomes necessary to free an obstructed tip from the arterial wall. The remainder of the catheter is secured to the patient's arm to avoid kinks in the catheter. The transducer and flush line are also taped to his arm so that he can move about freely without disturbing the monitoring assembly. The anterior aspect of the upper arm is often used because it can be easily observed and the patient is not likely to lie on it.

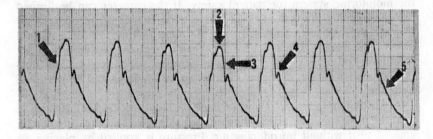

The initial rapid pressure rise in the artery (1) is usually accompanied by some turbulence and is the result of the contraction of the left ventricle forcing its bolus of blood through the open aortic valve into the aorta. As the ventricle empties and relaxes, a peak pressure in the artery is reached (2). A notch, called the anacrotic notch, often appears on the upstroke near the peak. Its origin is not well understood. The pressure drops sharply (3) as the bolus of blood moves downstream. Meanwhile, the pressure in the ventricle has dropped lower than that in the aorta, allowing aortic intravascular pressure to force the aortic valve closed. The tense aortic walls snap back to their resting mode. This phenomenon is seen on the pressure wave as the dicrotic notch (4). It appears whether pressure is measured in the aortic arch itself or far downstream, and is absent only when competent valve action is absent. Closure of the aortic valve is commonly considered the demarcation between the systolic and diastolic phases of the cardiac cycle. There is usually a change in slope (5) after the dicrotic notch, as the pressure continues to fall until the next systole.

The moment the catheter enters the artery, the monitor reveals the true nature of the patient's arterial pulse: the maximum (systolic) and minimum (diastolic) pressures, the rate, and an overall impression of his cardiovascular dynamics. The tracing on page 14 shows a well-defined recording of a typical arterial pulse (a wave of pressure passing any given point in the arterial tree).

ASSESSING PRESSURE

Because pressure waves differ in shape with the patient's anatomy and condition, the nurse needs criteria for determining that the signal reaching the monitor is accurate. Errors in technique can occur in direct pressure measurement as well as in indirect. Good criteria for accuracy are that the transducer is balanced at zero and the system calibrated to known units, as with any manometer, and that the pressure wave is well defined and shows the subtle fluctuations in the slopes.

Systolic pressure for each cardiac cycle is the maximum pressure reached by that pulse; diastolic pressure is the minimum level reached. In order to express these numerically, it is necessary to know the full scale (usually 0 to 200 mm. Hg) for the transducer and monitor, and the value of the divisions on the scope face. If the intra-arterial pressure is 120/80, the tops of the pulses will be at the 120 level on the scope, and the bottoms at 80; they can't be positioned anywhere else, as waveforms on an EKG often can be. With the scope calibrations clearly marked, it is possible to make instantaneous and continuous assessment of blood pressure without touching the patient.

The frequency of pulses, or heart rate, can also be counted by observing the monitor. Some monitors have automatic rate meters to make this calculation from the arterial pulse.

Cardiac output, or the volume of blood pumped by the left ventricle, can also be estimated by observing two aspects of the arterial pressure wave: mean pressure and area within the wave. Cardiac output is valuable to know; pumping blood is, after all, the very purpose of the heart. The relationship of the flow volume (cardiac output) to the arterial pressure wave is that: pressure equals flow times resistance. If resistance (dependent on size of the vascular bed) remains constant, then there is a greater volume of flow per heartbeat when pressure is high than when pressure is low. The area under the curve of the pressure wave is also correlated with cardiac output. This area will be greater when the pulse appears wide at the top, due to a sustained thrust of the myocardium through a greater part of the cardiac cycle. In both cases, flow from the heart is largely responsible for maintaining the level of the pressure wave.

INDICATIONS FOR INTRA-ARTERIAL MONITORING

Indication	Difference Between Intra-arterial and Cuff Pressures
Fluctuation in pressure from beat to beat due to arrhythmias and respiratory effect	Intra-arterial reading is continuous and the eye (or computer) averages the systolic levels; cuff reading measures only one beat
Shock: poor jet pulses and poor Korotkoff sounds	Intra-arterial reading higher than cuff reading
Arteriolar vasoconstriction or vasodilatation	Central reading higher or lower than peripheral
Obstruction in peripheral artery in patients with atherosclerotic disease or following diagnostic heart catheterization	Central reading higher than peripheral

In most cases, the arterial pressure changes somewhat from beat to beat in conjunction with the respiratory cycle. This is explained by the effect of respiration on the venous return from the lungs to the heart. Over a given time, the left ventricle can pump only as much blood as has been returned to it from the pulmonary system. Arterial pressure depends largely on this changing volume. Respiratory fluctuations in arterial pressure are most obvious when the blood pressure is low and when the patient is on a positive pressure respirator.

More erratic fluctuation are seen when the ventricular rate is irregular, as in atrial fibrillation. The longer the interval between ventricular beats, the more time the ventricle will have had to fill, and the stronger the pulse will be. Conversely, a very premature ventricular contraction will produce no pulse at all, due to lack of blood in the ventricle to be pumped, or to ineffective pumping action. If a nurse had to report such a blood pressure, what would she say? To report the highest systolic level would be misleading, especially when that pressure does not occur very often. Yet, when one is measuring only intermittently with a cuff, one strives to do just that. A truer expression of the patient's pressure status would be to select a median pulse from the sample observed, or to report the range of pressures.

Communication of observed data among the personnel managing the patient presents a problem when the blood pressure fluctuates from beat to beat. Computers are helpful in assigning the appropriate numerical values to the waveform. A consistent policy should be established for recording blood pressure when the pressure waves show it is fluctuating from beat to beat.

SOURCES OF INACCURACY

Agreement of a direct arterial pressure measurement with one made by cuff and sphygmomanometer is *not* a criterion for its accuracy. The cuff technique is a direct measurement of pressure *in the cuff*, and it is an effective technique only when the pressure is transmitted in full to the artery. Also, true differences may exist between central and peripheral pressures, due to vasomotor changes or vascular obstruction. Finally, cuff techniques depend on the quality of Korotkoff sounds and normal jet-like pulses. In low pressure states the sounds are lost, making the indirect technique ineffective in obtaining a correct measurement(9).

If a significant discrepancy between direct and indirect measurements is observed by the nurse, she should consider all possible problems, both in the cuff technique and in sources of error in the catheter-transducer-

SOURCES OF ERROR IN MEASURING BLOOD PRESSURES

Errors in Technique	Effect on Measurement	Remedy
Arterial catheter obstructed	False low direct measurement	Straighten arm; flush catheter; reduce kinks by pulling catheter back
Leak in catheter-transducer system	False low direct measurement	Improve connections; use sterile silicone grease prn; replace stopcock if cracked
Air in catheter-transducer system	False low direct measurement	Open system to air and flush bubbles out
Transducer not balanced	False low or high direct measurement	Balance when amplifier or transducer are exchanged
Pressure in cuff not reaching artery due to incorrect cuff size, faulty placement, arm not at heart level, etc.	Indirect measurement falsely high or low	Cuff diameter should be 20% greater than limb diameter; cuff bladder must be centered over artery; cuff must be snug, etc.
Errors in Equipment	*Effect on Measurement*	*Remedy*
Poor calibration of transducer amplifier or aneroid manometer due to damage	Measurement units unreliable	Obtain repair service
Too much or too little mercury in manometer.	Indirect measurement falsely high or low	

monitor system. Furthermore, she should consider any pressure wave attenuated, or damped, that lacks the usual cardiovascular dynamics if all other observations indicate that the heart is beating normally. Damped pressure waves appear to be narrowed in amplitude, and the notches and fluctuations are smoothed out. Damping occurs when something prevents the pulse from traveling through the fluid-filled catheter to the transducer so that full fluctuations in pressure are not sensed.

The nurse at the bedside should be able to identify possible causes for error in the direct pressure monitor and to correct them safely or seek appropriate assistance. Fortunately, most malfunctions, such as obstruction of the catheter due to its position or to tissue in the tip, a leak in the catheter-transducer assembly, or air in the system can be corrected quickly.

Electronic problems may affect the level of the pressure wave. Nurses necessarily depend on others to provide them with accurate measuring devices—mercury and aneroid manometers, thermometers, flowmeters, scales, and calibrated containers, for instance. The bedside nurse must be assured that reliable equipment has been selected for her use and, when appropriate, that periodic checks provide for its proper functioning, as errors in measurement attributable to the equipment are seldom obvious. The calibration of all instruments must be correct, and the zero level established at zero. Correct calibration means that the units of measurement represent what they are supposed to and that they are equal with one another throughout the scale.

Nurses who use a pressure monitoring system should learn the procedure for checking the zero baseline, or balancing the transducer to ensure accurate readings.

Invading the body in order to monitor cardiovascular variables is not done casually, but when other methods are inadequate it need not be dangerous. The risk of intra-arterial pressure monitoring must be recognized and minimized.

The most significant of these risks is thrombosis of the artery. Just as any indwelling catheter tends to be a focus for inflammatory changes, an arterial catheter may promote the clotting mechanism and thereby narrow or obstruct the channel. Nurses at the bedside can help protect the patient from impaired circulation by checking the pulses in his involved arm throughout the monitoring period and 24 hours after removal of the catheter, and calling signs of impaired circulation to the doctor's attention.

Arterial involvement should be distinguished from generalized reduction in perpheral circulation and paresthesias of the third and fourth fingers caused by pressure on the ulnar nerve within the elbow. If it appears that the artery is affected by the catheter, the catheter is usually removed. Armboards should not be taped to the skin, and intravenous infusion should be watched closely for signs of infiltration or avoided entirely in the same arm as the arterial catheter, if possible, to reduce the possibility of congestion of the vascular bed. The effect would be to close off the smaller vessels at a time when chances for the development of collateral circulation should be enhanced in every way possible.

Another significant hazard is the possibility of injecting air through the catheter. It is important that all personnel who open the catheter assembly to air be aware of this hazard and be capable of reassembling the system without introducing air.

Infection can be prevented by using good technique.

Rapid blood loss from the catheter is unlikely if the catheter is long and has a fine bore; flow through it is so slow that the blood tends to clot soon after the heparinized saline in the catheter is gone.

Electrical conductivity through the saline to the heart is lower than previously supposed. Although an invasion of the skin certainly breaks down electrical resistance of the body, it has been shown recently that a saline-filled Teflon catheter has far more resistance than do common metallic cardiac catheters and pacemaker leads(10).

How does the patient feel about his arterial catheter? The amount of anxiety experienced by patients as a result of the direct pressure monitoring apparatus is apparently small. This isn't surprising when one considers that most of the patients monitored in this way may be facing a life-threatening crisis. If the patient is alert, his anxiety level is already high. Although the needle represents a temporary threat, the pressure monitor offers the reassurance that he will be watched very closely. Observations of the pressure wave demonstrate objectively that the patient tends to relax quickly as soon as he knows that the catheter insertion has been accomplished. Interviews with patients several days after removal of the catheter revealed that many were not able to distinguish it from intravenous tubes.

The intra-arterial technique of pressure monitoring serves the patient well because it provides accurate, objective, and continuous data on which to base his management. Once the pressure signal is established, the monitoring equipment usually requires no further manipulation to obtain blood pressure measurements. The pressure signal that is visible from the entire bedside area allows the nurse to carry out lifesaving measures while watching the patient's blood pressure.

continued

REFERENCES

1. HALES, STEPHEN. *Statistical Essays Containing Haemostatics.* London, 1733, as reprinted in FREDERICK WILLUS AND THOMAS KEYS, EDS., *Classics of Cardiology.* New York, Dover Publications, 1961, pp. 129-155. (Originally published as *Cardiac Classics,* St. Louis, C. V. Mosby Co., 1941)
2. KOROTKOFF, N. S., *A Contribution to the Problem of Methods for the Determination of Blood Pressure.* St. Petersburg, 1905, as reprinted in RUSKIN, ARTHUR, *Classics in Arterial Hypertension.* Springfield, Ill., Charles C Thomas, Publisher, 1956, p. 126.
3. AMERICAN HEART ASSOCIATION AND CARDIAC SOCIETY OF GREAT BRITAIN AND IRELAND. *Joint Recommendation Standardization of Blood Pressure Readings.* New York, American Heart Association, July, 1939.
4. AMERICAN HEART ASSOCIATION, COMMITTEE TO REVISE STANDARDIZATION OF HIGH BLOOD PRESSURE READINGS. Statement. Recommendations for human blood pressure determination by sphygmomanometers. *JAMA* 147:632-636, Oct. 13, 1951.
5. BORDLEY, J., AND OTHERS. Recommendations for human blood pressure determinations by sphygmomanometers. *Circulation* 4:503-509, Oct. 1, 1951.
6. KERKENDALL, W. M., AND OTHERS. Recommendations for human blood pressure determination by sphygmomanometers. *Circulation* 36:980, Dec. 1967.
7. VAN BERGEN, F. H., AND OTHERS. Comparison of indirect and direct methods of measuring arterial blood pressure. *Circulation* 10:481-490, Oct. 1954.
8. WARNER, H. R. Experiences in computer-based patient monitoring. *Anesth.Analg.* 47:453-462, Sept.-Oct. 1968.
9. COHN, J. N. Blood pressure measurement in shock. Mechanism of inaccuracy in auscultatory and palpatory methods. *JAMA* 199:118-122, Mar. 27, 1967.
10. MONSEES, L. R., AND MC QUARRIE, D. G. Is an intravascular catheter a good conductor? *Med.Electronics Data* 2:26, Nov.-Dec. 1971.

From the *American Journal of Nursing* 73:1182-1186, July 1973.

Pulmonary Artery Catheterization

CAROLYN F. GERNERT • STEPHANIE SCHWARTZ

Critically ill patients frequently develop cardiopulmonary complications. Either right- or left-sided congestive heart failure may develop secondary to cardiac arrhythmias or fluid overload. Left ventricular failure may progress to pulmonary edema, or pulmonary edema may accompany acute pulmonary insufficiency. Acute pulmonary insufficiency, the "wet lung syndrome," often develops after severe shock and trauma, and may rapidly result in marked systemic hypoxemia. Untreated congestive heart failure may lead to cardiogenic shock(1).

Previously, it has been assumed that these complications could be diagnosed solely on the basis of central venous pressure (CVP) elevation. However, the CVP only provides information relating to the filling pressure of the right ventricle. Left ventricular failure, pulmonary edema, and pulmonary hypertension may occur independently of right ventricular failure(2). When this happens, CVP does not rise, and so no one is alerted to these developing problems. Therefore, a specific means of measuring left-sided heart pressure is used in conjunction with measuring the CVP when the possibility of cardiopulmonary complication exists.

Use of the balloon-tipped, flow-directed, pulmonary artery catheter for monitoring critically ill patients has become increasingly popular. The catheter can be inserted rapidly and safely, and it is an extremely useful tool in early diagnosis of complications. Along with the CVP, pulmonary artery pressures provide information about the patient's cardiodynamic

MS. GERNERT *is a research nurse at University Hospital, Boston, Massachusetts. She is a graduate of Arnot-Ogden Memorial Hospital School of Nursing, Elmira, New York.* MS. SCHWARTZ *is a research nurse at University Hospital, Boston, Massachusetts. She earned her associate and baccalaureate degrees at Northeastern University, Boston, Massachusetts. This work was supported in part by the U.S. Army Medical Research and Development Command Contract #DA 17-68-C-8132 and NIH Grant #5-PO1-GM17366-02.*

status that enables the physician to institute appropriate treatment before problems become full-bown or perhaps irreversible.

The three measurements which we have found to be of greatest value are the CVP, the mean pulmonary artery pressure (MPAP), and the mean pulmonary artery wedge pressure (MPAW). The CVP reflects the pressure in the right atrium, usually 0 mm. Hg(3). The MPAP indicates the pressure within the pulmonary vasculature, usually 13 mm. Hg(4). The MPAW reflects the left atrial pressure, usually 4 mm. Hg(5). Sudden changes in any of these pressures or a significant rise over a period of 24 hours or less, indicate impending problems which should be treated immediately with cardiotonic medications and diuretics.

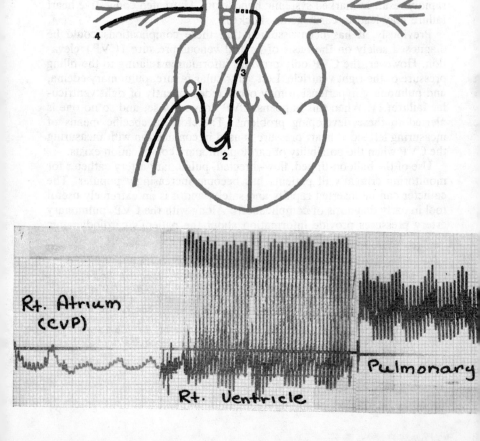

Patients in right ventricular failure show an increase in CVP without any significant change in MPAP or MPAW. Those with pulmonary artery hyptertension show an increase in MPAP only; the CVP and MPAW remain at normal levels. In left ventricular failure, the MPAW is elevated and there may be no increase in either CVP or MPAP. Pulmonary edema may be heralded by increases in any or none of the several pressures(6). In some cases, pulmonary edema is caused by a colloid osmotic effect due to a low serum albumin level(7).

Mixed-venous blood samples can be readily obtained through the pulmonary artery catheter. The measurements obtained can be used with other data to determine cardiac output, the amount of venous admixture

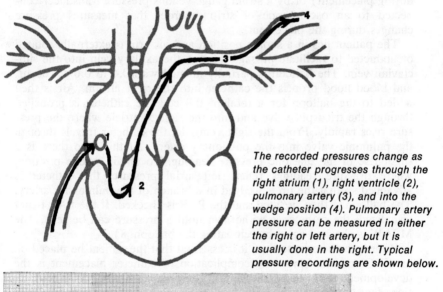

The recorded pressures change as the catheter progresses through the right atrium (1), right ventricle (2), pulmonary artery (3), and into the wedge position (4). Pulmonary artery pressure can be measured in either the right or left artery, but it is usually done in the right. Typical pressure recordings are shown below.

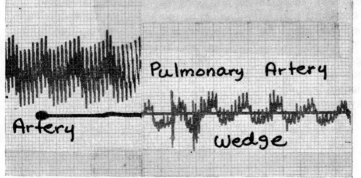

across the lungs, and the optimal rate for a temporary transvenous pacemaker. This information is similar to that obtained during right heart catheterization(8). For patients who might not tolerate cardiac catheterization, pulmonary artery catheterization is a simple means of assessing their hemodynamic status.

In the Trauma Unit at University Hospital, Boston, Massachusetts, pulmonary artery catheterization is performed for all patients with suspected cardiopulmonary complications. Insertion of the catheter is a minor surgical procedure and is easily done at the patient's bedside.

The catheter is placed through a peripheral cutdown. The basilic vein in the antecubital area is the usual site, but most peripheral veins can be used. The position of the catheter is observed through an image intensifier (a fluoroscopic device which allows visualization of the catheter during placement) or by a strain gauge venous pressure transducer connected to an oscilloscope or strip recorder that measures pressure changes during the placement.

The patient lies in a supine position and his arm is externally rotated or abducted to facilitate passage through the axillary vein into the subclavian vein. The balloon is partially inflated with 0.4 to 0.6 cc. of air, and blood flood propels the catheter into the right atrium. Air is then added to the balloon for a total of 0.8 cc. The catheter is propelled through the tricuspid valve and into the right ventricle where the pressure rises rapidly. From the right ventricle, the catheter travels through the pulmonic valve into the pulmonary artery. At this time there is a slight rise in the diastolic pressure reading. To obtain wedge position, where pressure readings reflect left atrial pressure, the catheter is advanced so that the tip is wedged in a branch of the pulmonary artery. The balloon is then deflated and the PAP is checked. If the PAP is not visualized, the catheter is withdrawn until a pressure can be seen. The MPAW is checked again by reinflating the balloon(8).

Prior to catheter insertion, it is essential that the patient be placed on an EKG monitor since one complication of catheter placement is the development of cardiac arrhythmias. The premature ventricular contractions that occasionally develop tend to be of short duration and subside spontaneously—without the need for medication or cardiac defibrillation(9).

Kinking of the catheter is the other complication that may occur during placement. This complication can be avoided by using a fluoroscopic device during placement or detected after placement by taking a chest x-ray immediately following catheterization. If the catheter is kinked, it is reinserted.

MEASURING PRESSURES

Pulmonary artery pressures can be measured with a strain gauge venous pressure transducer and oscilloscope or with a saline manometer. The transducer-oscilloscope technique is considered preferable since the information is continuously displayed on the oscilloscope screen. Less time and less technical skill are needed to obtain a reading. With the saline manometer, only MPAP and MPAW can be obtained. Pressure values measured by either method are most accurate if the patient is in a supine position and is not using any assisted ventilation device.

To obtain pressures using the transducer-oscilloscope technique, the catheter is connected to the transducer with a manifold. The transducer electrically transmits impulses to a specially designed oscilloscope. The manifold leads to the transducer, to a transpak of heparinized saline solution (5000 U.S.P. units of sodium heparin in one liter of normal saline), and to the patient's pulmonary artery line. To read systolic and diastolic pressures, a stopcock leading to the transpak is shut off and pressures are read directly from the screen. The MPAP is read from a gauge on the monitor. The MPAW is obtained by inflating the balloon with 0.8 cc. of air. The straight line which appears on the scope indicates the pressure value.

To prevent formation of microemboli at the tip of the catheter, it is essential to flush the line with 8 to 10 drops of flush solution every 30 to 60 minutes. To do this, a stopcock leading to the patient's line from the transpak line is opened and the appropriate amount of fluid is allowed to drip in. No pressures can be seen on the oscilloscope during the flushing period.

The saline manometer technique is similar to that used with a CVP line. After the catheter has been checked for patency, the manometer is placed at the level of the right atrium and filled with flush solution. The stopcock is then closed to permit the solution level to fall with pressure differences. Once the solution has reached its lowest level, and there is a steady fluctuation with respiration, the MPAP is recorded. The MPAW is obtained by inflating the balloon and reading the pressure at the lowest point of fluctuation. A constant, slow infusion of heparinized saline solution prevents the formation of microemboli.

COMPLICATIONS

In addition to the complications which can occur during placement of the catheter, and the formation of microemboli, there are other possible complications.

Air embolus secondary to balloon rupture can be prevented by pretesting the balloon before catheter insertion, and by checking the balloon for residual air prior to inflation. A syringe containing *only* the required amount of air always should be kept attached to the catheter. The balloon should *never* be inflated with more than the standard 0.8 cc. of air. Cardiac arrhythmias may develop if the balloon is left inflated so it is essential to deflate the balloon after each reading of MPAW. A related complication is ischemic damage to the lung. If the catheter remains in wedge position because the balloon has not been deflated or the catheter has migrated into one of the terminal branches of the pulmonary artery, diminution of blood flow to that portion of the lung will cause ischemia. Catheter position should be checked frequently by making sure that both systolic and diastolic pulse waves are present when using the transducer-oscilloscope technique, or by determining that good fluctuation is present when using the manometer technique.

Infection of the catheter site, indicated by gross redness, swelling, or foul drainage, can be prevented with daily care. The area is thoroughly cleansed with antiseptic solution, an antibiotic ointment and dry sterile dressing are applied. At the first sign of infection, the catheter should be removed, and the catheter site and catheter tip cultured.

Pulmonary artery catheterization has been performed for a number of patients in our unit, and we have encountered no complications. Catheters have remained in place for three to five days. When pulmonary artery catheterization is used, the nurse can make valuable, precise observations of the patient's cardiopulmonary status.

REFERENCES

1. GUYTON, A. C. *Textbook of Medical Physiology,* 4th ed. Philadelphia, W. B. Saunders Co., 1971, p. 343.
2. HECHTMAN, H. B. AND OTHERS. Independence of pulmonary shunting and pulmonary edema. *Surgery* (To be published).
3. GUYTON, *op cit.,* p. 271.
4. *Ibid.,* p. 302.
5. *Ibid.,* p. 303.
6. HECHTMAN AND OTHERS, *op. cit.*
7. SKILLMAN, J. J., AND OTHERS. Peritonitis and respiratory failure after abdominal operations. *Ann.Surg.* 170:122-127, July 1969.
8. SWAN, H. J., AND OTHERS. Catheterization of the heart in man with use of a flow-directed balloon-tipped catheter. *N.Engl.J.Med.* 283:450, Aug. 27, 1970.
9. *Ibid.,* pp. 447-451.

From the American Journal of Nursing 75:820-824, May 1975.

Central Venous Catheterization

JOHN M. DALY • BARBARA ZIEGLER
STANLEY J. DUDRICK

Central venous catheterization has been used in the research laboratory for many years, but only recently had it had common clinical application. The increased availability and improved quality of synthetic catheters, the development of a multitude of ingenious catheter placement devices, and the general recognition of the value of central venous pressure monitoring in critically ill patients are factors which have increased the clinical utilization of indwelling central venous devices.

More recently, the availability of potent antibiotics and other therapeutic agents that are caustic to the intima of peripheral veins and the development of parenteral hyperalimentation, which requires the use of irritating hypertonic nutrient solutions, have further promoted the use of central vein catheterization. A central venous catheter is virtually indispensable in treating any type of shock and can be used advantageously during major surgical operations when large amounts of blood and other fluids must be replaced rapidly.

Although many peripheral sites are available for insertion of catheters into central veins, only a few are used commonly. These are the saphenous, femoral, antecubital (cephalic or basilic), external jugular, internal jugular, and subclavian veins. Safe techniques and reliable devices for percutaneous insertion of catheters have reduced the need for surgical cutdown.

The saphenous and femoral veins are not satisfactory access routes to

JOHN DALY, M.D., is a resident in general surgery at Hermann Hospital-The University of Texas Medical School of Houston. BARBARA ZIEGLER, R.N., is a hyperalimentation specialist at the Hospital of the University of Pennsylvania, Philadelphia. STANLEY DUDRICK, M.D., is professor and director of the program in surgery at Hermann Hospital-The University of Texas Medical School at Houston.

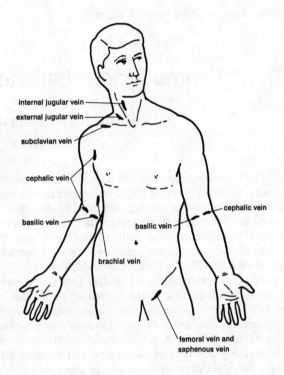

the central venous system except in dire emergencies, because of the high incidence of thrombophlebitis and thromboembolic disease associated with venous catheters placed in the lower extremities. Asepsis is extremely difficult, if not impossible, to maintain in these areas, as evidenced by the high incidence of infection and septicemia associated with long catheters inserted at these sites. Additional disadvantages of central venous catheters inserted via the lower extremities include the following:

- The relatively long distance that the catheter traverses the venous system increases the likelihood of intimal reaction, thrombophlebitis, and embolic phenomena.

- Such catheters cannot be used reliably to monitor central venous pressure because the readings obtained may be significantly affected by changes in intra-abdominal pressure.

- Diminished venous blood flow in the lower extremities and in the inferior vena cava is more likely to occur than in the veins of the upper half of the body during low flow states (shock, hypovolemia), predisposing to a higher incidence of intravascular clotting.

• In patients with major trauma to the lower abdomen or pelvis, the inferior vena cava or its tributaries may have been ruptured or lacerated, and fluid administered via the saphenous or femoral veins may leak into the peritoneal cavity or retroperitoneal space.

The antecubital veins (cephalic and basilic) maintain a fairly constant anatomic position but are small veins which tolerate indwelling catheters poorly. The outside diameter of the catheter and the inside diameter of the vein are similar, and the resulting postinsertion venospasm essentially occludes blood flow at the catheter site. Thus, a catheter placed percutaneously at this site has almost the same effect as a catheter inserted by cutdown. That is, a significant length of vein proximal to the entry site collapses around the catheter, creating dead space which is ideal for the growth of microorganisms. Pyophlebitis may ensue and result in septic emboli to the lungs and generalized sepsis. As with catheters inserted in the lower extremities, the distance between the insertion site and the central vein is quite long and increases the risk of intimal reaction and thrombophlebitis. Thrombosis, cellulitis, phlebitis, or sepsis rarely can be avoided for more than one week when these sites are used. On occasion, the cephalic or basilic vein has had to be stripped out to cure the suppurative thrombophlebitis.

In most adult patients and in the vast majority of children, the external jugular veins are sufficiently large for percutaneous insertion of large central venous catheters. For newborn infants or patients who are extremely obese, however, it may be necessary to insert catheters by cutdown. In approximately 75 percent of patients, the catheter can be directed into the superior vena cava. Failure usually occurs if the catheter cannot negotiate the acute angulation of the external jugular-subclavian vein confluence or if the catheter inadvertently enters one of the several small tributary veins in the lower neck or upper chest. Persistent, aggressive attempts to advance the catheter against moderate resistance usually result in perforation of the vein and development of a hematoma or extravasation of fluid. At times, catheters inserted through the external jugular vein are inadvertently directed into the venous branches in the shoulder girdle or into the arm veins. X-ray confirmation of correct central venous catheter placement should be obtained immediately after the procedure and prior to infusing irritating solutions or recording central venous pressure measurements.

The internal jugular vein is one of the most constant of all anatomic venous features. An adult who executes the Valsalva maneuver while in the Trendelenburg position can distend the internal jugular vein to a diameter of almost one inch. Its large size and high blood flow enable it to tolerate the catheter for long periods, if necessary. Using this site for central venous cannulation, Jernigan et al. report few, but serious, complications(1). All were preventable. Air embolism, thrombophlebitis of the internal jugular vein, and venous perforation with mediastinal infusion of fluids occurred in their series. Neck movement and close proximity of the hair-growing areas of the scalp and face make the jugular vein puncture site uncomfortable and confining for the patient, and difficult to keep clean.

In our experience, use of a subclavian vein for percutaneous insertion of a central venous catheter has yielded almost 100 percent success and minimal incidence of complications. Like the internal jugular vein, its large size and high blood flow favor tolerance of the catheter for long periods. The subclavian vein's anatomic position beneath the clavicle affords maximum stability and security for long-term use of a central venous catheter, and minimizes the risk of contamination.

Both the supraclavicular and infraclavicular approaches to the subclavian vein have been used for central venous catheterization. Barcia et al. believe that the supraclavicular approach causes less pain and is associated with a lower incidence of pneumothorax. Their impression is based on the theory that the pleura may be avoided if the vein is missed or pierced through and through because the direction of the needle is posterior-anterior and toward the mediastinum(2). We have found, however, that with rigid adherence to the technique described below, the infraclavicular approach also causes little discomfort and few complications(3).

CATHETER INSERTION

Successful percutaneous subclavian venous catheterization requires a thorough knowledge of thoracic and cervical anatomy, and familiarity with established techniques. Despite the many advantages of subclavian vein catheterization, it should only be attempted by an operator who observes the precautions necessary to ensure its safe performance.

Physician and nurse teamwork is essential for optimal success of subclavian catheterization. Before the procedure, accurate assessment of the patient's apprehensions and confident reassurance are very important. The patient is entitled to a careful, clear explanation of the steps in the procedure and their rationale. The equipment for central venous catheterization should be readily available to reduce delay and enhance efficiency.

Infraclavicular percutaneous puncture is done with the patient positioned with his head lowered 15 degrees (Trendelenburg position), and with a rolled sheet under his thoracic spine(4). Although the subclavian vein never collapses completely, the head-down position allows distention of the vein, making it a larger target. The roll under the spine allows the patient's shoulders to drop posteriorly. When his shoulders are depressed caudally (the movement opposite to shrugging the shoulders) and his head turned to the side opposite the insertion site, the subclavian vein becomes most easily accessible. Either subclavian vein may be used unless a specific contraindication is present, for example, unilateral apical bullous emphysema or a previously fractured clavicle.

The skin over the clavicle, shoulder, neck, and upper chest is shaved widely, defatted with ether or acetone, and prepared with an antiseptic solution, as in preparation for major surgery. Using aseptic technique, the infraclavicular area is draped and local anesthetic is infiltrated into the skin, subcutaneous tissue, and periosteum at the inferior border of the midpoint of the clavicle.

A 2-inch long, 14-gauge needle is attached to a two or three milliliter syringe, inserted bevel-down through the skin wheal, and advanced under the inferior border of the clavicle in a horizontal (frontal) plane aimed at the anterior margin of the trachea at the suprasternal notch. As the needle is advanced, a slight negative pressure applied through the syringe will help to indicate accurate venous puncture with a flashback of blood. The needle is advanced a few millimeters after blood first appears in the syringe to ensure that the entire bevel is within the lumen of the vein.

Free flow of blood through the needle should be obtained. The patient is asked to perform Valsalva's maneuver, that is, to expire against the closed glottis, much akin to "straining at stool." This minimizes the risk of air embolism. The syringe is removed carefully while the needle is held firmly in place. An 8-inch long, 16-gauge radiopaque catheter is introduced through the needle and threaded its full length into the vein. The catheter usually advances without difficulty if the needle tip is entirely within the lumen of the vein. It is then attached to a standard intravenous infusion set, and the catheter is flushed with isotonic fluid. The needle is withdrawn, and the catheter is sutured in place just lateral to the skin puncture site with 3-0 silk.

At this time, the solution bottle is lowered below the level of the patient and then quickly raised to confirm free flow in both directions, an indication that the catheter is properly placed within the superior vena cava. Antimicrobial ointment is applied to the puncture site, and a sterile gauze occlusive dressing is fixed to the skin with tincture of benzoin and adhesive tape. The I.V. tubing is looped over the top of the dressing and secured again with tape to guard against accidental traction on the catheter itself.

Conscientious adherence to this technique should ensure successful central venous catheterization, but several additional precautions must be taken to minimize complications.

As the needle is advanced under the clavicle toward the subclavian vein, a slight negative pressure should be applied through the syringe. If air is aspirated into the syringe, suggesting entry into the lung, the needle should be withdrawn. If the patient does not exhibit any respiratory distress, the airtight security of the needle-syringe connection should be examined.

If bright red blood fills the syringe without negative pressure having been applied, the needle has probably entered the subclavian artery, and the procedure should be terminated and pressure applied over the artery.

After the central venous catheter is inserted and secured, a portable chest x-ray should be obtained to verify proper placement of the catheter tip in the midsuperior vena cava and to rule out pneumothorax or hemothorax.

Percutaneous catheterization of large veins such as the subclavian involves potential hazards to adjacent anatomical structures. *Pneumothorax* is the most common complication of subclavian venipuncture, but is seldom dangerous. If the needle is introduced too far posteriorly, it may enter the pleural cavity. Each attempt at catheterization, successful or otherwise, should be followed by x-ray examination of the lungs.

Hydrothorax is a consequence of administering fluid through a catheter misplaced in the pleural cavity. This should not occur if the needle and catheter have entered the vein properly, as shown by a free flow of blood into the catheter.

Hemorrhage into the pleural cavity, *hemothorax*, may occur from laceration of the vein or puncture of the artery. To prevent laceration, the direction of the needle should never be changed in a sweeping motion if accurate venipuncture has not been accomplished on the first attempt. The needle should be withdrawn to the skin surface, redirected, and advanced with a straight thrust.

Brachial plexus injury can be avoided by not attempting to catheterize the subclavian vein lateral to the midpoint of the clavicle. Infusing fluid through a catheter directed outside the lumen of the subclavian vein but not penetrating the pleural cavity can result in a subpleural or mediastinal infiltration of the intravenously administered solution.

Due to an anatomical anomaly or some other cause, a catheter introduced by subclavian venipuncture may become misdirected and not properly positioned in the superior vena cava. Subclavian vein catheters have inadvertently entered an internal or external jugular vein, and occasionally have passed well up into the neck. The blood flow in these veins is insufficient to properly dilute the hypertonic fluid used for patients receiving parenteral hyperalimentation, and thrombophlebitis and other complications can occur. Infrequently, a misdirected catheter may curl or knot in the internal jugular, subclavian, or innominate vein. Misdirection of central venous catheters can be detected by using radiopaque catheters, and by confirming their intravenous position by x-ray.

Before the procedure, careful preparation of the patient is essential. He should be reassured that once the catheter is in place it will be no more uncomfortable than a regular I.V. and that it won't interfere with his breathing. He should be given a brief explanation of the purposes of central venous pressure monitoring.

Meticulous attention to an indwelling central venous catheter, regardless of its site, is essential for safe long-term use. Every two or three days, the nurse changes the intravenous tubing and carefully removes the dressing over the puncture site. Then, using aseptic technique, she cleanses the skin with acetone or ether, prepares it with antiseptic solution, and applies antimicrobial ointment and a sterile dressing. To prevent contamination of the intravenous solution or the administration tubing, extreme care must be exercised in adding intravenous medications. These precautions will help to ensure the long-term safety of central venous catheterization.

REFERENCES
1. JERNIGAN, W. R., AND OTHERS. Use of the internal jugular vein for placement of central venous catheter. *Surg.Gynecol.Obstet.* 130:520-524, Mar. 1970.
2. GARCIA, J. M., AND OTHERS. Percutaneous supraclavicular superior vena caval cumulation. *Surg.Gynecol.Obstet.* 130:839-841, May 1972.
3. COPELAND, E. M., III, AND OTHERS. Prevention of microbial catheter contamination in patients receiving parenteral hyperalimentation. *South.Med.J.* 67:303-306, Mar. 1974.
4. DUDRICK, S. J., AND OTHERS. General principles and technique of administration in complete parenteral nutrition. IN *Parenteral Nutrition*, ed. by A. W. Wilkinson. New York, Longman, 1972, pp. 222-233.

Section II Pathophysiology

Long-term and immediate therapy for any disorder is based on the underlying pathology. Anticipated and observed physiological events give clues to the prevention and treatment of cardiovascular diseases. While several of the articles in this section suggest methods for treating cardiac problems, the focus of each is on the reaction of body systems to these problems.

From the *American Journal of Nursing* 72:253-259, Feb. 1972.

Campbell Soup's Program to Prevent Atherosclerosis

MARYANN COX • ROLAND F. WEAR, JR.

By measuring blood fats and other factors involved in atherosclerosis for employees who wish to take part in the program, this company's medical department is actively helping employees at high risk to reduce their risk of heart disease.

"Would you believe I have lost eight pounds in the past two weeks?" asked Jim, an employee of the Campbell Soup Company. Jim weighed 210 pounds, approximately 50 pounds over his normal weight for a height of 70 inches. He has been participating in our atherosclerosis study, off and on, for the past three years. "Off and on" applies because Jim really never quite adhered to the low carbohydrate diet he was advised to follow by the medical director of the company.

The atherosclerosis study here at the Campbell Soup Company is strictly on a voluntary basis. Jim was among our first volunteers and was anxious to donate 15 cc. of blood to a study to measure blood fats and other factors involved in the development of atherosclerosis, which might eventually lead to a coronary occlusion or heart failure.

The results of his serum lipid study were an abnormal elevation of his triglycerides and a normal level of cholesterol. He was informed of the results of the test and was advised to start a diet low in simple carbohydrates (sugars) and adhere to the diet strictly for at least six weeks.

Simple carbohydrate restriction reduces calories without reducing bulk. Complex carbohydrates, vegetables and starches, are permitted in *normal* amounts. Since they are bulky they satisfy. Sugars are not bulky and thus supply many calories with little satisfaction of any duration.

Before Jim left the medical department that day, he stepped on the

35

scale and watched the needle soar to 210. We were assured this time he was definitely going to lose the excess weight—no more night snacks or other tempting goodies such as ice cream and candy. Jim had every reason to show concern about his recent laboratory results. His family history was not good: father—deceased, coronary, aged 52; one brother —coronary, aged 50 years; and one uncle on his father's side—deceased due to myocardial infarction.

Our plan is to do initial studies, follow-up observations, and needed diet manipulations on most of our employees who have been with the company five years or more. The Campbell Soup Company employees number about 25,000 in the United States; at least 10,000 of them have been with the company more than five years. These employees are located near approximately 30 plants throughout the United States or are salesmen in all states.

Communication concerning the study is by mail with each salesman or directly with our plant nurses. Serum specimens and medical observations are obtained by plant nurses, part-time or full-time plant physicians, or personal physicians. The entire study is directed and supervised by the authors. Data sheets and serum samples are sent to the corporate medical department in the general offices.

THE STUDY PLAN

The study is designed to evaluate (a) the prevalence patterns of lipoprotein and serum lipid (blood fat) abnormalities; (b) the relationship of lipid and various other factors to the subsequent development of atherosclerosis; and (c) the influence of changing some of these factors.

Atherosclerotic narrowing or occlusion occurs most commonly in the arteries of the heart, the brain (and sometimes the neck), and the aorta and its branches to the kidneys and the legs.

Initial observations on each individual include the date the blood sample is drawn, laboratory number (identification), sex, race, height, weight, year of birth, and age at menopause (when appropriate). Also included are current diet, presence or absence of diabetes or postprandial elevations of blood sugar, systolic and diastolic blood pressure, serum

MISS COX *is medical assistant in the Campbell Soup Company's Medical Department. Stationed at the General Office in Camden, N.J., she also travels to other plants of the company. She is a graduate of Philadelphia General Hospital School of Nursing, Pa.* DR. WEAR *is the corporate medical director of the Campbell Soup Company. His M.D. degree is from the University of Pennsylvania. He and Miss Cox direct the atherosclerosis program they describe in this article.*

triglyceride level (after a 12-hour fast), serum cholesterol level (after a 12-hour fast), and serum lactescence (absence, presence, degree). In some cases, plasma or serum electrophoresis is done.

History includes drug intake for hypertension (thiazides are specifically recorded), drugs for lipid elevations, or oral contraceptive agents; family history of diabetes; family history of angina or myocardial infarction prior to age 60 years; current smoking pattern; and past myocardial infarction or angina.

SERUM STUDY

The examinee must fast 12 hours or more prior to the venipuncture; only water is permitted. Fasting is required so that normal chylomicrons are cleared from the serum.

During the four days prior to the test, the examinee should observe his *usual* diet. He should not be more careful than usual, nor less careful. Pre-beta lipoprotein abnormalities (mostly triglcerides) may be quickly altered in some persons who are experiencing mild to moderate abnormalities.

At least 10 cc. of blood are drawn and allowed to clot for one to three hours at room temperature. The sample of blood is spun in a centrifuge at 3,000 rpm for 10 minutes. Blood-cell-free serum (approximately 5 cc.) is drawn off the top using a 5 cc. syringe with a 1½-inch needle. Serum lactescence should be estimated and recorded before the specimen is refrigerated.

There must be no suspended red blood cells, because they would give a smoky appearance that may be confused with lactescence. The serum tubes are spun in the centrifuge a second time (after removing the serum from the clotted blood) and then examined before any agitation has occurred, which might stir up the sediment.

We determine the degree of lactescence by holding the Vacutainer of serum below an incandescent lamp. An opaque shield is placed between the lamp and the examiner's eyes. A fluorescent light is not satisfactory.

A second observation is made one or more days later of sera with more than a trace of lactescence. Since chylomicrons are large particles of high fat content, they will come to the surface and form a creamlike layer. Chylomicrons are normally present in the serum for several hours following a meal containing fat, but they are cleared from the serum within 12 hours unless the person has the extremely rare type I hyperlipoproteinemia or the type V hyperlipoproteinemia, which will be described later. Type I serum has a creamy top (supernate) and a clear bottom (infranate) after standing for a few days refrigerated, then

GLOSSARY

ADIPOSE: Animal tissue in which fat is stored in the cells of adipose tissue.

CHOLESTEROL: A steroid alcohol important in physiologic processes, found in bile, gallstones, brain, blood cells, plasma, egg yolk, seeds, and animal tissues generally in varying amounts, with 150 to 250 mg./100 ml. a normal value for human serum.

ELECTROPHORESIS: Application of electric current to a suspension of protein molecules suitably buffered causes their migration to the positive pole, and the various protein fractions can be recorded and analyzed because they differ in rate of movement and in refractive index.

ESTERIFIED: Converted into an ester, a compound formed from an alcohol and an acid by the removal of water. Normally, 68 to 76 percent of the serum cholesterol is esterified.

FATTY ACID: Obtained from the lipids of most plants and animals, these saturated or unsaturated monocarboxylic acids are used by tissues as a major source of energy, and some are believed to aid in the transport of fat from the depots to various tissues for oxidation. Normal serum values are 190 to 420 mg./100 ml.

HETEROZYGOUS: Containing genes for both members of at least one pair of allelomorphic characters. If one gene produces its effect in the presence of the other, it is called dominant and the other recessive.

HOMOZYGOUS: An organism is said to be homozygous for a given character when all the germ cells transmit identical genes for this character. When a condition such as hyperlipoproteinemia is involved, the person with homozygous heredity is more at risk of heart disease than one with heterozygous heredity.

HYPERLIPOPROTEINEMIA: An excess of lipoproteins in the blood.

LACTESCENCE: Milky in appearance. In tests of serum lipids, lactescence suggests that triglycerides will be elevated due to an increase of pre-beta lipoproteins or chylomicrons.

LIPID: A group of fats and fatlike compounds that vary widely and that constitute a major class of tissue components and a major foodstuff. They are defined operationally as the portion that dissolves in the solvent when plant or animal material is crushed and ground with nonpolar solvents such as benzene, chloroform, or carbon tetrachloride. They are not water soluble. Normal range: 450-850 mg./100 ml.

LIPOPROTEIN: A combination of lipid and protein possessing the general properties of proteins. Lipids are not water soluble or free in the blood stream, but can be dissolved and transported when combined with protein. Various fractions can be analyzed by electrophoresis, which separates the lipoproteins into bands:

1. *Alpha lipoproteins:* These are tiny particles, rich in protein, apparently unrelated to atherosclerosis.

2. *Beta lipoproteins:* This type is rich in cholesterol and is, therefore, significant in serum studies related to atherosclerosis. Particles are smaller than pre-beta lipoproteins or chylomicrons.

3. *Pre-beta lipoproteins:* The particles are large, yet are smaller than the chylomicrons and are produced in the body from carbohydrates and perhaps from short-chain fatty acids, butter and coconut being examples. Abnormalities respond quickly to diet change.

4. *Chylomicrons:* These very large particles—about 1 micron in diameter—are found in the serum during digestion of fat and usually are cleared from serum 12 hours after eating.

PHENOTYPE: The outward visible expression of the hereditary constitution of an organism.

PHOSPHOLIPID: These lipids that contain phosphorus are the most dominant type in the body other than the adipose or storage fat. Normal values in serum are 6 to 12 mg./100 ml. as lipid phosphorus.

TRIGLYCERIDES: Sometimes called the "neutral fat" or "simple lipids," they are triesters (three ester groups) of glycerol with one, two, or three acids, and are found in such substances as lard, tallow, butterfat, olive oil, coconut oil, and soybean oil. They are carried to adipose tissue cells in the form of chylomicrons and low-density lipoproteins. Normal ranges in serum are 0 to 150 mg./100 ml.

XANTHOMA: A condition in which skin and tendons have small, flat yellow plaques due to deposits of lipids.

---

warmed to room temperature before reading. Type V has a creamy supernate and a milky infranate after standing.

An important step of our atherosclerosis study is to have each plant nurse record all data in code for computer processing. Several forms are used to facilitate counseling, review, subsequent studies, and record keeping on each employee.

All employees are notified of the results of the test. Our upper limit of normal is considered to be about 260 mg./100 ml. for cholesterol, and about 150 mg./100 ml. for triglycerides. (In Japan, where there is a low incidence of coronary heart diease, most Japanese have cholesterol levels below 220 mg./100 ml.) A variety of forms are used to notify employees of results. Some of these forms advise repeat testing and special test diets. In order to reduce our correspondence, an employee is asked to inform his personal physician of the results.

ADDITIONAL OBSERVATIONS

Occasionally other blood serum analyses are done such as electrophoresis of the serum lipoproteins. Periodic health examinations may also be used to add information about the blood vessels, blood pressure, electrocardiogram, and so forth.

The serum lipids are retested periodically. At those times, the current diet and body weight are recorded.

Through many of these observations during the next several years, valuable information regarding the usefulness of diet should be accumulated. The relative importance of various factors thought to be associated with atherosclerosis may be further clarified.

Some individuals in the study are asked to remain on experimental diets for long periods, if their personal physicians agree.

LIPID AND LIPOPROTEIN ABNORMALITIES

The following is a brief summary of serum lipid and lipoprotein abnormalities, their relationship to disease, particularly atherosclerosis, and their responses to dietary and drug treatment. About 35 percent of the employees in our study appear to have an elevation of serum lipids.

Elevation of any of three classes of lipids—triglycerides, cholesterol, and phospholipids—in the serum are associated with an increased risk of having a heart attack. The *triglycerides* are sometimes called neutral fat. *Cholesterol* may be in a so-called "free" form or chemically combined (esterified) with a fatty acid. *Phospholipids* all contain phosphoric acid and are the dominant type of lipid in the body tissue other than adipose or storage fat. Since phospholipids are not elevated unless either triglycerides or cholesterol or both are elevated, it is not necessary to measure phospholipids to find persons with higher risk of heart attacks.

To further understand the various serum lipid disorders, other types of analyses have been made, analyses of the lipoproteins. Lipids are not free in the blood stream, they are not water soluble, but when they are combined with protein (lipoprotein), they are dissolved and can be transported in the blood.

When the lipoproteins in the blood serum are placed in solution in an electrical field, they separate into four different bands, since each of the four classes of lipoproteins moves at a different speed and therefore a different distance from the origin after 15 to 20 hours. These lipoprotein classes that separate on electrophoresis are as follows:

CHYLOMICRONS: These are very large particles, very high in triglycerides that have been absorbed from digested fats in the intestinal tract and not yet altered by the liver or other body tissues. The presence of chylomicrons in the blood is not associated with an increased incidence of atherosclerosis or heart attacks. These are classified as very low-density lipoproteins (VLDL).

Density relates to the weight of particles in relation to their size. Thus, the greater the percentage of protein in the particle, the bigger the relative weight. Conversely, the greater the fat percentage, the lower the relative weight and the greater the tendency to float in salty solutions—just as fat persons float in water more easily than lean persons. An ultracentrifuge can be used to effect separations similar to the electrical separations of electrophoresis.

PRE-BETA LIPOPROTEIN: This band, which separates on electrophoresis, is made up of large particles that are smaller than chylomicrons. They are also rich in triglycerides (five times as much as cholesterol). These lipoproteins are produced in the body from carbohydrate or excess calories and perhaps from short-chain fatty acids as in butter and coconut. They are increased in types III, IV, and V hyperlipoproteinemia (see hyperlipoproteinemia phenotypes which follow). These, too, are classified as VLDL.

BETA LIPOPROTEIN: This electrophoretic band is made up of lipoprotein particles that are much smaller than chylomicrons or pre-beta lipoproteins. These particles are rich in cholesterol. The classical elevation of this lipoprotein is in the type II hyperlipoproteinemia or in the persons with cholesterol levels well above 300 mg./100 ml. These are classified as low-density lipoproteins (LDL).

ALPHA LIPOPROTEIN: This electrophoretic band is made up of very small particles that are rich in protein. These are considered to be high-density lipoprotein (HDL), and there appears to be no relationship between these particles and atherosclerosis.

These chemical and physical studies of the serum lipids and lipoproteins are an attempt to discover those persons with metabolic defects that lead to an increased risk of coronary heart disease and to determine the exact type of that metabolic defect (phenotype) for better understanding of the degree of risk and of the best corrective measures.

HYPERLIPOPROTEINEMIA PHENOTYPES

Roman numerals from I to V are used to designate each of these inherited and inherited-acquired defects.

TYPE I: This rare familial disorder is not associated with atherosclerosis. Chylomicrons are markedly increased and, therefore, serum triglyceride levels are very high. When it is diagnosed, the patients are usually children who have repeated attacks of abdominal pain. This disease is controlled by a low fat diet.

TYPE II: This is a common familial disorder that can be diagnosed at birth in most cases by analysis of the baby's blood serum. Both sexes are equally affected. In heterozygous type II, it is transmitted to half the couple's offspring. The patient's serum cholesterol levels are high, usually above 300 mg./100 ml., and one parent will be found to have the same defect. Tendon xanthomata may be present. These small, yellow, flat plaques may be found in the Achilles tendon and the tendons of the back of the hands. The risk of heart attack is of the order of 50 percent by age 50 years.

If both parents have this defect, their offspring may be homozygous type II, with the risk of heart attack being more on the order of 50 percent by age 30 years. Some have attacks prior to age 20 years. However, women with type II seem to have a lower risk.

Serum triglyceride levels are usually normal and the serum is grossly clear. Rarely, the total serum cholesterol level is not significantly elevated, but the amount of the cholesterol in the LDL fraction on ultracentrifugation (and beta band on electrophoresis) may be higher than normal (above 170 mg./100 ml. in children or 210 mg./100 ml. in adults). For this reason the person with only slight cholesterol elevation but with a strong family history of early heart attacks may need detailed studies to determine risk.

There are apparently many "spontaneous" or acquired cases of type II that develop in persons without demonstrable defects in either parent, and these may have a lower risk. A high percentage of postmenopausal women have elevated cholesterol levels, but it takes, perhaps, 20 to 30 years for this elevation to produce much atherosclerosis. This would then explain the favorable difference for this group.

Treatment of type II is by diet, but quite frequently a cholesterol-lowering drug is also needed to significantly lower the levels of serum cholesterol. The cholestyramine resins are the newest of these agents and appear to be the most potent.

TYPE III: This is a very much less common disorder, usually familial, that may be present if there is elevation of both cholesterol and triglycerides. On electrophoresis there is a wide band in the beta position or a combined beta and pre-beta band. (This abnormal "floating beta" is of-lower density than beta.) The serum may be clear or lactescent.

In addition to premature coronary disease, these persons have a high incidence of premature peripheral vascular disease. Treatment is primarily by diet, which reduces body weight to ideal (lean) level. The diet should be reduced in simple carbohydrate (sugar), and in butter and coconut (short-chain saturated fats) and cholesterol. Clofibrate appears to be a useful drug in the therapeutic program.

TYPE IV: This appears to be a common lipoprotein disorder that seems to be familial and associated with several mutations. Serum triglycerides are elevated, so the serum is usually lactescent. Serum cholesterol is normal or elevated. A pre-beta band is seen on electrophoresis.

This disorder is not commonly seen prior to age 20 years. We are finding an increased prevalence with increased age. Premature atherosclerosis occurs, and diabetes or abnormal glucose tolerance tests are fairly commonly associated. Elevation of serum uric acid is not uncommon. When triglycerides are very high, eruptive xathomata of the skin over the knees, elbows, or buttocks may occur. Our study suggests that this disorder is not common in premenopausal females.

The response to a weight-reducing, low sugar (and low butter and coconut) diet is excellent. In fact, the response is so prompt in many that moderate to mild triglyceride elevations may drop to the normal range in a few days after starting a reducing diet. For this reason, diagnostic testing should not be done while persons are reducing their weight or are on any temporary restricted diet. We want to know what their lipid levels or lipoprotein patterns are while on their *usual* diets.

Once a diagnosis has been made, patients can be retested while on restricted diets, as long as the diet is their usual restricted diet, not one that was more strict for a few days prior to the test. Since diet is so effective, there should be no need for drugs in most cases.

TYPE V: Some cases are familial and some are secondary to diabetic acidosis, pancreatitis, alcoholism, and nephrosis. The patient with the familial type may have attacks of abdominal pain, pancreatitis, and enlargement of liver and spleen. Triglycerides are markedly elevated (usually above 1,000 mg./100 ml. and sometimes above 5,000 mg./ 100 ml.).

On electrophoresis there is a prominent pre-beta band and a chylomicron band suggesting a double defect—one related to abnormal fat absorption (chylomicrons) and the other related to abnormal (pre-beta) triglyceride synthesis from carbohydrate or from excess calories. Cholesterol elevation is secondary to the increase in chylomicrons and pre-beta lipoprotein and returns to normal with diet. Abnormal glucose tolerance is common.

Treatment is a combination of the treatment of type IV and type I with emphasis on type IV treatment, since this has the potential atherosclerotic complications. However, fat must also be restricted to prevent episodes of abdominal pain or pancreatitis.

The normal pattern of the various lipoprotein bands on paper electrophoresis would show only a light narrow beta band and the alpha band after 12 hours fasting.

By measuring only the serum cholesterol and serum triglycerides, we are not able to make a definite diagnosis of the phenotype of those who are abnormal, but we have a good start. Types I and V are separated from the others by the creamy layer on the serum top for both and a relatively clear bottom for type I, and a milky bottom for type V. These finding are associated with high triglyceride levels. The remainder of those with high triglyceride levels and homogeneous serum lactescence are mostly type IV. If high triglyceride levels are also associated with cholesterol elevation that does not return to normal on a low sugar, reducing diet, the person may have type II or a mixed type II and type IV or possibly type III.

Electrophoresis has been a helpful additional study, but does not appear to be an essential test in most cases. There is no clear-cut difference between the densities of some of the normal and abnormal beta bands and pre-beta bands on the electrophoresis, just as there is no certainty about the normality or abnormality of triglyceride levels in the range of 130 to 190, or cholesterol levels in the range of 220 to 280. It appears that all of those abnormal and borderline test results may represent degrees of risk.

DIET HELP AND RESISTANCE

Our basic reducing diet, low in both sugar and short-chain fat, is shown on p. 45. Besides this form, we used additional handouts to help insure adequate intake of vitamins and minerals and to assist patients to estimate the carbohydrate content of various common mixtures. This diet is used for most of those with elevated triglyceride levels, with or without cholesterol elevations.

A "prudent diet" (reduced in sugars, cholesterol, and saturated fats) is often used for employees with cholesterol elevations alone or those

LOW CARBOHYDRATE—NO SUGAR DIET
(Limit carbohydrate intake to maximum of 150 Gm. daily)

This experimental diet is designed to reduce weight in those who are overweight, and lower serum triglyceride levels by lowering serum pre-beta lipoprotein levels. Serum cholesterol may also fall in those with high triglyceride levels. Bulky vegetables, meat, and most fats are permitted so that the diet is physically satisfying. Sweets, alcohol, and dairy and coconut fat are severely restricted. Cholesterol intake is reduced.

The following foods are NOT allowed, or quantities are SEVERELY limited:

Sweets. Maximum of one small serving of fresh fruit per day (= 15 Gm. carbohydrate). No sugar, candy, pastry, ices, desserts, soft drinks, fruit drinks, jellies, jams.

Milk, butter and milk products. Includes cheese, ice cream, and ice milk. One cup of cottage cheese is permitted; 2 cups of skim milk are permitted (= 10 Gm. carbohydrate).

Coconut oil. Pastry, most cream substitutes, some margarines.

Alcohol. In most cases intake is limited to maximum of 1½ ounces whiskey or gin, 4 ounces wine, or 1 bottle of beer per day; many persons can not have that much. Each portion = 20 Gm. carbohydrate.

The following foods are permitted in NORMAL amounts:
(Each portion = about 5 Gm. carbohydrate)

Vegetables.

Asparagus	Cauliflower	Dandelion	Mushrooms	Pickles	String Beans
Beets	Celery	Eggplant	Mustard	(Dill or	Tomatoes
Broccoli	Chard	Escarole	Okra	Sour)	Water Cress
Brussels	Chicory	Green	Onions	Radishes	Winter Squash
Sprouts	Collard	Peas	Peppers	Rutabagas	Tomato Juice
Cabbage	Cucumbers	Kale	Pumpkin	Sauerkraut	"V/8" Juice
Carrots		Lettuce		Spinach	

Meat, poultry, and fish.

Fats. Margarine (corn oil), cooking oils, mayonnaise, "Coffee-Rich."

The following foods must be MODERATELY limited:

Liver, shell fish, and egg yolks (maximum of 4 per week in most cases).

Starches are moderately limited: A maximum of 8 portions per day of the list below is permitted. Each portion contains approximately 15 Gm. of carbohydrate:

Baked beans—¼ cup	Crackers, Graham—2	Potatoes, baked
Beans, dry Navy,	Crackers, Oyster—20	or boiled—1
Lima—½ cup	Crackers, Round—6-8	Potatoes, mashed—
Biscuit, muffin, } 1	Crackers, Saltine—5	½ cup
roll, cornbread }	Crackers, Soda—3	Potatoes, sweet or
Bread—1 slice	Flour—2½ tbsp.	yams—¼ cup
Cereal, cooked—½ cup	Parsnips—⅔ cup	Rice or grits (cooked)—
Corn—⅓ cup	Peanuts—½ cup	½ cup
Cereal, flakes } ¾ cup	Peas, dry split—	Spaghetti, noodles—
or puffed }	½ cup	½ cup

Remember that excess intake of any foods must be avoided so that you carry no excess weight. Regular use of a scale can help you determine your needs.
Blood serum tests of triglyceride and cholesterol levels may need to be repeated periodically to be sure that your dieting is adequate for your particular needs.

who have reduced their weight and their triglycerides, but not cholesterol on the reducing diet. If cholesterol levels remain significantly elevated despite adequate dieting, the employee is sometimes referred for consideration of a cholestyramine resin.

Cooperation with diet restrictions is poor unless the person is highly motivated. Intelligence correlates slightly, but many intelligent employees seem to be unable to diet adequately on a continuing basis. A *permanent change in eating habits* is required for continuing adequate control.

We have found that at least 90 percent of employees placed on a test diet for a few weeks and then retested have been cooperative, as measured by significant reduction in weight and serum triglycerides. But longer periods of dieting are less successful. Only about 10 percent are dieting *adequately* and only 50 percent are dieting at all at the end of a year.

When restimulated by new tests, many once again become cooperative for varying periods of time. If a friend or relative has a heart attack, the degree of cooperation increases. If the employee himself has a heart attack, the degree of cooperation subsequently is usually excellent.

Since the mortality rate from the first heart attack is so high, we are aiming at preventing the first heart attack by trying to favorably modify *all* positive risk factors that we find, including cigarette smoking, hypertension, diabetes, serum lipid abnormalities and inadequate exercise. While doing this, we are hopeful that careful record keeping that uses machine systems will permit evaluation of the influence of various risk factors and of various forms of intervention.

From the *American Journal of Nursing* 73:277-279, Feb. 1973.

Serum Enzymes in Myocardial Infarction

AYNSELY M. SMITH • JUDITH A. THIERER

SHELIA H. HUANG

The serum levels of cardiac enzymes can be correlated with the patient's clinical course. Accurate interpretation of their significance is based on knowing when changes begin to occur, when they peak, and when they return to normal.

The diagnosis and management of an acute myocardial infarction are based primarily on the patient's clinical picture, alterations in the electrocardiogram, and changes in the serum levels of specific cardiac enzymes. The relationship between the clinical and the electrocardiographic course has been well documented. The usefulness of cardiac enzyme changes in evaluating a patient's condition, however, is quite controversial. But when such data are available, it is important for the nurse to be able to correlate changes in the serum levels of myocardial enzymes with the clinical course.

Cardiac enzymes are proteins formed by the protoplasm of the cell. They act as catalysts, which are substances capable of accelerating a reaction without themselves being altered. One of their most interesting qualities is their specificity of action which, due to their structural configuration, allows combination with only one particular substance. Enzyme chemists have stated that as many as 1,000 separate enzymes may exist in the cytoplasm, mitochondria, or bound to a cell(1).

ENZYMES IN MYOCARDIAL INFARCTION

The three most frequently studied enzymes in patients with acute myocardial infarction are lactic dehydrogenase (LDH), serum glutamic oxaloacetic transaminase (SGOT), and creatinine phosphokinase (CPK). These enzymes are useful diagnostically because they are present in large amounts in cardiac cells; because they are released by injured or dead myocardial cells, which raises their serum levels significantly following myocardial infarction; and because they can be easily and reliably quantitated and standardized.

LACTIC DEHYDROGENASE (LDH) This enzyme is important because the heart uses lactate as a source of energy. LDH catalyzes the oxidation of lactic acid to pyruvic acid which is then either converted to glucose or enters the Krebs cycle to produce adenosine triphosphate or ATP(2).

As cells break down in an infarcted area, LDH is released from the leaking cell membrane into the blood. The serum level of LDH usually becomes elevated within 24 hours after myocardial cell breakdown, peaks at approximately 72 hours, and returns to normal within 5 to 14 days(3).

Lactic dehydrogenase is present in tissue other than heart muscle; for this reason, elevations of serum LDH may result from diseases of other organs. Acute injury to red blood cells, liver, skeletal muscle, kidney, and skin frequently increases the serum LDH. Therefore, further enzyme differentiation is needed.

Lactic dehydrogenase can be separated by electrophoresis of plasma into five isoenzymes. The five are alike in enzymatic activity, but, because of minor structural differences, they are dissimilar in their migration characteristics in an electromagnetic field. These dissimilar patterns make it possible to measure the quantity of each of the five isoenzymes in various body tissues.

Cardiac muscle has a distinctly different isoenzyme composition from other tissue and contains a preponderance of the isomer LDH_5. Thus, assays of LDH_5 would seem more informative about myocardial damage than total LDH determinations(4). Increased LDH_5 levels may also occur in renal infarction, hyperthyroidism, pernicious and hemolytic anemias, and cancer of the stomach. But it has been suggested that, because of the relatively low incidence of these problems, serum LDH_5 level may

MS. SMITH *is a staff nurse in the surgical cardiovascular unit at St. Mary's Hospital in Rochester, Minn. She was graduated from Winnipeg General Hospital School of Nursing in Canada.* MS. THIERER *directs a course for coronary care nurses, sponsored by the Minnesota Heart Association and Northlands Regional Medical Program at the Rochester Methodist Hospital in Minnesota. She was graduated from Allen Memorial Lutheran School of Nursing in Waterloo, Iowa.* MS. HUANG, *a staff nurse in the CCU at Group Health Hospital in Seattle, Washington, received her B.S.N. degree from the University of Taiwan in the Republic of China and her M.S. degree in nursing from the University of Maryland in Baltimore.*

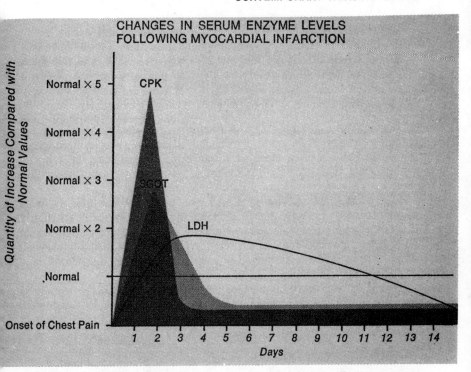

CHANGES IN SERUM ENZYME LEVELS FOLLOWING MYOCARDIAL INFARCTION

be more valuable in diagnosing an acute myocardial infarction than either total LDH or SGOT(5). However, because of the lack of absolute specificity, the isoenzyme elevation must still be correlated with the patient's clinical signs and symptoms of myocardial infarction.

SERUM GLUTAMIC OXALOACETIC TRANSAMINASE (SGOT) All transaminase enzymes catalyze the reaction between an amino acid and a keto acid to form both a new keto and a new amino acid. SGOT specifically catalyzes the transfer of the alpha amino group of aspartic acid and of glutamic acid, which results in the synthesis of oxaloacetic acid. This is important because oxaloacetic acid is a key point of entry in the Krebs cycle. Thus, SGOT is an important enzyme in carbohydrate and protein metabolism.

The SGOT may rise as early as six hours following infarct. It usually peaks in 24 to 48 hours and returns to normal in about four days(6). Relatively high concentrations of SGOT are found in the heart muscle skeletal muscle, brain, liver, and kidney (listed in descending order of concentration). It is apparent that the plasma levels of SGOT will be elevated whenever there is necrosis or injury to any transaminase-rich tissue. Consequently, an elevation of plasma SGOT levels is certainly not limited to myocardial infarction.

CREATININE PHOSPHOKINASE (CPK) This enzyme catalyzes the reversible conversion of creatine phosphate to creatinine, which combines with the adenosine triphosphate (ATP) in cardiac muscle to furnish energy for cardiac contraction. In acute myocardial infarction, the plasma concentration of CPK is often elevated within three to five hours of ischemic onset, peaks at approximately 33 hours, and returns to normal within three days if no extension of the ischemic area occurs.

Inasmuch as the plasma level may rise, peak, and fall quickly to its normal value, the precise degree of elevation may be missed, particularly if relatively long intervals elapse between laboratory determinations of CPK levels. For this reason, the test for CPK is most meaningful when done as soon after the suspected infarction as possible and then assayed daily during the critical period of cardiac recovery.

Outside of myocardial muscle, creatinine phosphokinase usually is found only in skeletal muscle and brain tissue(7). Due to this limited distribution, the CPK level is considered a more specific indication of myocardial damage than the LDH and SGOT levels.

CLINICAL APPLICATIONS

Since all three major enzymes are present in tissue other than heart muscle, there is no enzyme activity measurable in serum which is specifically diagnostic of myocardial infarction. Despite this lack of specificity, enzyme activity is an important quantitative indication of myocardial injury when the levels of the three enzymes are scrutinized and compared simultaneously for several days following a possible myocardial infarction. They may be helpful in distinguishing between crescendo angina and myocardial infarction. When coordinated with other clinical findings, the relationship between the rise in plasma levels of these enzymes and the extent of myocardial damage may be of clinical significance in determining the patient's prognosis after a myocardial infarction(8).

Not all patients develop the classical manifestations of an acute myocardial infarction. In addition to persons who experience unusual symptoms are those who have painless infarctions during anesthesia, postoperative narcosis, or illnesses like diabetic acidosis where consciousness is impaired(9). For these patients, correlation of serum enzyme levels with EKG changes may show that myocardial injury has occurred.

On the other hand, though the electrocardiogram often is useful in determining the presence and location of myocardial infarction, occasionally, the EKG does not demonstrate changes consistent with acute ischemic myocardial injury. The trace may be affected by drugs such as digitalis, quinidine, or procainamide (Pronestyl). It may also be distorted by previously existing dysrhythmias, electrolyte imbalance, or conduction defects. Under such conditions in which myocardial damage cannot be detected by EKG but clinical signs are suggestive, serum enzyme levels may indicate that the myocardium has been injured. The usefulness of enzyme levels is shown by two examples.

PATIENT CASE REPORTS Two men—59-year-old Mr. A. and 69-year-old Mr. B—were admitted to the coronary care unit with continuous chest pain. Mr. A.'s EKG showed a left bundle branch block. Mr. B's EKG showed ST-segment depression with T-wave inversion on leads II, III, and AVF. Serum enzymes of each man were studied to determine whether the diagnosis was crescendo angina or acute myocardial infarction.

The enzyme profiles of both patients for a three-day period are shown below. Although the clinical pictures of both patients were similar and neither electrocardiogram was diagnostic of acute injury. Mr. A's enzyme profile clearly demonstrates that he had sustained myocardial cell necrosis.

NURSING JUDGMENTS

Several nursing judgments may be made on the basis of enzyme results, but only if the nurse is able to use this information in the context of the total clinical picture.

Normal Enzyme Levels	MR. A				MR. B			
	12 hr.	24 hr.	48 hr.	72 hr.	12 hr.	24 hr.	48 hr.	72 hr.
LDH 127 I.U.	100	110	110	105	129	126	127	129
SGOT 24 I.U.	30	120	110	90	21	24	26	24
CPK 71 I.U. (m) 55 I.U. (f)	124	330	190	106	73	75	71	70

Mr. A.'s SGOT and CPK indicate ischemia. Mr. B.'s levels are normal.

The continued presence of injured and ischemic myocardial cells, as shown by elevated enzymes, predisposes to electrical instability. Therefore, the nurse will observe the patient with special vigilance throughout this critical period. The decline or return to near normal enzyme levels may be an indication that the patient has passed the first, most critical phase of the myocardial infarction. Again, the levels must be evaluated in light of the patient's entire clinical picture.

Cardiac enzyme determinations offer nurses a third guide in planning a patient's care. Even when he "feels fine" and his EKG is normal, the elevation of serum enzymes dictates caution in permitting activity. Injudicious activity during the acute injury phase places greater strain on an already embarrassed pump and can lead to left ventricular failure.

Even in such matters as the progression of diet, enzyme results may be helpful. Because digestion of a large meal requires a large cardiac output, it increases cardiac work and may place excessive demand on an injured heart. Therefore, particularly for a patient with serum enzyme levels that indicate injury, smaller, more frequent meals may be appropriate.

Enzyme results are helpful, too, in establishing priorities for transferring patients in or out of the CCU, especially when one must plan patient care with a limited number of nursing staff and a limited number of cardiac monitors.

In summary, the nurse working with cardiac patients needs to differentiate between benign and potentially fatal changes in EKG rhythms and patterns, and to assess the alterations in enzyme levels. An adequate understanding of cardiac enzymology enables the nurse to explain to the patient why repeated blood samples are drawn. By correlating the rise and fall of enzymes with EKG alterations, the nurse will be aware that a decline in the level of serum enzymes means the cessation of myocardial cell breakdown, one indication that conditions now are conducive to healing and myocardial recovery.

REFERENCES

1. ROUTH, J. L., AND OTHERS. *Essentials of General Organic and Biochemistry*. Philadelphia, W. B. Saunders Co., 1969, p. 600.
2. COHEN, L. Contributions of serum enzymes and isoenzymes to the diagnosis of myocardial injury., 1. *Mod.Concepts Cardiovasc.Dis.* 36:43-47, Aug. 1967.
3. WEST, M., AND OTHERS. Serum enzymology in the diagnosis of myocardial infarction and related cardiovascular conditions. *Med.Clin.North Am.* 50:171-191. Jan. 1966.
4. HARPER, H. A. *Review of Physiological Chemistry*. 10th ed. Los Altos, Calif., Lange Publications, 1965, pp. 126-128.
5. HURST, J. W., AND LOGUE, R. B. *The Heart*. 2nd ed. New York,

Blakiston Division, McGraw-Hill Book Co., 1970, pp. 965-966.
6. BRAINERD, HENRY, AND OTHERS, EDS. *Current Diagnosis and Treatment.* 4th ed. Los Altos, Calif., Lange Publications, 1965, p. 206.
7. TODD, J. C., AND SANFORD, A. H. *Clinical Diagnosis by Laboratory Methods.* 14th edition edited by Israel Davidson and J. B. Henry, Philadelphia, W. B. Saunders Co., 1969, p. 736.
8. WROBLEWSKI, FELIX. Serum enzyme and isoenzyme alterations in myocardial infarction. *Progr.Cardiovasc.Dis.* 6:63-83, July 1963.
9. HARRISON, T. R., AND OTHERS, EDS. *Principles of Internal Medicine.* 4th ed. New York, Blakiston Division, McGraw-Hill Book Co., 1962, p. 1453.

BIBLIOGRAPHY

U.S. CENSUS BUREAU. *World Vital Statistics. The United States. 1967 Volume 2, Parts A and B, Mortality.* Washington, D.C., U.S. Government Printing Office, 1969.

LITTAUER, D. Welcome address. In *Aggressive Nursing Management of Acute Myocardial Infarction,* a symposium presented at Cedars-Sinai Medical Center, Los Angeles. Philadelphia, Charles Press, 1968, p. 1.

MORRIS, D. G. The patient in cardiogenic shock. *Cardiovasc.Nurs.* 5:15-17, July-Aug. 1969.

PAGE, D. L., AND OTHERS. Myocardial changes associated with cardiogenic shock. *N.Eng.J.Med.* 285:133-137, July 15, 1971.

ADDENDUM to ARTICLE

Isoenzymes of creatine phosphokinase (CPK) have been identified, and measurements of these isoenzymes (MM, MB, and BB) are clinically available at the present time. The isoenzyme MB is found primarily in myocardial tissue. Therefore, measurement of CPK-MB activity has clinical significance in differentiating whether increased total CPK activity is due to skeletal muscle injury (i.e., trauma, surgical procedures, intramuscular injections) or myocardial infarction.

The reader is referred to Roberts, et al: Quantification of Serum CPK Isoenzymes. American Journal of Cardiology 33:650-654, 1974.

From the *American Journal of Nursing* 72:1597-1600, Sept. 1972.

Arrhythmias and Cardiac Output

GLORIA GILBERT MAYER • **PATRICIA BUCHHOLZ KAELIN**

Almost any physiologic disturbance in any body system can initiate cardiac arrhythmias or complicate existing ones. Cardiac arrhythmias are clinically significant for two reasons: first, minor cardiac arrhythmias may evoke more serious ones; second, any arrhythmia may lead to subsequent hemodynamic alterations. Thus, even "minor" arrhythmias may lead to morbid circumstances.

A major factor in the hemodynamics of the body is the cardiac output. Cardiac output is determined by the stroke volume, the amount of blood ejected with each ventricular contraction, and by the heart rate; it is calculated by multiplying these two factors together. Cardiac arrhythmias may either increase or decrease the heart rate, and alterations in rate can significantly affect cardiac output.

With a slower heart rate, diastolic filling is increased, which increases stroke volume. But, with progressively slower heart rates, the effect of an increased stroke volume eventually levels off and, with the decreased rate of contractions, cardiac output falls.

Studies have proved that patients with complete heart block can partially compensate for increasing metabolic demands by increasing stroke volume or by increasing arteriolar oxygen extraction. However, compensation is limited. In experiments increasing the heart rate of patients with heart block from 30 to 50 beats a minute to 60 to 80 beats a minute, using cardiac pacing and drugs, resulted in a 50 to 150 percent increase in cardiac output(1).

While an increased heart rate increases the number of ventricular ejections, it reduces the period of diastolic filling, which decreases the stroke volume. Thus, with increasing heart rates, a point is eventually reached when cardiac output falls.

Unsynchronized atrial and ventricular systoles can also alter hemodynamics in a number of ways. In particular, they affect the stroke volume. The atrium functions as a booster pump. About 70 percent of blood in the atria flows directly to the ventricles before atrial systole; the remaining 30 percent is ejected during atrial systole. With such asynchrony as occurs in atrial fibrillation, atrial contraction may be incomplete. Very little of this 30 percent will be ejected into the ventricles and, hence, the output from the ventricles will be less. This is not always crucial, but that additional volume may be significant during exercise or in a severely decompensated heart. In addition, atrial-ventricular synchrony which is necessary for the normal closure of the A-V valves may be affected. The asynchrony of such arrhythmias as atrial fibrillation often leads to mitral and tricuspid insufficiency.

While a certain amount of blood will still flow into the ventricles with total asynchrony of atrial muscle contraction, this same asynchrony in the ventricles, as occurs in ventricular fibrillation, will result in no cardiac output. Degrees of asynchrony, such as in bundle branch block, result in a decrease in cardiac output.

The consequences of any arrhythmia are influenced by the underlying pathologic condition of the heart and by the integrity of the vasomotor control mechanisms. Hemodynamic alterations may be more severe depending on the degree of pathology in the myocardium or coronary arteries. Many patients with atrial fibrillation may remain asymptomatic, except in the presence of such myocardial pathology as congestive heart failure. It is also true that cardiac disease can increase in severity with the presence of an arrhythmia. For example, a patient with angina pectoris may have increasingly severe attacks in the presence of sinus tachycardia.

If a patient with an arrhythmia has normal vasomotor control, his body can alter peripheral resistance in an attempt to compensate for a decrease in cardiac output. However, a patient with essential hypertension may not be able to compensate. The same inability to maintain adequate perfusion can occur with any condition in which there is a decreased venous return.

MS. MAYER *is an instructor at St. Mary's Junior College in Minneapolis, Minnesota. She was graduated from the Miami-Dade Junior College department of nursing in Florida, received her B.S. degree in nursing from the University of Miami, her M.S. degree in nursing from the University of Maryland, and her M.Ed. from Teachers College, Columbia University in New York City.* MS. KAELIN *was an assistant professor of nursing at Columbia University at the time this paper was prepared. She was graduated from St. Joseph School of Nursing in Flint, Mich. and received both her B.S. and M.S. degrees in nursing from Wayne State University in Detroit, Mich.*

EXTRACARDIAC FACTORS IN CARDIAC OUTPUT

The major and lethal arrhythmias may all cause a decrease in cardiac output. Careful examination of the patient, interpretation of laboratory data, and EKG monitoring can help a nurse determine the presence and estimate the severity of decreased cardiac output.

All nurses must be cognizant of various factors which may further decrease the cardiac output either by initiating arrhythmias or increasing their severity. Such extracardiac factors as alcohol, tobacco, certain drugs, and such acute emotional states as anxiety, pain, fear, and depression, especially in the chronically stressed individual, may produce or aggravate arrhythmias. It has been shown that initially nicotine slows the heart rate due to vagal stimulation and later, with repeated or increasing

DRUGS TO REVERSE ARRHYTHMIAS

	Quinidine	procaine amide (Pronestyl)	propranolol (Inderal)	diphenylhydantoin (Dilantin)	lidocaine (Xylocaine)
Routes of administration	oral, I.M.	oral, I.M., I.V.	oral, I.V.	oral, I.V. (bolus)	I.V.
Arrhythmias	atrial: premature contractions (APC), paroxysmal tachycardia (PAT), fibrillation (AF). atrioventricular junctional tachycardia and premature contractions. ventricular: premature contractions (PVC).	atrial: premature contractions (APC), paroxysmal tachycardia (PAT), fibrillation (AF). ventricular: premature contractions (PVC), tachycardia (VT).	digitalis-induced arrhythmias (atrial and ventricular). atrial: paroxysmal tachycardia (PAT).	ventricular: premature contractions (PVC), tachycardia (VT). digitalis-induced arrhythmias (atrial and ventricular).	ventricular: premature contraction (PVC), tachycardia (VT). digitalis-induced arrhythmias (atrial and ventricular).
Dosage:					
Total oral/day	1.2-3.2 gm.	1.0-4.0 gm.	10-100 mg.	300-600 mg.	
Frequency	q6h (q4h)	q6h (q4h)	q6h	qid	
I.V., initial		100 mg./5 min. to 1 gm. total	1 mg./min. to 5 mg. total	100 mg./5 min. to 1 mg. total	1 mg./kg. 3-5 min. to 200-300 mg. total
I.V., maintenance		20-80 mcg./kg./ min. (1.5-5.0 mg./ min.)			20-50 mcg./kg./ min. (1.0-3.5 mg./ min.)
Plasma level					
Peak (single oral dose)	1.5-2 hour	1-1.5 hour	1-4 hours	6-12 hours	Onset of action within 2 min.
Duration of effect	6-8 hours	6 hours	3-6 hours		20 min.
Metabolism	liver	liver	liver	liver	liver
Excretion via kidney of unmetabolized drug	20-50%	50-60%		less than 5%	less than 10%

doses of nicotine, cardiac rate is increased due to sympathetic ganglia stimulation.

Experimental studies show that coffee also stimulates the myocardium and, if the stimulation is great enough, it may actually produce cardiac irregularities. Alcohol, on the other hand, seems to have minimal and inconsistent cardiac effects. Finally, various drugs and hormones—amphetamines, phenothiazines, and thyroid hormones—have been known to engender cardiac arrhythmias(2).

Certain electrolytes affect the electrophysiologic properties of the heart. Hyperkalemia, for example, decreases cardiac irritability and may produce cardiac standstill. Hypokalemia increases ventricular irritability and may lead to ventricular fibrillation. Hypercalcemia increases ventricular irritability and can produce fibrillation, whereas hypocalcemia

	Quinidine	procaine amide (Pronestyl)	propranolol (Inderal)	diphenylhydantoin (Dilantin)	lidocaine (Xylocaine)
Side effects and Toxic effects	anorexia, nausea, vomiting, diarrhea, ventricular tachycardia, ventricular fibrillation, and ectopic beats with high doses.	decreased BP; ventricular tachycardia, ventricular fibrillation, and ectopic beats; anorexia, nausea, vomiting, flushing, weakness, psychosis, agranulocytosis.	nausea, vomiting, light-headedness, diarrhea, constipation, mental depression.	CNS toxicity: drowsiness, nystagmus, diplopia, vertigo, nervousness, tremors, slurred speech.	CNS toxicity: drowsiness, disorientation, apprehension, parathesias, decreased hearing, visual disturbances, muscle twitching, convulsions.
	idiosyncratic effects: decreased BP, vertigo, tinnitis, visual disturbances, rash, fever, thrombocytopnea purpura, headache, confusion, vascular collapse.	hypersensitivity: fever, chills, urticaria.	contraindications: bronchial asthma, allergic rhinitis, sinus bradycardia, second degree or total heart block, cardiogenic shock, CHF, anesthetics or adrenergic-augmenting psychotropic drugs.		
	precautions: Because excreted by kidney essentially unmetabolized, caution should be exercised in administering to patients with renal insufficiency.			precautions: Because of metabolism in liver, caution should be exercised in administering to patients with hepatic damage.	
EKG:					
PR interval	unchanged or increased	unchanged or increased	unchanged or increased	unchanged or decreased	unchanged
QRS interval	increased	increased	unchanged	unchanged	unchanged
QT interval	increased	increased	decreased	decreased	decreased
Treatment of toxicity	successfully *treated* with I.V. molar sodium lactate and catecholamines. partially *ameliorated* with 1-5 mg. glucagon I.V.				discontinuation of drug or, if patient convulsing, administration of short-acting barbiturate.

Adjusted from J. T. Bigger and R. H. Heissenbuttel, "Clinical use of Antiarrhythmic drugs," Postgraduate Medicine, January 1970.

may produce cardiac standstill. Alterations in sodium and magnesium concentrations also affect electrophysiologic properties and may produce arrhythmias. Therefore, the nurse must keep abreast of changing electrolyte status so that replacement therapy, either medicinal or nutritional, can be given if indicated.

Acid-base imbalance and poor oxygenation may also alter cardiac activity. Oxygen and pH affect the rate of spontaneous depolarization of automatic cells. Hypoxemia or any alterations of carbon dioxide tension, especially in combination with respiratory alkalosis, are, therefore, arrhythmogenic. These changes are particularly evident in the critically ill patient.

How do so many patients get into this problem? Diffuse atelectasis with venoarterial shunting is the most frequent cause of hypoxemia and is due to a number of factors in hospitalized patients. Normal individuals sigh four to ten times an hour which opens any collapsed alveoli. In hospitalized patients, Ayres and Grace point out:

> *General anesthesia, sedation, chest pain, general debility, pulmonary congestion and the shock state decrease the frequency of sighing and also interfere with both the production of surfactant and the function of the vascular scaffolding. These two factors, decreased deep breathing and decreased antiatelectasis properties, interact to produce alveolar collapse in most critically ill patients.(3)*

There are factors other than hypoxemia which can have potentially dangerous effects. Hyperventilation and hypoventilation can alter arterial carbon dioxide tension and pH. Although hypoxemia is a major stimulus to hyperventilation, such other factors as pain, anxiety, metabolic acidosis, and pulmonary congestion also appear to be instrumental. Hypoventilation commonly accompanies oversedation or ischemic brain damage. The nurse must appreciate the importance of proper positioning and prescribed humidified oxygen therapy; maintain a schedule of pulmonary physiotherapy, especially coughing and deep breathing; and avoid injudicious use of sedatives. The nurse must take special precautions when caring for the patient on a respirator because of the danger of faulty ventilation. Suctioning must be done with utmost care to remove secretions without inducing hypoxia.

Because of the relationship of hypoxemia to cardiac irregularities and decreased output, the nurse needs to consider the energy expenditure demanded by various types of activities. Archibald and Gefter emphasize the energy expenditure needs to be selected on the basis of cardiac reserve, which decreases as the work load increases(4). Therefore, gradually increasing selected activities in progressive phases of hospitalization is important. During any activity, the nurse must carefully observe the patient's tolerance, using such clues as vital sign changes, increasing arrhythmias, pain, respiratory distress, pallor, cyanosis, or diaphoresis. She must then decide whether regression or progression of the rehabilitative regimen is indicated or whether activity should be maintained at the same level.

There are three major modes of treating patients with arrhythmias: drugs, cardiac pacing, and precordial shock. The desired mode of therapy will depend upon the physician and the patient.

Choice of an antiarrhythmic drug is contingent upon several factors: natural history of the arrhythmia, the patient's clinical status, electrocardiographic and hemodynamic effects of the drug, and knowledge of the specific mechanism by which an arrhythmia is initiated and maintained, if this information is known(5). Five of the more common drugs in use include quinidine, procaine amide, propranolol, diphenylhydantoin, and lidocaine.

There are two major methods by which controlled electricity can be employed in the management of the cardiac patient. Low voltage current in the form of pacemakers can be applied to the myocardium when the heart stops abruptly or slows to such a rate that it can no longer maintain an effective cardiac output. Although pacemakers are primarily used for bradyarrhythmias, they are occasionally used to overdrive the heart in tachyarrhythmias.

The second method in which electricity is used is countershock therapy which requires a somewhat higher voltage current. This includes cardioversion and defibrillation and is used to treat tachyarrhythmias.

Though the mode of therapy differs, each has the same general goal —to return the heart to its optimal rate and force of contractions so that it can effectively maintain circulation.

REFERENCES

1. McIntoch, H. D., and Morris, J. J. Jr. Hemodynamic consequences of arrhythmias. *Progr.Cardiovasc.Dis.* 8:348-349, Jan. 1966.
2. Dreifus, L. S., and Watanabe, Y. Tension, drugs and premature systoles. *Am.Heart J.* 70:291-294, Set. 1965.
3. Ayres, S. M., and Grace, W. J. Abnormal alveolar gas exchange

in acute myocardial infarction; theory and therapy. *Vull.Acad.-Med.N.J.* 15:192-196, Sept. 1969.
4. ARCHIBALD, K. C., AND GEFTER, W. I. Rehabilitation of the elderly cardiac patient. *Geriatrics* 25:133-141. Mar, 1970.
5. BIGGER, J. T. JR., AND HEISSENBUTTEL, R. H. Clinical use of antiarrhythmic drugs. *Postgrad.Med.* 47:119-125, Jan. 1970.

BIBLIOGRAPHY

ACKER, J. E. Exercise and rehabilitation; role of the nurse in rehabilitation of the myocardial infarction patient. *J.S.C.Med.Assoc.* 65(Suppl.1): 65-66. Dec. 1969.

ANDREOLI, KATHLEEN G. Cardiac monitor. *Am.J.Nurs.* 69:1238-1243, June 1969.

BUCHOLZ, PATRICIA K., AND GILBERT, GLORIA H. Understanding the ECG. *RN* 35:38-42, Feb. 1972.

CASSEM, N. H., AND OTHERS. Reactions of coronary patients to the CCU nurse. *Am.J.Nurs.* 70:319-325. Feb. 1970.

GILBERT, GLORIA. Electrical hazards in the use of monitors and defibrillators. *Nurs.Clin.North Am.* 4:615-619, Dec. 1969.

HUNN, VIRGINIA K. Cardiac pacemakers. *Am.J.Nurs.* 69:749-754, Apr. 1969.

JENKINS, ADELINE C. Successful cardiac monitoring. *Nurs.Clin.North Am.* 1:537-547, Dec. 1966.

UNGER, P. N. Target, heart disease; electrical conversion of cardiac arrhythmias. *Am.J.Nurs.* 66:1962-1965, Sept. 1966.

From *Nursing Research* 23:489-491, Nov.-Dec. 1974.

Cyclic Occurrence of Premature Ventricular Contractions in Acute Myocardial Infarction Patients: A Pilot Study

JUDITH M. HOCKENBERGER • MARILYN B RUBIN

To determine if an association exists between premature ventricular contractions and the time of day in which they occur, a systematic comparison was made between the occurrence of the contractions and the time in ten male postmyocardial infarction patients over a four-day period in a coronary care unit. Findings indicated that fewer premature ventricular contractions occurred between 12:00 MDNT. and 6:00 A.M.; on the fourth day there were fewer premature ventricular contractions than on any other day; administration of antiarrhythmic drugs may be indicated during peak time of premature ventricular contraction occurrence.

Premature ventricular contractions have been associated with lethal arrhythmias and the new postmyocardial infarction patient. Both clinical experience and a review of the literature suggested that premature ventricular contractions might display a rhythm in their occurrence during the day.

Cardiac arrhythmia is one of the most severe complications of myocardial infarction(1). About 75 percent of such patients show premature ventricular contractions(2). Premature ventricular contractions are forerunners of ventricular fibrillation, one of the most dangerous arrthythmias. Clearly, detection and management of the arrhythmia are basic to the treatment of myocardial infarction.

On the premise that lethal arrhythmias in the postmyocardial infarction patient may be prevented if the time during a 24-hour period in which premature ventricular contractions are most likely to occur is known, the specific aim of this investigation was to determine any relationship between the time of day and the occurrence of premature ventricular contractions in the postmyocardial infarction patient.

REVIEW OF THE LITERATURE

Myocardial infarction occurs when blood flow to the myocardium is obstructed(3). The myocardium is similar to other kinds of muscle in that it can respond to abnormal stimuli as well as normal stimuli. It differs from skeletal muscle in that its refractory period is relatively long(1), thus protecting the heart from remaining in a continuous state of contraction and thereby stopping the circulation.

Bruce stated that one of the most important characteristics of heart muscle is its capacity to contract independently of neural control(4).

The properties automaticity and rhythmicity facilitate survival when there is an interruption of the conduction of impulses in the muscles of the ventricle. When a myocardial infarction occurs, one or more groups of muscle cells become abnormally irritable and initiate ectopic beats or premature ventricular contractions.

The various parts of the circulatory system are regulated in relation to one another. Integration of the activity of the heart with the activity of the body is under the control of the autonomic nervous system(1). Brown pointed out that when a myocardial infarction occurs, there is a desynchronization of the electrical conductivity of the heart(5). Frequently, premature ventricular contractions occur during the refractory period or immediately thereafter. The effects upon the individual depend on the frequency with which the contractions occur and on the extent to which they interfere with the heart's capacity to function adequately. Romhilt and Fowler noted that premature ventricular contractions lead to a decrease in cardiac efficiency and predispose to cardiac failure(6).

Premature ventricular contractions may be the first indication of sub-

JUDITH M. HOCKENBERGER (*St. Vincent Hospital School of Nursing, Toledo, Ohio; M.S.N., Saint Louis University, St. Louis, Missouri*) *is an instructor in nursing at Saint Louis University School of Nursing and Allied Health Professions, St. Louis, Missouri.* MARILYN RUBIN (*Lutheran Hospital School of Nursing, St. Louis, Missouri; Ph.D., Southern Illinois University, Carbondale, Illinois*) *is associate professor and chairman of Medical-Surgical Nursing, Saint Louis University School of Nursing and Allied Health Professions, St. Louis, Missouri.*

sequent myocardial damage, precipitating ventricular tachycardia and ventricular fibrillation. These events culminate in death unless there is medical intervention(7). Identification of premature ventricular contractions is thus important for the nursing staff.

Many concepts have been developed about the cause of premature beats. The theory considered here is one in which ventricular premature beats occur in association with various types of myocardial abnormalities(8). If the effects of drugs and electrolyte alterations are excluded, the serious ventricular arrhythmias occur in postcoronary patients with muscle tissue damage. To make clinical diagnosis, the nurse should be familiar with the cardinal features of premature ventricular contractions: prematurity of the beat, bizarre deviation from the normal configuration, and compensatory pause following the beat(3).

Hurst also showed that ventricular fibrillation may be initiated by ventricular premature contractions(3). These usually occur early in diastole, at the end of the T wave, which frequently leads to ventricular fibrillation. This is particularly apt to occur in the presence of myocardial infarction.

Wolff *et al.* stated that the first beat which follows the pause after a premature beat may show a shorter time of isometric contraction and an augmentation of stroke volume(9). Failure of such compensation to occur acts as a trigger mechanism for ventricular tachycardia or fibrillation.

Cyclic processes exist in all living organisms and medical interest at present has focused on the circadian rhythm(10,11). Periodicity has been noted in many circulatory functions. The average frequency with which many rhythmic variations recur under normal conditions of life is that of one cycle in 24 hours, which is referred to as 24-hour periodicity(12). Yamamoto and Brobeck found that the heart rate has been known to vary along a 24-hour time scale(13). Brown suggested that all circulatory values follow a similar periodicity(5). Detailed studies by Kleitman and Ramsaroop of six subjects examined at two-hour intervals showed that the heart rate shows periodicity with lowest values during late evening. These rhythms can change by a few minutes or a few hours(14).

Research at the German Air Force Institute of Aviation Medicine revealed that the greatest frequency of premature ventricular contractions occurred during periods of rest and sleep. In their studies 52 subjects showed premature ventricular contractions. These arrhythmias appeared in two-thirds of the examinees without signs of cardiac damage and appeared only at one time, during periods of rest and sleep(15). In addition to this, Smith *et al.* determined that premature ventricular contractions have a tendency to occur more frequently during the sleep-wake transitions than during sleep.(16).

HYPOTHESIS

On the basis of the studies by Dietz and Kirchoff and Smith *et al.* it was hypothesized that premature ventricular contractions will occur more frequently from 6:00 P.M to 12:00 MDNT. in the postcoronary patient.

METHOD

The data were collected in the 15-bed coronary care unit (CCU) of a 1,100-bed hospital in St. Louis. Ten males who entered the CCU with a diagnosis of both premature ventricular contractions and myocardial infarction were included in the sample. The first patient was chosen on the basis of the time the investigator arrived in the CCU, in that the first male patient admitted after the investigator's arrival was the first patient admitted to the study. The investigator then eliminated patients who did not experience premature ventricular contractions or have a myocardial infarction. Only patients who were being treated with Xylocaine hydrochloride were included in the study.

The diagnostic enzymes elevated in concentration included lactic dehydrogenase, serum glutamicoxaloacetic transaminase, and creatine phosphokinase. Documentation of myocardial infarction was also evidenced by the abnormal repolarization pattern in the electrocardiogram. Documentation of premature ventricular contractions was accomplished by two methods: First, a Mennen-Greatback computer recorded electrocardiographic events in all patients within this unit. The information obtained included the total number of premature ventricular contractions per minute and per 24 hours. Second, each patient's monitor was observed by the nursing staff on a 24-hour basis. The staff was familiarized with purpose and methods of the study. The nurses charted the time and number of the premature ventricular contractions that occurred. Coder reliability in identification of premature ventricular contractions was presumed because of the special training of the CCU nurses. In addition, electrocardiogram rhythm strips from patients with premature ventricular contractions were reviewed by the resident staff of the hospital for further reliability.

The patients were studied for four consecutive days. The time and number of premature ventricular contractions were recorded from the hour of admission, continued for the first 24 hours, and then continued for the second, third, and fourth days postadmission. The contractions were observed for time, number, and possible patterns and the information was compared to ascertain if premature ventricular contractions occurred more frequently at any particular time of day. In the CCU utilized in this study, frequent interruptions were made by the nursing staff, medical staff, and family. There was no set routine for visiting hours nor for medical or nursing rounds—activities which are stress producing for the patient and may lead to premature ventricular contractions.

The 24-hour computer readout obtained on each patient was divided into six-hour periods (6:00 A.M.—12:00 NOON, 12:00 NOON—6:00 P.M., 6:00 P.M.—12:00 MDNT., 12:00 MDNT.—6:00 A.M.) and gave the following information: premature ventricular contractions, heart rate, and data loss percentage. The average highest number and lowest number of premature ventricular contractions that occurred in a minute during a six-hour period were utlized as the significant numbers of premature contractions in a given time period.

RESULTS

When compared with the hypothesized time of greatest occurrence of premature ventricular contractions, that is, between 6:00 P.M. and 12:00 MDNT., the data indicated that: On day one, the most frequent occurrences were between 12:00 MDNT. and 6:00 A.M. and 6:00 A.M. and 12:00 NOON; on day two between 12:00 MDNT. and 6:00 A.M.; on day three between 12:00 NOON and 6:00 P.M. (see Table 1).

More premature ventricular contractions per minute occurred in the postmyocardial infarction patients on day two (2.5) following admission to the hospital than on the other days (day one, 2.0; day three, 1.5; day four, 1.0).

DISCUSSION

Findings in this study did not support the hypothesis that premature

Table 1. Frequency of Mean Premature
Ventricular Contractions per Minute in
Four Postadmission Days for Ten Patients

DAY	TIME OF DAY			
	12 MDNT.- 6:00 A.M.	6:00 A.M.- 12 NOON	12 NOON- 6:00 P.M.	6:00 P.M.- 12 MDNT.
1	1.0	1.5	2.5	2.0
2	2.0	2.5	3.5	2.5
3	1.5	2.5	1.0	1.5
4	1.0	1.0	1.0	1.0

ventricular contractions occur more frequently between 6:00 P.M. and 12:00 MDNT. or during resting periods.

If further research should reveal a time of day that premature ventricular contractions occur with greater frequency, nursing staff could give closer attention to the patient during those times, normal activity periods and the timing of medications could be altered, and visitors to the patient's room could be prohibited. Lethal arrhythmias might thus be avoided.

Recommendations. This pilot study should be followed up, employing a larger, randomly selected sample. It is also recommended that the number of interruptions to the patient during day and night be controlled.

A more accurate way of obtaining the number of premature ventricular contractions occurring should be sought. If the abnormal beats were counted on a per minute basis, the reliability would be greater than in this study. In the six-hour intervals, the investigator arbitrarily counted the number per minute of premature ventricular contractions. Data loss occurred for reasons which included the patient's leaving the floor, electrodes being removed, and inaccurate readings of the computer readout in regard to premature ventricular contractions. More sophisticated equipment, such as 24-hour 12-lead electrocardiograms, should be used.

Some asymptomatic patients could be used for comparison in a future study. These samples should include both men and women, various age levels, and various races.

Medications should be controlled for the hospitalized patients treated for premature ventricular contractions. Although in this study patients were not accepted into the sample if the premature ventricular contractions were being treated with any medication other than Xylocaine hydrochloride, the study showed that during a 24-hour period premature ventricular contractions would occur even if the symptoms were abated with intermittent injections of Xylocaine hydrochloride.

An additional dimension for study in an investigation of premature ventricular contractions might include occurrence on a seasonal or yearly basis. Such information would allow for greater awareness about the expectation of onset. Additional research might also lead to greater knowledge regarding the rhythms of the heart and its electrical activity.

Another dimension might be a study of type of people who are more prone to premature ventricular contractions, including such factors as family history, personality traits, and response to stress. Further analysis of an individual's biorhythms in relation to the occurrence of their premature ventricular contractions may be worthwhile.

REFERENCES

1. GUYTON, A. C. *Textbook of Medical Physiology,* 4th ed. Philadelphia, W. B. Saunders Co., 1971.
2. DENBOROUGH, MICHAEL, AND OTHERS. Arrhythmias and late sudden death after myocardial infarction. *Lancet* 1:386-388. Feb. 24, 1968.
3. HURST, J. W., ED. *The Heart.* 3d ed. New York, McGraw-Hill Book Co., 1973.
4. BRUCE, T. A. Cardiac adaption. IN *Pathophysiology,* ed. by E. D. Frohlich. Philadelphia, J. B. Lippincott Co., 1972, p. 11.
5. BROWN, F. A., JR. Living clocks. *Science* 139:1535-1543, Dec. 4, 1959.
6. ROMHILT, D. W., AND FOWLER, N. O. Physical signs in acute myocardial infarction. *Heart Lung* 2:74-80. Jan.-Feb. 1973.
7. ROTHFELD, E. L., AND OTHERS. Idioventricular rhythm in acute myocardial infarction. *Circulation* 37:203-209. Feb. 1968.
8. BELLET, SAMUEL. *Clinical Disorders of the Heart Beat.* 3d ed. Philadelphia, Lea and Febiger, 1971.
9. WOLFF, G. A., AND OTHERS. Vulnerable period for ventricular tachycardia following myocardial infarction. *CardiovascFes.* 2:111-121, Apr. 1968.
10. REIMANN, H. A. *Periodic Diseases.* London, F. A. Davis, Co., 1963.
11. ———. Medical importance of long biorhythms in acromedicine. *Aerosp Med.* 42:1086-1087, Oct. 1971.
12. MILLS, J. N. Human circadian rhythms. *PhysiolRev.* 46:128-171, Jan. 1966.
13. YAMAMOTO, W. S., AND BROBECK, J. R., EDS. *Physiological Controls and Regulations.* Philadelphia, W. B. Saunders Co., 1965.
14. KLEITMAN, N., AND RAMSAROOP, A. Periodicity in body temperature and heartrate. *Endocrinology* 40:1-20, 1948.
15. DIETZ, A., AND KIRCHHOFF, H. W. *Cardiac Rhythm Disturbances in Flying Personnel.* Paper presented at Aerospace Medicine Conference. Bal Harbour, Florida, May 8-11, 1972.
16. SMITH, RICHARD, AND OTHERS. Sleep and cardiac arrhythmias. *Arch Intern Med* 130:751-753, Nov. 1972.

From the *American Journal of Nursing* 74:1830-1834, Oct. 1974.

Pump Failure

SUE B. FOSTER

Efforts by the failing heart to augment cardiac function may lead to further decompensation.

The heart's function is to pump enough blood to the body's cells to satisfy their metabolic needs. Blood is propelled through the blood vessels by the gradient of pressure generated by the cardiac output. The less efficient the heart is as a pump, the lower is the cardiac output and, consequently, the amount of blood that reaches the cells. Clinically, a decreased cardiac output causes a fall in perfusion pressure. The end result is cardiac decompensation.

The cardiac output is calculated by multiplying the heart rate per minute by the stroke volume. Thus, any condition that significantly decreases stroke volume or heart rate reduces cardiac output. Factors influencing the heart's ability to pump blood are cardiac disease, cardiac rhythm disturbances, pharmacological agents, autonomic nervous system disturbances, fluid, electrolyte, and acid-base imbalances, and endocrine disorders.

CARDIAC DISEASE Ischemic heart disease involves injury and death to segments of the myocardium. Myocardial tissue cannot regenerate. In acute myocardial infarction caused by coronary artery disease, death of heart muscle limits the total area available for effective contraction. If the functioning, viable myocardium cannot compensate for this loss and for

MS. FOSTER *(Rex Hospital School of Nursing, Raleigh, N.C.; B.S.N., University of North Carolina, Chapel Hill; M.S.N., Catholic University, Washington, D.C.) is an instructor in nursing, St. Louis University School of Nursing and Allied Health Professions, St. Louis, Mo., and a nurse clinician at the St. Louis University Hospitals.*

the subsequent dysynergy and noncompliance, the volume of blood ejected from the left ventricle is reduced and heart failure develops.

Heart failure can be a consequence of other pathophysiological events. For example, in hypertensive heart disease, the heart must propel blood against an elevated mean aortic pressure. In valvular heart disease, such as mitral stenosis, the left atrium must contract more forcefully to propel blood through an immobile bicuspid valve.

Another pathophysiological condition which may lead to pump failure is diversion of oxygenated blood through a shunt. In a ventricular-septal defect characterized by a left-to-right shunt, the left ventricle hypertrophies in an effort to eject a sufficient amount of oxygenated blood into the aorta. At the same time, blood flows through the intraventricular-septal defect and mixes with unoxygenated blood in the right ventricle. The shunt may remain left to right, become reversed, or function in both directions, but heart failure will occur eventually.

As a complication of heart disease, heart failure is signalled by sinus tachycardia, cardiac dilatation and hypertrophy, pulmonary rales, and pathological heart sounds (S_3 or ventricular-diastolic gallop; and S_4 or atrial-diastolic gallop). The sinus tachycardia and cardiac dilatation and hypertrophy result from compensatory mechanisms to increase cardiac output. They become signs of decompensation when the body's metabolic needs at rest exceed the available blood supply. Cardiac reserve is gradually lost and catecholamine stores become depleted[1]. As circulation slows and cardiac output falls, a greater amount of oxygen is extracted from the blood[2]. Ventilation-perfusion abnormalities, anatomical right-to-left shunting, atelectasis, and diffusion abnormalities, if present, further contribute to hypoxemia[3].

The larger the heart, the more muscular tension is required to produce a given systolic pressure[1]. Therefore, the failing heart must work to maintain a given systolic aortic pressure at a time when it is also attempting to satisfy the increased metabolic demands of a hypertrophied myocardium. Eventually, myofibril overstretch and slippage occur, the left ventricular end-diastolic pressure (LVEDP) rises, and cardiac output is compromised[1]. Pump failure results in a lowered arterial pressure and this leads ultimately to inadequate perfusion throughout the body.

CARDIAC RHYTHM DISTURBANCES Arrhythmias are a major source of ineffective mechanical pumping[4]. An arrhythmia is a sign or symptom of a primary or secondary disorder. It is a sign if found during an examination of the patient, as in an EKG reading, and a symptom if reported by the patient as palpitations or shortness of breath, for example. Primary disorders include cardiac conditions, such as myocardial infarction, viral myocarditis, rheumatic heart disease, and hypertensive heart disease. Among the extracardiac disorders involving the heart are thyrotoxicosis, pheochromocytoma, and pulmonary emphysema. Rhythm disturbances are often associated with fever, exertion, and emotional excitement.

Extremes in heart rate normally alter cardiac output, but can cause serious problems in a person with heart disease. Tachycardia shortens ventricular diastolic filling time, and thereby decreases the stroke volume. As heart rate increases, stroke volume falls, and cardiac output finally is diminished. Coronary artery filling is concomitantly reduced because diastole, the period when the coronary arteries normally fill, is shortened.

Sinus bradycardia prolongs ventricular diastolic filling time, and thereby increases stroke volume. However, this augmented stroke volume is insufficient to compensate for the reduction in heart rate at extremely slow rates. Cardiac output falls and the perfusion pressure necessary to fill the coronary arteries is inadequate to meet myocardial metabolic demands. In patients with acute myocardial infarction a heart rate as low as 40 beats per minute or as high as 130 beats per minute can precipitate angina and left ventricular failure.

Arrhythmias characterized by non-sequential atrioventricular conduction also produce derangements in pumping ability. The absence of sequential atrioventricular conduction results in a mechanical loss of atrial kick, reduced left ventricular volume, and decreased cardiac output. Atrioventricular dissociation is always secondary to a primary rhythm disturbance, for example, accelerated idioventricular rhythm with intermittent capture by the sinus node, third-degree heart block, and ventricular tachycardia.

PHARMACOLOGICAL AGENTS Medications may have an inotropic (affecting the strength of myocardial contractility), chronotropic (affecting the rate of firing of the sinus node), or dromotropic (affecting impulse conduction) effect on the heart. Drugs given for their direct cardiac effect include adrenergic agents, cholinergic agents, and antiarrhythmics. In addition, patients without cardiac disease may be taking medications which may have an untoward cardiac effect. Certain hormones and antihistamines can produce a dromotropic response(5). Morphine may elicit vagomimetic response, a slowing of the heart rate accompanied by hypotension(6).

70

One drug may potentiate the effects of another drug and cause an enhanced or undesired cardiovascular response(7). For example, the strong hypotensive drug guanethidine may interact with an amphetamine to precipitate a hypertensive crisis. Digitalis taken with calcium may result in arrhythmias. In the presence of liver or renal disease, accumulation of drugs may lead to toxicity. Retention of digoxin in oliguric patients can cause dangerous rhythm disturbances, including tachyarrhythmias with or without block, ventricular ectopic beats, and varying degrees of atrioventricular block.

AUTONOMIC NERVOUS SYSTEM DISTURBANCES Sympathetic and parasympathetic responses are elicited by emotional stimulation and pharmacological agents. Emotional responses, particularly extreme fright or profound dejection, can lead to autonomic nervous system inhibition, and this can cause arrhythmias and sudden death(8). Vagal stimulation, causing bradycardia and hypotension, may be a response to severe pain. In anxiety states, sinus tachycardia and a rise in blood pressure are characteristic of a sympathoneural and sympatho-adrenal response to stress.

Antihypertensive and psychotropic agents may alter autonomic nervous system balance. Reserpine, an anti-hypertensive drug, depletes body stores of catecholamines. This may slow the heart rate and inhibit cardiovascular adaptations to stressful states. Phenothiazines, such as chlorpromazine (Thorazine) and thioridiazine (Mellaril), also can cause various cardiac arrhythmias(9).

ELECTROLYTE AND ACID-BASE BALANCE Imbalance of electrolytes and disturbances in the pH may be sufficient to depress the contractibility of the myocardium. Hypoxia, acidosis, and deficiencies in magnesium and calcium are examples of conditions that may give rise to arrhythmias and hinder contractility.

ENDOCRINE DISORDERS An endocrine disorder can affect the pumping of the heart by speeding metabolism, as in hyperthyroidism; or by secreting sympathomimetic substances, as with pheochromocytomas, which release epinephrine and norepinephrine; serotonin-secreting tumors; and adrenal crisis, which increases the secretion of catecholamines.

REGULATION AND CONTROL OF THE PUMP

The stoke volume is an outcome of three interacting factors, the left ventricular end-diastolic volume (LVEDV), ventricular afterload, and myocardial contractility(1). The heart abides by Starling's law: the force

ASSESSMENT OF PUMP FAILURE

I. Patient History
   Present symptoms
   Past illnesses
   Social history
   Family history
   Allergies
   Medications
   Diet

II. Data Related to Perfusion
   Heart rate
   Cardiac rhythm
   Blood pressure
   Heart murmurs or thrills
   Urinary output
   Pulse:
      thready
      bounding
      mechanical (pulsus) alternans
      pulsus paradoxus
   Cerebral manifestations:
      restlessness
      confusion
      disorientation
   Respiration:
      rate
      shallow or deep
      retractions
      flaring of nostrils
      rales, ronchi, or wheezes
      breath sounds
   Skin:
      color
      condition

Liver:
   palpable
   tender
   Temperature

III. Data Related to Cardiac Filling
   Pressure and volume
   Central venous pressure (CVP)
   Pulmonary artery diastolic pressure
      (PADP)
   Pulmonary capillary wedge
      pressure (PCWP)
   Left ventricular end-diastolic
      pressure (LVEDP)
   Jugular venous distention
   Jugular venous pulsations
   S_3 gallop
   S_4 gallop
   Edema

IV. Laboratory Findings
   Blood gases
   Serum electrolytes
   Enzymes
   Urinary specific gravity
   Complete blood count
   Electrocardiogram
   X-ray

V. Tentative Diagnosis
   Etiological
   Anatomical
   Physiological
   Functional ability

of cardiac contraction is related to the degree of filling of the ventricles. The more the ventricles fill (also affected by the length of the muscle fibers at the end of diastole, by left ventricular and end-diastolic volume, or by pre-load), the more vigorous is the subsequent contraction, within physiological limits. When these limits are exceeded, contractility diminishes. Failing hearts have lower physiological end points than healthy hearts, and therefore operate on a depressed Starling curve(10).

The LVEDV approximates the amount of blood delivered to the normal heart(11). When cardiovascular alterations occur, such as changes in the total blood volume, redistributions of blood volume, and absence of atrial contribution to ventricular filling, the LVEDV rises or falls(1). If the rise in LVEDV exceeds the pumping ability, an increment in residual volume stretches the end-diastolic myofibril. If the myofibril is overstretched, the heart fails. The LVEDP rises, and, in persons without pulmonary disease, the pulmonary artery diastolic pressure (PADP) also rises.

The LVEDV may be reduced if total blood volume is low. In acute myocardial infarction, hypovolemia may mimic cardiogenic shock when in reality the patient's blood volume is depleted due to diaphoresis or nausea and vomiting. Vasopressor therapy for patients in hypovolemic shock may worsen the clinical picture. Drug-induced constriction of the vasculature may cause further loss of fluid from the capillary bed. For all these reasons, the patient's total blood volume is a significant variable to be assessed in determining his cardiac output(12).

Closely related to decreased intravascular volume is the redistribution of blood. Loss of venous tone, an increase in thoracic or abdominal pressure, body position, and intrapericardial pressure may reduce venous return to the heart, diminish ventricular filling, and compromise cardiac output(1).

The amount of blood reaching the ventricles is decreased further when the atria no longer actively contribute to ventricular filling. Loss of the atrial kick occurs in many rhythm disturbances (atrial fibrillation, and junctional and ventricular rhythms) and in patients with artificial pacemakers implanted in the ventricle. The atria contribute a minimal amount of blood by contraction. Most blood actually reaches the ventricles passively. However, in some pathological states—mitral stenosis, for instance—the atrial kick assumes greater importance and is responsible for a significant amount of the blood received by the ventricles. If the atrial kick is lost, the patient's condition may deteriorate.

A second factor governing the performance of the pump is ventricular afterload. Left-ventricular stroke volume is a function of aortic impedance. Therefore, hypertension, alpha-adrenergic stimulators (Levophed, Neo-Synephrine), increased systemic vascular resistance due to sympathetic stimulation, and increased blood viscosity raise the energy demands on the myocardium(1).

The third component of the pump triad is myocardial contractility. If the myocardium is intrinsically depressed, even with adequate blood volume and sufficient systemic resistance, the perfusion pressure falls. Contractility is enhanced by digitalis and other inotropic agents (calcium, caffeine, theophylline), circulating catecholamines, sympathetic nerve impulses, and post-extrasystolic potentiation—the augmented contraction of the beat following an extrasystole. Contractility is inhibited by anoxia, hypercapnia, acidosis, such pharmacological depressants as lido-caine and quinidine, loss of myocardium secondary to infarction, and by the depletion or deficiency of any of the agents that enhance contractil-ity(1).

THERAPY

The obvious causes of pump failure must be eliminated first. Fever

---

SELECTED THERAPEUTIC INTERVENTIONS

LEFT VENTRICULAR END-DIASTOLIC VOLUME

To increase
- elevate legs
- administer intravenous fluids and/or plasma expanders
- remove or alleviate any impairment to venous return (for example, thoracentesis for ascites; nasogastric tube drainage for gastric distention)
- initiate active or assisted exercises for skeletal muscle contraction
- administer anti-arrhythmic agents as indicated
- provide elastic leg supports, gravity suits

To decrease
- apply rotating tourniquets
- decrease circulating volume by phlebotomy
- restrict fluid intake
- restrict dietary sodium
- administer IPPB treatments
- administer diurectics

MYOCARDIAL CONTRACTILITY

To augment
- relieve pericardial pressure (pericardial paracentesis for cardiac tamponade)
- administer positive inotropic agents and observe for untoward myocardial depressant effects of drugs
- observe for early signs of hypoxia and acidosis
- maintain normal fluid-electrolyte and acid-base balance (IPPB, oxygen, alkalizing agents)
- manage arrhythmias

AFTERLOAD

To increase
- administer vasopressors (titrate with blood pressure carefully; excessive vasoconstriction reduces cardiac output)
- intra-aortic balloon pump

To decrease
- administer antihypertensive agents
- administer anticoagulant agents
- administer fibrinolytic agents
- administer viscosity-reducing agents (dextran)
- reduce anxiety (psychotropic agents and therapeutic communication)

FACTORS THAT ALTER
BLOOD VOLUME DISTRIBUTION

Position
When person stands, gravity causes blood to pool in dependent areas.

Example: orthostatic hypotension.

Intrathoracic Pressure (ITP)
The less negative the ITP, the greater is the thoracic interference with venous return. This reduces artial and then ventricular filling. Cardiac output is diminished.

Examples: intermittent positive pressure respirator, ascites.

Intrapericardial Pressure
Pressure within the pericardial sac restricts cardiac filling and contraction, with a resulting fall in cardiac output and blood pressure.

Examples: cardiac tamponade, constrictive pericarditis.

Venous Tone
Lack of venous tone promotes venous stasis and limits blood return to the heart.

Example: varicose veins.

Pumping Action of Skeletal Muscle
Contraction of skeletal muscle assists movement of blood through the veins to the heart. Without this assistance, circulation slows and atrial filling is reduced.

Example: immobility.

---

and hypoxemia are corrected and depressant drugs are discontinued. If ventricular filling pressure and arterial pressure are low, intravenous fluids are infused. If perfusion pressure is low, norepinephrine (Levophed) or dopamine, a precursor of norepinephrine, is the agent of choice. If cardiac output is low and systemic vascular resistance and filling pressure are elevated, isoproterenol (Isuprel) and digitalis are frequently employed(12).

Accurate hemodynamic assessment and precise recordings are of the utmost significance in identifying the patient's response to therapy. If the patient does not improve clinically with one therapeutic agent, another agent or mode of therapy is used.

Nursing responsibilities depend on the severity of decompensation. The nursing diagnosis of inadequate cardiac pump function must be made on the basis of a complete history and assessment, including observable patient data, a clinical examination, laboratory findings, and data from the physician's assessment. Clinical evaluation is ongoing, and essential in determining the patient's condition and response to therapy.

A hemodynamic assessment should provide specific data about cardiac filling pressure and volume, perfusion problems, and laboratory results. For visualization and delineation of trends in data, the information should be presented graphically when possible and consistently measured in the same units. Notations of increments, decrements, or changes in therapy should be made on the graphic sheet or in the nurses' notes.

Once a diagnosis is established and its etiology known or suspected, the nurse can plan specific interventions for the identified problem. Nursing care can be directed to modify afterload, to alter the LVEDV, and to improve inotropy. The success of an intervention can be determined by comparing actual results with the expected outcomes. For example, sinus rhythm is the expected result of administering intravenous atropine to a patient with a junctional escape rhythm due to sinus bradycardia. Another example: if a patient has a vasovagal reaction, a rise in blood pressure would be the expected result of elevating his legs.

The failure of the heart to pump sufficient blood may respond to therapy if the patient is treated early and aggressively. In order to recognize pump failure and assist in its management the nurse must know the signs and symptoms of a poorly functioning heart and the operant mechanisms for effective cardiac contraction.

REFERENCES

1. BRAUNWALD, EUGENE, AND OTHERS. *Mechanisms of Contraction of the Normal and Failing Heart.* Boston, Little, Brown and Co., 1968.
2. RAMO, B. W., AND OTHERS. Hemodynamic findings in 123 patients with acute myocardial infarction on admission. *Circulation* 42:567-577, Oct. 1970.
3. DAVIDSON, R. M., AND OTHERS. Blood-gas and hemodynamic responses to oxygen in acute myocardial infarction. *Circulation* 47:704-711, Apr. 1973.
4. MAYER, G. G., AND KAELIN, P. B. Arrhythmias and cardiac output. *Am.J.Nurs.* 72:1597-1600, Sept. 1972.
5. GOODMAN, L. S., AND GILMAN, ALFRED. *Pharmacological Basis of Therapeutics.* 4th ed. New York, Macmillan Co., 1970.
6. ZIPES, D. P. Treatment of arrhythmias in myocardial infarction. *Arch. Intern.Med.* 124:101-109, July 1969.
7. DRUG interactions that can affect your patients. *Patient Care,* Oct. 31, 1970, 3-11.
8. WOLF, STEWART. Central autonomic influences on cardiac rate and rhythm. *Mod.Concepts Carciovasc.Dis.* 38:29-34, June 1969.
9. ALEXANDER, C. S., AND NINO, ALFREDO. Cardiovascular complications in young patients taking psychotropic drugs. *Am.Heart J.* 78:757-769, Dec. 1969.
10. SPANN, J. F., AND OTHERS. Recent advances in the understanding of congestive heart failure: Part 1. *Mod.Concepts Cardiovasc.Dis.* 39:73-78, Jan. 1970.
11. FOLKOW, BJORN, AND NEIL, ERIC. *Circulation.* New York, Oxford University Press, 1973.
12. LOEB, H. S., AND OTHERS. The failing myocardium: Part 1. Drug management. *Med.Clin.North Am.* 57:167-185, Jan. 1973.

From the *American Journal of Nursing* 74:1636-1640, Sept. 1974.

Cardiogenic Shock

CAROL STUDE

Cardiogenic shock occurs in approximately 10 to 25 percent of all persons admitted to hospitals with the diagnosis of myocardial infarction. Eighty percent of these patients die(1,2,3). It shock could be detected and treated early in even a few of these patients, many lives would be saved each year.

Shock can be recognized by the clinical findings of acute circulatory failure: rapidly developing mental confusion, lassitude, and physical weakness; cold extremities; cool, moist skin; rapid, weak pulse; oliguria; and a fall in arterial blood pressure.

Essentially, shock develops when cellular oxygenation is impaired or has failed because there is an inadequate flow of blood to vital organs or because the cells fail to use oxygen. Shock can be diagnosed on the basis of three interdependent factors: the clinical situation, including causative factors, the nature of the disease process, and its severity and duration; an arterial blood pressure lower than 80 mm. Hg systolic, or a drop of 30 mm. Hg or more below the patient's normal systolic pressure; and the patient's clinical signs and symptoms.

Because all forms of shock are related to low-flow states and, consequently, to impaired tissue perfusion, shock can be classified according to the primary cause of failure. The blood flow to any body system is directly proportional to cardiac function and the volume of fluid in the system, and inversely proportional to the resistance throughout the system(4).

Cardiogenic shock may be an isolated phenomenon or it may be a complication of another form of shock. For example, hypovolemic shock can precipitate heart failure or myocardial infarction and result in cardiogenic shock. However, in this article cardiogenic shock is discussed exclusive of other pathological states.

MS. STUDE (B.S.N., University of Minnesota, Minneapolis) is a staff nurse at Hillcrest Hospital, Pittsfield, Mass.

Three progressive stages occur as cardiogenic shock proceeds. In the initial stage, clinical signs reflect a decrease in cardiac output and resultant tissue anoxia. In the compensatory stage, generalized vasconstriction is a paramount sign. Eventually, untreated cardiogenic shock progresses to an irreversible stage, and death is inevitable(5).

In cardiogenic shock, the profound decrease in effective blood flow is the result of a progressive inability of the left ventricle to pump blood throughout the body. Oxygen perfusion to the brain and other vital organs becomes inadequate to sustain life. Except for those persons whose shock is precipitated by a cardiac arrhythmia that impairs cardiac filling or contractility, the cause of the ventricular failure associated with acute myocardial infarction is unknown. However, two mechanisms are suspected: either the left ventricle is so damaged by the infarction that it cannot generate enough force to pump blood into the systemic circulation, or myocardial ischemia leads to metabolic derangements that inhibit effective contraction. This uncertainty about the physiological mechanisms involved in the development of cardiogenic shock makes definitive treatment difficult(3).

Because of the vicious circle it creates, *cardiogenic shock is especially dangerous in persons suffering from an acute myocardial infarction.* The decreased pumping action of the heart causes hypotension. Hypotension compromises coronary blood flow to an already damaged heart, causing additional myocardial damage, even more diminished pumping action, and so on.

The mechanisms of cardiogenic shock can be explained by the formula: SVR=MAP-CVP/CO.

SVR (systemic vascular resistance) is normally maintained by vasodilation and vasoconstriction of blood vessels and capillaries.

MAP (mean aortic pressure) is the pressure measured in the aorta as blood leaves the heart. The coronary vessels branch from the aorta, so a diminished aortic pressure leads to a diminished blood supply to the heart.

CVP (central venous pressure) measures the pressure of the blood entering the right atrium and is a good indicator of the amount of blood entering the heart. Therefore, a low CVP often indicates hypovolemia.

CO (cardiac output) is the amount of blood pumped each minute. Cardiac output is directly related to stroke volume, the amount of blood pumped with each contraction. In a damaged myocardium, a decrease in effective contractions results in a diminished stroke volume and, subsequently, a lowered cardiac output. A patient in cardiogenic shock has a cardiac output estimated at 60 to 80 percent of normal. Stroke volume is approximately 30 to 50 percent of normal(3).

The severity of cardiogenic shock can be equated with the decrease in cardiac output. Decreased cardiac output also lowers metabolism and leads to an increase in anaerobic metabolism, lactic acid production, and acidosis. The classical signs of shock are seen when cardiac output is so depressed that the systemic vascular resistance cannot compensate sufficiently to maintain an adequate mean aortic pressure.

Arrhythmias which are often seen in patients with myocardial infarctions and which are associated with the development of shock have the following characteristics:

• A rapid ventricular rate, as in atrial tachycardia, fibrillation, and flutter; and nodal and ventricular tachycardias. These arrhythmias compromise diastolic filling and so decrease cardiac output and coronary blood flow.
• Replacement of the sinus node by the atrioventricular node as the origin of impulses, with consequent slowing or acceleration of the ventricular rate, as in nodal rhythms.
• Blocked transmission of supra-ventricular impulses to the ventricles with take over by a slow ventricular pacemaker, as in complete heart block. This decreases perfusion to an already damaged heart.

The body's primary compensatory response to cardiogenic shock is generalized vasoconstriction. Nerve endings in the aortic arch and carotid body respond to a drop in arterial pressure by stimulating the adrenal medulla and sympathetic nerve endings to release epinephrine and norepinephrine. These cause generalized vasoconstriction, which confines the circulating blood volume to a smaller area by redistributing blood from the skin and muscle to vital organs. The adrenal cortex releases cortisol and aldostersone, which conserve salt and water and fortify the body for stress(6). The posterior pituitary secrets antidiuretic hormone in a similar effort to conserve water and so increase the circulating volume.

Initially, vasoconstriction increases the blood pressure and cardiac output, and enhances perfusion in a normal heart. However, in a damaged heart, vasoconstriction increases the heart's workload by increasing resistance. Cardiac output is not increased because the damaged heart cannot pump effectively. Although vasoconstriction is helpful in other forms of shock, such as hypovolemia, its role in cardiogenic shock is uncertain.

Because vasoconstriction increases perfusion to the vital organs by depriving other tissues, these tissues employ an anaerobic form of metabolism in order to preserve cellular function. The end product of anaerobic metabolism is lactic acid. Lactic acid accumulates in the blood and results in acidosis. The body attempts to compensate for this with hyperventilation, which lowers pCO_2 and decreased renal excretion of nonvolatile acids. Usually the body in shock cannot compensate sufficiently, and acidosis leads to cellular death and lethal arrhythmias.

As compensatory mechanisms begin to fail and tissue anoxia and necrosis increase, a generalized vasodilatation develops. Shock becomes irreversible and death is inevitable. A fine line divides reversible and irreversible shock, but there is a direct relationship between the duration of inadequate tissue perfusion and the onset of irreversible shock. Some researchers believe that certain enzyme systems involved with tissue oxidation are irreparably damaged during cardiogenic shock and that this is the cause of death[1]. Others suggest that failure of the adrenal gland contributes to the irreversibility of shock[1]. Neither theory has been proved.

CLINICAL SIGNS

The earliest indication of impending shock is a change in the patient's mental condition or general behavior. He is often very restless, agitated, and confused, which indicates decreased cerebral oxygenation. As the shock state worsens, the patient becomes listless, apathetic, extremely weak, and may eventually slip into coma.

Initially the skin is pale and cold due to vasoconstriction and lowered cardiac output. Pallor and cyanosis develop as cardiac output and oxygen perfusion decrease.

The blood pressure is low or unobtainable. Although a systolic blood pressure of less than 80 mm. Hg or a drop of more than 30 mm. Hg from the patient's normal systolic pressure usually defines shock, it is not the only criterion. A low blood pressure in conjunction with other clinical features, such as cyanosis, oliguria, and lethargy, *is* indicative of shock. As cardiogenic shock progresses, the systolic pressure usually falls before the diastolic. Therefore, a decrease in pulse pressure, the difference between the systolic and diastolic pressures, is considered an early manifestation of shock. Because accurate blood pressure measurement is crucial to treatment, many physicians introduce an arterial catheter to reduce the hazard of false readings and to record direct arterial pressures.

In cardiogenic shock, the peripheral veins constrict and eventually collapse. This increases the CVP, which is a function of the volume of blood in the central veins; the distensibility and contractility of the right heart chambers; the constriction and dilatation of central veins; and intrathoracic pressure. Monitoring the CVP is very important. Myocardial damage and decreased pumping action cause an elevated CVP. Therefore, a rising CVP may herald congestive heart failure and pulmonary edema. Fluid intake is usually prescribed on the basis of CVP readings.

Tachycardia, clinically evident in the characteristic rapid and thready pulse, is noted as the body attempts to compensate for a decreased stroke volume. As shock worsens, especially when there is myocardial damage, bradycardia eventually develops and proceeds to ventricular standstill.

Urine volume is a good indication of the effectiveness of compensatory mechanisms and therapeutic effort. Vasoconstriction decreases blood flow to the kidneys and perfusion pressure drops. Coupled with a falling blood pressure, this lowers output to less than 25 cc./hour. Blood urea nitrogen (BUN) and creatinine (CR) levels rise. Severe, prolonged, renal ischemia damages the kidneys, acute tubular necrosis ensues, and the patient becomes anuric.

As shock progresses, numerous arrhythmias develop. Arrhythmias are common in cardiogenic shock secondary to myocardial infarction because the damaged myocardium is already irritable. These arrhythmias, notably ventricular fibrillation, are highly resistant to treatment. Acidosis and electrolyte imbalance also contribute to the incidence of arrhythmias.

TREATMENT

Because of the uncertainty about the cause of cardiogenic shock, specific treatment is not yet available. Most patients who develop cardiogenic shock die. Therefore, treatment is aimed at early detection. Therapy seeks to correct the hemodynamic disturbances which accompany shock, by improving the heart's pumping action in order to improve tissue perfusion.

Inotropic agents are given to improve the strength of myocardial contraction. Digitalis and isoproterenol (Isuprel) increase cardiac output without raising systemic resistance. Digitalis should be used with caution because toxicity develops rapidly in damaged hearts. Isuprel (usually given in titrated doses after dilution of 2 mg. in 500 cc. 5% dextrose in water) increases the heart rate and, consequently, the oxygen needs of the damaged myocardium. Also, the narrow range between therapeutic and toxic doses increases the danger of myocardial irritability.

Vasopressor drugs are given to sustain the blood pressure and so maintain blood flow to the coronary arteries. Some researchers believe that the systemic release of norepinephrine and epinephrine constricts blood vessels and that vasopressors merely introduce the risk of arrhythmias(1,5). Others believe that vasopressors help maintain adequate perfusion(1,5).

When these drugs—levaterenol (Levophed), metaraminol (Aramine) mephentermine (Wyamine)—are used, blood pressure must be monitored frequently. A sharp rapid rise in blood pressure can overwork the heart and impair perfusion. A systolic pressure of 100 mm. Hg is usually adequate. Urine output is a good measure of the adequacy of treatment. The patient's ECG should be monitored closely. Vasopressors can cause significant myocardial irritability and arrhythmias, such as tachycardia and premature ventricular contractions. The continuous use of vasopressors for more than two or three hours can increase blood vessel permeability. Hypovolemia can result as fluid is lost into the extravascular spaces. Also, the longer a patient receives vasopressor drugs, the more difficult it is to wean him from them.

Special caution must be exercised when Levophed is infused. It can cause tissue damage and necrosis if it infiltrates. Five to 10 mg. of Regitine added to each 1,000 cc. of fluid prevents tissue reaction without inhibiting Levophed's vasopressor action.

Some vasodilating drugs, such as phenoxybenzamine (Dibenzyline) and chlorpromazine (Thorazine), have been used experimentally with some success(7). The rationale for their use is that excessive vasoconstriction and consequent ischemia in the splanchnic circulation causes release of toxins which aggravate shock. Vasopressors increase cardiac work and so increase the oxygen demands of an ischemic heart. When vasodilators are administered, blood pressure and CVP must be carefully monitored. These drugs can induce hypotension, further hypoxia, and arrhythmias.

Sodium bicarbonate is administered to combat the effects of acidosis.

Glucocorticoids (hydrocortisone, Solu-medrol), in massive doses of as much as 100 mg./Kg. of body weight, are now being used with some success. They may restore the structural integrity of smooth muscle which has been damaged by prolonged shock(5,7).

Anticoagulants are given because irreversible shock may be caused by progressive clot formation(4).

Glucagon, a pancreatic hormone, increases the contractility of isolated muscle by activating the adenyl cyclase enzyme system(8). Glucagon is most effective when used in combination with Isuprel. It increases cardiac output and heart rate without decreasing systemic vascular resistance or aggravating arrhythmias(9).

Because of the serious defect in pulmonary ventilation and cardiac perfusion which occur during cardiogenic shock, oxygen therapy is important. One hundred percent oxygen is usually administered by nasal catheter or mask at six to eight liters/min. Arterial blood gas levels must be monitored frequently to guide further medical treatment. The arterial pO_2 should be maintained above 60 mm. Hg. Oxygen therapy increases oxygen perfusion to ischemic tissues, causes some vasoconstriction, and increases heart rate(3).

Pain and anxiety frequently precede cardiogenic shock, and their relief can prevent a major shock crisis. Morphine sulfate, 5-10 mg. I.V., is administered with extreme caution because it causes hypotension, increases the heart rate, and depresses respirations.

MECHANICAL DEVICES

Because cardiogenic shock may be the result of extensive left ventricular muscle damage, several mechanical devices have been designed to decrease the heart's workload, augment coronary blood flow, and thus increase cardiac output.

The permanent mechanical auxiliary ventricle was one of the first devices. A flexible silicone, rubber chamber encased in a rigid plastic shell is implanted across the aortic arch. During systole, this device receives blood from the left ventricle through the silicone chamber. When the aortic valve closes at the beginning of diastole, the chamber collapses into the space between it and the shell. The auxiliary ventricle is powered by an external, compressed-air source and regulated by a circuit timed to coincide with the patient's ECG. Blood is ejected from the chamber into the coronary arteries and on to the systemic circulation. The net result is a 50 to 54 percent increase in aortic flow and an increased coronary flow. The device decreases the workload of the left ventricle by 47 percent. Although the auxiliary ventricle is effective, its use has been limited by the fact that most patients suffering from acute left ventricular failure or shock are too ill to undergo the major surgery required to implant it(10).

Veno-arterial pumping devices draw blood from the heart's venous circulation and pump it into the arterial system. Ordinarily, the femoral veins and arteries are used for this procedure. Venous blood is artificially oxygenated in a cardiopulmonary bypass machine. This decreases cardiac workload and augments arterial circulation. Because elaborate equipment is required to provide this assisted circulation, it is not practical for most circumstances. A similar procedure is left-heart bypass. Oxygenated blood from the left atrium is removed and returned to the arterial circulation through peripheral cannulas. This decreases flow to the left ventricles while sustaining adequate systemic circulation(7).

Another available treatment is counterpulsation. This technique is based on the premise that, if the aortic blood pressure falls during ventricular systole and the diastolic pressure is mechanically increased, cardiac workload will be decreased and coronary blood flow will be augmented. A catheter is passed into a central artery. During ventricular systole, blood is removed to a single-ended, plastic pouch which serves as an artificial ventricle and returned to the aorta in a retrograde fashion during diastole by a pump which is activated by the R wave on the ECG(5).

Intra-aortic, phase-shift, balloon pumping is perhaps the most significant development in assisted circulation(7,10,11). A polyurethane pumping chamber and catheter are introduced through the femoral artery into the descending thoracic aotra to a point just behind the heart. Heparin, 50-75 mg., is administered through the venous line before pumping begins. The pumping chamber of the catheter is actively expanded with compressed helium during diastole. This increases aortic pressure and so increases coronary flow as well as augmenting the systemic circulation. The chamber passively deflates during systole when the aortic valve opens. This decreases left ventricular work because the ventricle need overcome only the resistance of the collapsing balloon instead of the greater pressure of the blood in the aorta.

The balloon pump is controlled by an electronic timing device which is triggered by the R wave of the patient's ECG. The device provides a 50 percent increase in the amount of blood flowing to the coronary arteries, an increase of approximately 50 percent in cardiac output, and a decrease of 38 percent in peripheral resistance(7,11). The patient is monitored until all signs of shock are absent. Then, the inactive pumping chamber is left in place for several hours before being removed.

A study of 16 patients who were unresponsive to other medical therapies before they were treated with the balloon pump revealed a short-term survival rate of 81 percent; the long-term survival rate was 44 percent. A survival rate of 5-15 percent would be anticipated if the pump were not used(10).

The balloon pump permits speedy application (total time for preparation and introduction of the catheter is usually 20 to 25 minutes);

mobility of all system components; and freedom from complication. There is no evidence of depression of distal circulation, arterial wall damage from the pump, or trauma to blood elements. Aortic-valve incompetence is the only contraindication for this procedure. The pumping chamber may be difficult to insert in patients who have severe sclerosis or aneurysms of the aorta, or iliac or femoral arteries.

Surgery has been attempted to correct severe cardiogenic shock resulting from myocardial infarction. Emergency infarctectomy is done to resect large infarcted areas and repair any ventricular septal defects resulting from infarction. By excising infarcted muscle, the focus of myocardial irritability can be removed, and the hazard of fibrillation reduced. Infarctectomy also eliminates the paradoxical systolic expansion of the ventricles and so enhances left ventricular function. Large sections of left ventricular muscle can be excised without markedly impairing ventricular function. Candidates for this procedure are those who have sustained a first infarction associated with shock or pulmonary edema. The procedure is most successful in the patient whose infarction is due to occlusion of the anterior descending coronary artery(10).

Techniques to assist circulation mechanically are performed to achieve adequate tissue perfusion with a minimum expenditure of energy. Techniques that require surgical intervention pose problems associated with the logistics of patient care, and are limited to short-term procedures. Synchronous, external-assist methods have evolved in response to these problems(12,13).

Blood volume is normally distributed as follows: 15 percent in the arterial system, 5 to 10 percent in the capillary system, and 75 to 80 percent in the venous system(12). The venous system acts as a large reservoir. It can compensate for the changes which occur in blood-volume distribution when cardiovascular equilibrium is disturbed. External-assist devices are used to passively activate the arterial portion of the vascular system. External energy is introduced during diastole by synchronous pulsation of extramural pressures. Energy is stored during systole by decreasing extramural pressure rather than increasing intravascular pressure, which only increases ventricular work. By modifying extramural pressure synchronously with cardiac action, an effective driving-pressure differential is created(13).

The patient is placed in a pneumatic chamber which electronically synchronizes pressures with his ECG. The result is an increased cardiac output, decreased left-ventricular work, and control of blood-volume distribution. This external device can be used for prolonged periods of time because there is no need for cannulation or anticoagulation. Also, the external-assist device is quickly and easily applied to the patient.

The experimental use of hypothermia has been proposed on the principle that a lowered body temperature reduces metabolic demands of tissues and, therefore, reduces cardiac work(1).

A final treatment of cardiogenic shock is the use of hyperbaric oxygen. Normally, we are exposed to 21 percent concentration of oxygen at one atmosphere of pressure. During treatment with hyperbaric oxygen, the patient intermittently receives 5 to 100 percent oxygen at 2 to 3 atmospheres of pressure. He usually remains in the hyperbaric chamber for two hours and is taken out for 20 to 30 minutes. Oxygen tension of the blood is increased, and this increases the rate of oxygen diffusion into underperfused anoxic tissues. This prevents the irreversible damage of tissue anoxia(13). Some authorities doubt the effectiveness of this treatment, believing that increased oxygen tension cannot benefit an individual as long as perfusion is impaired by coronary occlusion(5).

Several problems arise with hyperbaric therapy. The most significant is oxygen toxicity, manifested by pulmonary complications, retinal abnormalities, and central nervous system disturbances. Other adverse effects of hyperbaric oxygen therapy include headaches, eardrum perforation, euphoria, nitrogen narcosis, decompression sickness, and possible air embolism. The physical and environmental problems also pose a major obstacle in the practicality of this form of treatment. The equipment is expensive and cumbersome and requires highly skilled technicians.

Despite ongoing efforts to clarify and treat the mechanisms involved in the development of cardiogenic shock, mortality rates remain extremely high. Medical, surgical, and mechanical treatment of cardiogenic shock seek to correct the basic problem—a heart which is pumping so ineffectively that an insufficient supply of blood and oxygen is delivered to vital organs. The crucial means to reduce mortality from cardiogenic shock is still prevention through early detection.

REFERENCES

1. MELTZER, L. E., AND OTHERS. *Intensive Coronary Care—a Manual for Nurses.* rev. ed. Philadelphia, Charles Press, 1970, pp. 93-100.
2. CLARK, N. F. Pump failure. *Nurs.Clin.North Am.* 7:529-539, Sept. 1972.
3. LEAVITT, M. A., AND POLANSKY, B. J. Cardiogenic aspects of shock and coma. *Surg.Clin.North Am.* 48:273-285, April, 1968.

4. GUYTON, A. C. *Textbook of Medical Physiology.* 4th ed. Philadelphia, W. B. Saunders Co., 1971, pp. 204-217, 325-335, 342-343.
5. FRIEDBERG, C. K. *Diseases of the Heart.* 3d ed. Philadelphia, W. B. Saunders Co., 1969, pp. 444-463, 882-891.
6. CHANDLER, J. C. Physiology and treatment of shock. *RN* 34:42-43, June 1971.
7. WHIPPLE, GERALD, AND OTHERS. *Acute Coronary Care.* Boston, Little, Brown and Co., 1971, pp. 55, 60-68, 136-139, 238-243, 267.
8. LOEB, H. S., AND OTHERS. The failing myocardium, Part 1. *Med.Clin.North Am.* 57:167-185, Jan. 1973.
9. LYOFF, R., AND WILCKEN, D. Glucagon in heart failure and in cardiogenic shock: experience in fifty patients. *Circulation* 45:534-542, Mar. 1972.
10. STEPHENSON, J. E., JR. *Cardiac Arrest and Resuscitation.* 3d ed., St. Louis, C. V. Mosby Co., 1969, pp. 232-237, 242, 306-307, 320-321, 525.
11. LANE, CLETA. Intra-aortic phase-shift balloon pumping in cardiogenic shock. *Am.J.Nurs.* 69:1654-1661. Aug, 1969.
12. SCROFF, H., AND OTHERS. Assisted circulation. IN *Cardiac Surgery,* ed. by J. C. Norman. New York, Appleton-Century-Crofts, 1967, pp. 558-565.
13. GIRON, F., AND OTHERS. Assisted circulation by synchronous pulsation of extramural pressure. *Surgery* 60:894-901, Oct. 1966.

Section III Cardiac Care: Intervention

Therapeutic interventions—ranging from the application of basic resuscitation techniques to the operation of sophisticated machinery —demand broad nursing expertise. The first article in this section describes the new standards for providing basic life support to victims of sudden death. Following articles explain the use of a wide range of mechanical devices used to support and augment heart function in patients with cardiovascular disease. Finally, the establishment and maintenance of interpersonal relationships and approaches to the rehabilitation of the cardiac patient are discussed.

From the American Journal of Nursing 75:236-247, Feb. 1975.

CPR: Current Practice Revised

PETER J. UNGVARSKI • NINA T. ARGONDIZZO • PATRICIA K. BOOS

*The trained, skilled rescuer is the key to resuscitating
victims of sudden death.*

Each year over one million people in the United States have acute
myocardial infarctions. More than half of these people (650,000) die.
One half of those who die expire within the first two hours, never having
received the emergency care or the definitive treatment they needed.

To help counteract this awesome number of deaths, many of them
among persons in their most productive years, the American Heart Association, in cooperation with the National Academy of Sciences-National
Research Council, has issued new guidelines and standards for cardiopulmonary resuscitation (CPR) and emergency cardiac care (ECC).
These standards were published recently as a special supplement to the
*Journal of the American Medical Association.** Reprints of the supplement are available through local heart associations and should be studied.

Basic life support is the emergency first aid procedure which begins
with the recognition of cardiac and respiratory arrest and the application
of cardiopulmonary resuscitation to support the person's life until he can
be transported or until advanced life support is operable. To be effective,
CPR must begin as soon as the need for it is recognized. The *trained,
skilled* person at the scene is the key.

Basic life support is indicated for cardiac arrest caused by ventricular
fibrillation, ventricular asystole, cardiovascular collapse or electrome-
chanical dissociation, or respiratory arrest. Death from these causes is
called "sudden death"—the *immediate* and *unexpected* cessation of functional circulation and respirations. The death of a person who has a
long-term, lingering, fatal illness cannot be called a "sudden death."

---

* AMERICAN HEART ASSOCIATION, CARDIOPULMONARY RESUSCITATION AND EMERGENCY CARDIAC
CARE COMMITTEE AND NATIONAL ACADEMY OF SCIENCES-NATIONAL RESEARCH COUNCIL, MEDICAL
SCIENCES DIVISION, EMERGENCY MEDICAL SERVICES COMMITTEE. Standards for cardiopulmonary
resuscitation (CPR) and emergency cardiac care (ECC); Part 1. Introduction. *JAMA* 227:
Feb. 18, 1974, p. 838.

When the expected outcome of an illness is death, patients, families, and health personnel must agree about resuscitative efforts. Compassion must prevail and the person's right to live with dignity up to and including the moment of death must not be violated. When such a patient is hospitalized, an order should be written in the progress notes indicating that he is not to be resuscitated. This order must be communicated to everyone having the responsibility to perform cardiopulmonary resuscitation.

Basic life support skills maintain the viability of the vital centers of the central nervous system until the functional integrity of the body has been restored. No adjunctive equipment is necessary in basic life support. The trained person is the instrument. Waiting or searching for bag-masks, airways, and other equipment diverts attention from the prime effort, which is to begin resuscitation immediately.

When the rescuer does not actually see the victim collapse but is called to the scene of the incident, the situation is called an "Unwitnessed Arrest." The rescuer should take these steps:
- Open the victim's airway.
- If breathing is absent, deliver four quick ventilations.
- If the person's chest does not rise when ventilations are delivered, clear airway. Attempt to ventilate again.
- Palpate the carotid pulse.
- If pulse is absent, begin external cardiac compressions.

When the rescuer is present and sees the victim collapse, the situation is termed a "Witnessed Cardiac Arrest." The rescuer should:
- Open the victim's airway. Simultaneously palpate his carotid pulse.
- If pulse is absent, deliver one precordial thump.
- If breathing is absent, deliver four quick ventilations.
- If pulse and breathing are not immediately restored, begin cardiopulmonary resuscitation.

The following step-by-step instructions review the principles and techniques of CPR to be applied in cases of sudden death.

MR. UNGVARSKI (*Bellevue-Mills School of Nursing, New York, N.Y.; B.A., Marymount Manhattan College, New York*) *is an assistant director of nursing at Bellevue Hospital Center.* MS. ARGONDIZZO (*St. Elizabeth's School of Nursing, Dayton, Oh.; B.S.N., St. John's University, New York, N.Y.; M.A., Columbia University, New York, N.Y.*) *is assistant dean for continuing education, Cornell University-New York Hospital School of Nursing.* MS. BOOS (*Providence Hospital School of Nursing, Detroit, Michigan; B.S.N., Hunter College-Bellevue School of Nursing, New York*) *is an assistant in instruction, Division of Continuing Education, Cornell University-New York Hospital School of Nursing.*

basic life support

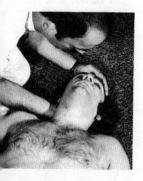

Action

Opening the Airway
☐ Ask someone else to summon assistance.
☐ Position patient on his back. Tilt his head back as far as possible. Place one hand beneath the victim's neck and lift it. Use the other hand to press forehead backward.

Ventilation
☐ To begin mouth-to-mouth ventilation the resuscitator should
- Tilt the head back as far as possible by lifting up the neck with one hand and pushing on the forehead with other.
- Pinch nostrils closed with thumb and finger of hand used to press forehead down.
- Open his mouth wide.
- Take a deep breath
- Make an airtight seal over the victim's mouth.
- Exhale forcefully into patient's mouth.
- Remove mouth and allow victim to exhale passively.

- Repeat steps to ventilate the patient *four times initially*.

☐ Mouth-to-nose ventilation
The resuscitator should:

- Keep the victim's head tilted back with one hand on the forehead and lift the victim's lower jaw with the other hand.

- Open his mouth wide.
- Take a deep breath.
- Make an airtight seal around the victim's nose.
- Exhale forcefully into the victim's nose.

Principles and Points to Consider

☐ This simple maneuver sometimes is all that is required for breathing to resume spontaneously.

- This moves the tongue and mandible upward, preventing them from obstructing the air passage.

- Adequate ventilation is ensured on every breath when the rescuer sees the chest rise and fall, feels his own airway resistance and compliance of the victim's lungs as they expand, and hears and feels air escape during exhalation.
- The initial ventilatory maneuver should be four quick, full breaths without allowing time for full lung deflation between breaths.
☐ This technique is recommended when it is impossible to open the victim's mouth, impossible to ventilate through his mouth, the mouth is seriously injured, or it is difficult to achieve a tight seal around the mouth.
- This position will keep the neck maximally extended and the mouth closed. Pressure should be exerted on the bony portion of the lower jaw, not on the soft tissue.

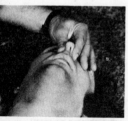

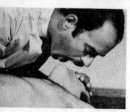

Action

- Remove mouth and let the victim exhale passively.

☐ Mouth-to-stoma ventilation
The resuscitator should
- Open mouth widely.
- Take a deep breath.
- Make an airtight seal around the stoma and exhale forcefully.

☐ For infants and small children:

- The resuscitator covers the mouth and nose of the victim with his mouth.
- Use *less* volume to inflate the lungs.

☐ Accident Victims:

- The resuscitator opens airway by placing hands on either side of the victim's head so that the head is maintained in a fixed, neutral position and not in extension.
- Uses the index fingers to displace the mandible forward.
- Continues mouth-to-nose or mouth-to-mouth ventilations.

☐ Foreign bodies

- If obstruction is suspected, the resuscitator should roll the victim onto his side, place a knee under the victim's shoulder, and force his mouth open with crossed-finger technique:
  Run index and middle fingers along inside of the cheek toward base of tongue, deep into victim's throat.
  With a sweeping motion move fingers across the back

Principles

- When mouth-to-nose ventilation is used, the victim's mouth must be opened or his lips separated to let air escape during exhalation because the soft palate may obstruct the nasopharynx.

☐ This technique is used for persons who have had a laryngectomy. The head tilt or jaw maneuvers are not required for mouth-to-stoma resuscitation.

☐ An infant's neck .is very malleable. Forceful backward tilting of the head may obstruct breathing passages. Do not exaggerate the tilt position.

☐ When resuscitating accident victims, use caution to avoid extension of the neck when there is a possibility of neck fracture. A fractured neck should be suspected in diving or automobile accidents when the victim has lacerations of the face or forehead. If a fracture is suspected, avoid all forward, backward, lateral, or turning movement.

- This should be done without tilting the head backward or turning it from side to side.

☐ The resuscitator should not search for foreign bodies in the upper airway unless he knows or strongly suspects they are present. The first effort to ventilate will determine whether airway obstruction is present.

Repeated attempts may be required.

Action	Principles

Action

of the throat, removing any foreign matter.

If unable to dislodge the foreign body, or if it is impacted below the epiglottis, roll the victim onto his side to face resuscitator. Deliver sharp blows with the heel of hand between victim's shoulder blades.

If still unsuccessful, repeat mouth-to-mouth resuscitation, blows to back, and probing of upper airway with fingers.

If a small child has an obstructed airway, pick him up quickly, invert him over resuscitator's arm, and deliver blows with flat of palm between child's shoulder blades.

☐ Gastric distention

When distention is noted:
- Turn victim's head and shoulders to one side.

- Use one hand to exert moderate pressure over the victim's epigastrium.

☐ *Artificial Circulation*
(external cardiac compression)

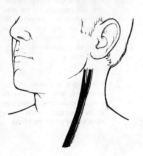

☐ Palpate the carotid pulse:

- Use the tips of the index and middle fingers.
- Locate the larynx.
- Slide the finger tips laterally into the groove between the trachea and the muscles at the side of the neck.

Principles

☐ Artificial ventilation frequently causes distention of the stomach. This occurs most often in children, but it is not uncommon in adults. It is most likely to occur when excessive pressures are used for inflation or if the airway is obstructed. Marked distention is dangerous because it promotes vomiting.

- Aspiration of gastric contents during this maneuver is prevented.
- The epigastrium is located between the umbilicus and rib cage.

Cardiac arrest is recognized by pulselessness in large arteries (carotid or femoral) in an unconscious victim who has a death-like appearance and is not breathing.

☐ The kind of arrest, witnessed or unwitnessed, indicates the sequence in which the carotid pulse is palpated. The carotid pulse is recommended rather than other pulses because the resuscitator is already at the victim's head to perform artificial ventilation, the victim's neck is accessible, and clothing need not be removed. Carotid pulses are central and may persist when peripheral pulses are no longer palpable.

- The carotid pulse can be felt at this point.

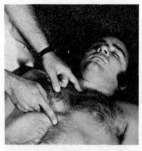

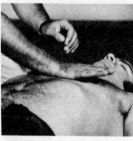

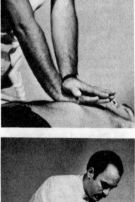

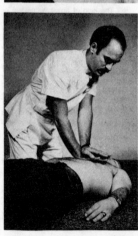

- The pulse area must be palpated gently and must not be compressed. Absence or questionable presence of the pulse is the indication for starting artificial circulation.

☐ Perform artificial circulation (adults)

External cardiac compression consists of the rhythmic application of pressure over the lower half of the sternum, but not over the xiphoid process. Performed properly, external cardiac compression will produce:

Pulsatile artificial circulation.

Systolic blood pressure peaks of over 100 mm. Hg. The diastolic pressure is zero and the mean pressure seldom exceeds 40 mm. Hg in the carotid arteries.

Carotid artery blood flow of about one quarter to one third of normal flow.

- Place victim supine on the ground or floor. If he is in bed, place a board, preferably extending the full width of the bed, under his back.
- Locate the lower half of the sternum by feeling the tip of the sternum (xiphoid process).
- Apply long axis of the heel of one hand over lower half of the sternum 1-1½ inches above the tip of the sternum, toward patient's head.
- Keep fingers off chest wall.
- Place the second hand on top of the first one, bringing shoulders directly over the victim's sternum.
- Keeping arms straight and elbows locked, apply firm, heavy pressure so that the sternum is depressed vertically 1½-2 inches.

- The patient must be on a firm surface so that pressure is not dissipated.

- Resuscitator may have to get onto the bed to achieve correct position.
- For the average adult, a pressure of 80 to 120 pounds is required. The compressions must be regular, smooth, and uninterrupted.
- The heel of the resuscitator's hand should not be removed from the chest during relaxation, but pressure on the sternum should be completely released so that the sternum returns to its normal resting position between compressions.

Artificial circulation for infants and children:
- Provide a firm support under the victim's back.

- If the victim is a small child or an infant, one hand can be placed under child's back as a firm support, while other hand compresses the chest.

Action	Principles

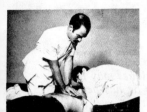

- Apply compression to the midsternum of infants and small children.

- For a small child use only the heel of one hand to depress the sternum; depress sternum ¾-1½ inches.
- For an infant use only the tips of index and middle fingers; depress sternum ½-¾ inch.
- Compress the chest 80-100 times per minute; deliver breaths as quickly as possible after each five compressions.

- The ventricles of infants and small children lie high in the chest. Therefore, the external pressure should be exerted over the midsternum.

- The ratio of compressions to ventilations is 5:1.

Resuscitation by one resuscitator

The ratio of compressions to ventilations is 15:2.

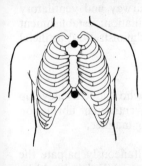

☐ Administer two very quick lung inflations after each 15 chest compressions. The compression rate is 80 per minute.

☐ The two full lung inflations must be delivered in rapid succession within five seconds, without allowing for full lung exhalation by the victim between breaths.

Resuscitation by two rescuers

The ratio of compressions to ventilations is 5:1.

☐ One rescuer performs external cardiac compression and the other ventilates.

☐ Artificial ventilations are interposed, *without pause*, between fifth and next compressions.

Precordial thump

This technique is indicated only if the cardiac arrest is witnessed. It is *not recommended for unwitnessed cardiac arrests, nor is it recommended for children.*

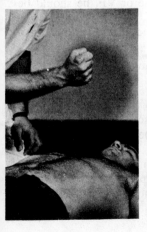

☐ Locate the midportion of the sternum, between the sternal notch and the xiphoid process.

☐ Deliver a sharp, quick, single blow over the midportion of the sternum with the bottom, fleshy portion of the fist. Strike the blow from 8 to 12 inches over the chest.

☐ The thump should be delivered within the first minute after the arrest. The precordial thump is not useful for anoxic asystole and cannot be depended upon to convert an established ventricular fibrillation. It is not useful for electro-mechanical dissociation associated with exsanguination. It should not be used for a ventricular trachycardia that is providing adequate circulation.

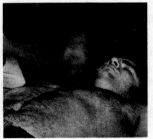

☐ If there is no immediate response, begin basic life support at once.

☐ If the precordial thump is effective, a carotid pulse will be palpable.

Advanced Life Support

*Adjunctive equipment, drugs, and techniques may be
needed to maintain a person's life after he has been
revived or when sustained CPR is required.*

Advanced life support involves the use of special equipment to prevent
cardiopulmonary arrest or to supplement basic life support measures.
Adjunctive equipment is not needed to initiate and perform CPR.
Rather, it is used when it becomes available, by adequately trained persons
who are skilled in using the specific devices and techniques. Basic
life support should not be delayed until equipment arrives; nor should
the use of adjunctive equipment divert attention or effort from basic
CPR.

Advanced life support consists of cardiac monitoring for dysrhythmia
recognition and control; adjunctive therapy for airway and ventilatory
maintenance and for artificial circulation; defibrillation; establishment
and maintenance of intravenous infusions; drug administration; artificial
pacing; and stabilization of the patient's condition.

MONITORED PATIENTS

Patients who are monitored continuously and who suddenly develop
ventricular tachycardia (VT) without a pulse, ventricular fibrillation
(VF), or asystole should be treated in the following manner:
- Give a single precordial thump.
- Observe monitor for cardiac rhythm and simultaneously palpate the
carotid pulse. If patient is in VT without a pulse or VF, he should be
countershocked as soon as possible.
- If the pulse is absent, tilt the patient's head back and give four quick
ventilations.
- Palpate the carotid pulse again.
- If the pulse is absent, begin CPR.

VENTILATORY ADJUNCTS

The exhaled air ventilation provided by rescue breathing delivers
about 16 or 17 percent oxygen to the patient. The oxygen concentration
of air is about 21 percent. Therefore, exhaled air ventilation should
deliver sufficient amounts of oxygen to the patient. Oxygenation can be
improved by using certain airway adjuncts and supplemental oxygen.

Oropharyngeal airways should be used whenever a bag-valve-mask system or an automatic breathing device with a mask is used. An oropharyngeal airway should be inserted only in deeply unconscious patients. If it is placed in an alert or semiconscious patient, the airway invariably stimulates the gag reflex and induces vomiting. Extreme care must be exercised when the airway is inserted so that the mucous membrane is not traumatized. Incorrect insertion can also displace the tongue back into the pharynx and cause airway obstruction.

To use an oropharyngeal airway, first select the proper size. Open the person's mouth and place a tongue blade on the dorsal portion of the tongue. Gently press the tongue down and out toward the lips. Gently insert the airway with your free hand. Once the airway is inserted, check it for patency. Check the person's lips to be sure that they are not caught between the teeth and the airway. Patients who have large lips or who are edentulous may occlude the airway. Therefore, the flange should be outside the lips. An airway that is too short is of no value. It cannot lift the tongue away from the oropharynx(1).

Nasopharyngeal airways may be used to maintain a patent airway in a semiconscious patient. Again, the proper size must be selected; if the airway is too short, it will not reach the oropharynx and will not push the tongue forward. Before inserting a nasopharyngeal airway, lubricate it with water-soluble jelly to ease its passage and minimize trauma. If insertion is obstructed, rotate the tube. If resistance persists even after you have rotated the tube, remove it and insert it in the other nostril. Check the patency of the nasopharyngeal airway after insertion. The nasal airway's proximal end should be flared to prevent it from slipping past the nares. However, some nasopharyngeal airways are not flared, and for these a safety pin should be inserted through the exposed tip at the nares to prevent it from slipping.

S-tube airways have certain limitations and are rarely effective when used for artificial ventilation. They do not provide an adequate airway seal, may induce vomiting if used improperly, and require repositioning between chest compressions when only one rescuer is doing CPR. S-tubes do, however, assist in maintaining a patent airway and in keeping the victim's mouth open.

Mouth-to-mask devices that fit well are effective, simple adjuncts for respiratory resuscitation. All personnel who use these devices should practice with mainikins to develop the dexterity required for this technique. Oral airways should be used whenever a mask is placed on the patient. Mouth-to-mask devices should be made of a transparent material, have a well-sealing cuff, headstraps, and an oxygen insufflation outlet. The coupling size should be 15 mm./22 mm. One standard size should be available for adults, and additional sizes available for infants and children.

The mouth-to-mask technique of respiratory resuscitation is most effective when the rescuer is positioned at the top of the patient's head and uses the jaw-thrust maneuver to maintain airway patency(2).

Bag-valve-mask devices usually produce less ventilatory volume than mouth-to-mouth or mouth-to-mask ventilation because it is difficult to provide a leakproof seal to the face while maintaining a patent airway. Therefore, self-inflating bags should be used only when the patient has a cuffed endotracheal tube or esophageal obturator airway in place.

Bag-valve-mask units should be self-refilling devices without sponge rubber inside. Sponge rubber is difficult to cleanse and disinfect, retains ethylene oxide, and is subject to fragmentation. The device should have a non-jam valve system with a 15 liter/minute oxygen inlet flow. The face mask should be constructed of transparent plastic and have an air-filled or contoured, resilient cuff. Except for pediatric models, it should have a non-pop-off valve. Standard 15 mm./22 mm. fittings are recommended. A system for delivery of high concentrations of oxygen should be provided through an ancillary oxygen inlet at the back of the bag or through an oxygen reservoir. The valve should be a true nonrebreathing valve.

All bag-valve-mask devices should be satisfactory for practice on manikins and should perform satisfactorily under all common environmental conditions and extremes of temperature. They should be available in adult and pediatric sizes(2).

Any bag-valve-mask device should be used only when it meets these criteria, and then only by a rescuer who has had extensive training and manikin practice. Two rescuers must do CPR when this mask is used.

When a bag-valve mask is applied, an oral airway should be inserted. The rescuer should position himself at the top of the victim's head, maintain the victim's head in extension, and secure an optimum fit of the mask with one hand while squeezing the bag with the free hand. The external cardiac compression to ventilation ratio should be 5:1, with a ventilation interposed after every fifth compression, without interruption.

Supplemental oxygen should be used with both the bag-valve-mask and bag-valve-tube systems. Low cardiac output and ventilation-perfusion abnormalities are encountered during CPR, with development of marked discrepancies between the alveolar and arterial oxygen tension, causing hypoxemia. Hypoxemia leads to anaerobic metabolism and metabolic acidosis, which will impair the beneficial effects of drugs and countershock. Supplemental oxygen increases myocardial and cerebral oxygenation and enhances the effects of treatment modalities used during resuscitative efforts.

Esophageal obturator airways are relatively new devices. A cuffed endotracheal tube is mounted through a face mask. A soft, plastic obturator blocks the distal orifice. Multiple openings are found in the upper one third of the tube at the level of the pharynx. After the obturator is passed into the esophagus, the mask is placed on the face and the cuff is inflated. Because the esophagus is blocked, air is forced into the tube and passes down the trachea. The esophageal obturator airway should be used only on patients who are apneic or deeply unconscious. Suction must be readily available when this device is used, especially when the person is extubated. Vomiting frequently occurs when the tube is removed. This device should be used only by people who have had extensive training and practice with it. The potential for damage to the esophagus is ever present.

Endotracheal intubation with a cuffed tube isolates the airway, maintains its patency, prevents aspiration, and ensures the delivery of a high concentration of oxygen to the lungs. The main problem with endotracheal intubation is that it is frequently attempted by medical personnel who are not trained in this technique. As a result, precious time is lost while CPR is interrupted. CPR should *never* be interrupted for longer than 15 seconds during intubation attempts. Faulty intubation can result in regurgitation and aspiration; laryngeal edema and pharyngeal bleeding from the trauma sustained during repeated, unskilled attempts at intubation. Endotracheal intubation should be restricted to medical personnel and professional allied health personnel who are highly trained and use endotracheal intubation frequently or are retrained frequently.

Conventional, pressure-cycled, automatic devices, such as IPPB respirators, positive-negative pressure resuscitators, and resuscitator-inhalators, should not be used in conjunction with CPR. External cardiac compression will trigger the termination of the inflation cycle prematurely and result in inadequate ventilation.

Manually triggered, time-cycled devices have flow rates that allow ventilations to be interposed between compressions during CPR. Manually triggered, oxygen-powered resuscitators should provide instantaneous flow rates of 100 liters/minute or more and an inspiratory pressure safety release valve that opens at 50 cm. of water. This high, instantaneous flow rate usually will cause gastric distention unless a cuffed endotracheal tube or cuffed esophageal obturator airway is used.

The respirator should provide 100 percent oxygen. It must operate satisfactorily under varied environmental conditions, including all North American temperature extremes. A standard 15 mm./22 mm. coupling should be available for attachment to a mask, endotracheal tube, esophageal airway, or tracheostomy tube. Portable devices should be rugged, breakage-resistant, compact, and easy to hold. The trigger should be positioned so that the rescuer can keep both hands on the mask to hold it in position while he supports and tilts the victim's head and keeps his jaw elevated(2).

Portable or installed suction equipment should be available for resuscitation emergencies. Suction should be powerful enough to provide an air flow of more than 30 liters/minute at the end of the delivery tube and a vacuum of more than 300 mm. Hg when the tube is clamped.

After the airway has been isolated by endotracheal intubation, a nasogastric tube should be inserted to provide for gastric decompression. However, if gastric distention interferes with adequate ventilation, a nasogastric tube should be inserted before endotracheal intubation. External cardiac compression should not be interrupted during this procedure.

CIRCULATION ADJUNCTS

Cardiopulmonary resuscitation should be performed wherever the victim is found. If the patient arrests in bed, a firm support should be placed beneath his back. The best support is a bedboard that extends from the shoulders to the waist and across the full width of the bed. Metal or heavy-duty serving trays may be used, but these do not provide the ideal, evenly distributed support of a bedboard.

Simple, hinged, manually operated chest compressors can be used for effective external cardiac compression. These devices should provide an adjustable sternal-depression depth of one-and-a-half to two inches. Application of the device should be accomplished without interrupting CPR for more than five seconds.

Automatic mechanical chest compressors provide the most consistently effective cardiopulmonary resuscitation during prolonged resuscitative

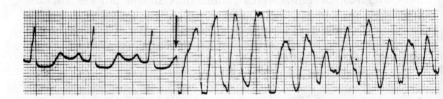

PVC on T wave (arrow) triggered VF. VF and VT can be terminated by defibrillation.

efforts. Because they are heavy and relatively hard to move, it is difficult to transfer the patient to the device without losing time during CPR. With a chest compressor in place, the patient's position must be watched constantly because changes in position may cause the plunger to depress the epigastric region or ribs, causing further complications. These devices should be used only by personnel who have had extensive training and manikin practice in the manual method, as well as practice in the proper technique for changing from manual to automatic compression without interrupting CPR for more than five seconds at any one time.

DEFIBRILLATION

Defibrillation, or emergency countershock, synchronously depolarizes the myocardium. After this, spontaneous, coordinated, electrical activity can resume. Direct-current countershock should be delivered as soon as possible when the heart is known to be in ventricular tachycardia without a peripheral pulse or in the presence of ventricular fibrillation. The usefulness of emergency countershock in the treatment of asystole has not been established.

Effective defibrillation is achieved when one paddle is placed to the right of the upper sternum, below the right clavicle, and the other paddle just to the left of the cardiac apex or left nipple. Electrode paste, covering the entire paddle surface, or saline-soaked gauze pads that are large enough to accommodate paddle size should be used as conductive media. The defibrillator usually is set at its maximum voltage, commonly 400 watt seconds.

Ineffective results usually can be traced to one of several causes:
• The electrode paddles are too small, or of different sizes. This interferes with current flow.
• Insufficient pressure is used to apply the paddles to the chest wall. Approximately 20 pounds of pressure are required.
• The entire surface of the paddles is not in contact with the skin.
• Excessive conductive media are on the chest wall surface. This will cause the current to arc, and deter its flow to the myocardium.
• Defibrillation in the presence of hypoxemia and acidosis usually is ineffective. Adequate ventilation, supplemental oxygen, and sodium bicarbonate may reverse these conditions.
• Defibrillation is seldom effective in the presence of fine ventricular fibrillation manifested by slow, irregular ECG activity of low amplitude. Epinephrine may convert this to a coarser fibrillation and also may lower the defibrillation threshold.
• The amount of current selected may be insufficient.

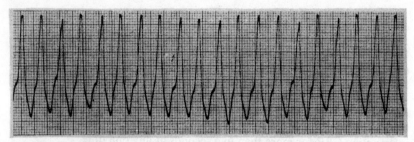
A rapid ventricular tachycardia usually does not stimulate effective cardiac pumping.

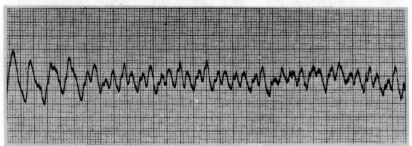
The gross irregularity of ventricular fibrillation is recognized easily.

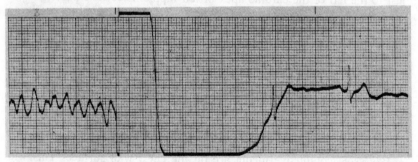
Fibrillation is terminated by countershock, and normal conduction is established.

- The person defibrillating the patient does not wait for the capacitator to charge fully. Charging time—the time required for energy to build up in the defibrillator—varies from model to model and takes from nine to 30 seconds.
- The defibrillator may be defective.
- The electrode surface of paddles may be defective due to oxidation of metal or pitting.

A single emergency countershock does not cause serious functional damage to the myocardium. If a direct-current defibrillator is available, an emergency countershock should be delivered to any adult who is unconscious, pulseless, and unmonitored. Adelhardt, Rigney, and Grace call this "blind" or "unmonitored" defibrillation, and have incorporated it as immediate intervention in basic life support. This treatment has increased survival rates(3). Unmonitored defibrillation is not recommended for children.

The defibrillator as well as all other emergency equipment should be checked by a trained person at the beginning of every tour of duty.

INTRAVENOUS THERAPY

Establishing an intravenous infusion route is essential to provide intermittent or continuous rapid administration of drugs and fluids. If the central line is inserted peripherally, through the basilic vein, the tip of

DRUGS FOR CARDIOPULMONARY RESUSCITATION AND ADVANCED LIFE SUPPORT

Drug and Dose Range	Reasons for Use and Precautions
PRIMARY Sodium Bicarbonate	Counteracts metabolic acidosis.
Adult: 1 mEq./kg. I.V.	After initial dose, continued administration should be governed by arterial blood gas and pH measurements.
Child: 0.9 mEq./kg. I.V. (dilute 1:1 with sterile water)	When blood gases and pH determinations are not available, *one half* the initial dose may be administered at *10-minute* intervals. Metabolic alkalosis and hyperosmolality from excesses must be avoided.
	When asystole or persistent ventricular fibrillation is present, sodium bicarbonate should not be used alone. Rather, repeated doses of sodium bicarbonate and epinephrine should be administered while performing CPR. This may convert asystole to ventricular fibrillation, which can be defibrillated, or may improve myocardial status during ventricular fibrillation and enhance the effectiveness of defibrillation.
Epinephrine	May restore electrical activity in asystole.
Adult: 0.5 ml. of 1:1000 solution I.V. 5 ml. of 1:10,000 solution intracardially	May enchance effectiveness of defibrillation in ventricular fibrillation.
Child: 0.3 to 2 ml. of 1:10,000 solution intracardially (0.1 ml./kg.)	Epinephrine will increase myocardial contractility, elevate perfusion pressure, lower defibrillation threshold, and, in some instances, may restore myocardial contractility in electro-mechanical dissociation. Should be given every 5 minutes during CPR.

Drug and Dose Range	Reasons for Use and Precautions
SECONDARY **Atropine Sulfate** Adult: 0.5 mg. I.V. Repeat at 5-minute intervals until pulse rate is greater than 60. TOTAL DOSE SHOULD NOT EXCEED 2 mg.	Indicated for sinus bradycardia with a pulse of less than 60 beats/min. when accompanied by premature ventricular contractions or when systolic blood pressure is less than 90 mm.Hg. Indicated for high-degree atrioventricular block accompanied by bradycardia. Is of no value in ventricular ectopic bradycardia if there is no atrial activity.
Lidocaine (Xylocaine) Adult: 50 to 100 mg. I.V. bolus Repeat as needed TOTAL DOSE SHOULD NOT EXCEED 300 mg./hr. Child: 5 mg. I.V. bolus Repeat as needed Infant: 0.5 mg./kg. I.V. bolus TOTAL DOSE SHOULD NOT EXCEED 100 mg./hr.	Raises the fibrillation threshold. Exerts antidysrhythmic effect by increasing the electrical stimulation threshold of the ventricle during diastole. Depresses irritability when successful defibrillation repeatedly reverts to ventricular fibrillation. Controls premature ventricular contractions (coupled, multiform, PVC on T, or more than 5/min.), and recurrent bouts of ventricular tachycardia. Is of no value in asystole.
Calcium Chloride 10% Adult: 2.5 ml. to 5 ml. (3.4 to 6.8 mEq.) I.V. bolus. Repeat at 10-minute intervals Child: 1 ml./5 kg. I.V. bolus Maximum dose 1 ml./5 kg. Intracardially: dilute 1:1 with saline	Indicated for profound cardiovascular collapse. May enhance electrical defibrillation. May restore electrical rhythm in asystole. Calcium increases myocardial contractility, prolongs systole, and enhances ventricular excitability. Calcium can suppress sinus impulse formation. Sudden death has been reported following a rapid intravenous injection, especially in fully digitalized patients. Calcium mixed with sodium bicarbonate forms a precipitate.
Isoproterenol (Isuprel) Adult: 2 to 20 micro mg./min. I.V. infusion (1 to 10 ml. of solution with 1 mg./500 cc. 5% D/W)	Indicated for profound bradycardia caused by complete heart block and for profound sinus bradycardia refractory to atropine. Dose should be adjusted to increase heart rate to approximately 60 beats/min. Use with extreme caution in the patient with myocardial infarction.
Propranolol (Inderal) Adult: 1 mg. I.V. Repeat to total of 3 mg.	The antidysrhythmic properties of the beta adrenergic blocking agents have proven useful in the treatment of repetitive ventricular tachycardia or repetitive ventricular fibrillation when maintenance of a rhythmic heartbeat cannot be achieved with lidocaine. Use with extreme caution in the patient with congestive heart failure or chronic obstructive pulmonary disease.
Vasoactive Drugs **Levarterenol (Levophed)** Adult: 16 micro mg./ml. I.V. infusion **Metaraminol (Aramine)** Adult: 0.4 mg./ml. I.V. infusion	The selection of a vasoconstrictor or a positive inotropic agent remains controversial in the treatment of cardiac arrest and the immediate post resuscitation period. However, during cardiac compression and the post resuscitation period, blood pressure must be supported when low blood pressure and inadequate cerebral and renal perfusion give evidence of shock. The selection of therapy is dictated by the patient's clinical state. Extravasation of these drugs can cause tissue necrosis and sloughing.

the catheter will lie in the superior vena cava or right atrium. This will preclude the need for transthoracic cardiac injections. The use of the intracardiac route to administer drugs is strongly discouraged. "Blind" attempts at using this route may result in rupture of a coronary artery, further insult to an infarcted area of tissue, pneumothorax, or injection of the drug into the muscle instead of the chamber and consequent increased myocardial irritability. Adequate external cardiac compression will circulate any medication given intravenously, even those administered through peripherally inserted plastic catheters.

EMERGENCY PACING

Patients who develop a bradycardia associated with a significant decrease in cardiac output, as in acute heart blocks, may require immediate insertion of a temporary cardiac pacemaker by a transvenous or transthoracic approach. This treatment is used after it has been determined whether the condition is transient or chronic and whether the disturbance is in rhythmicity or conduction. Once it is inserted, the pacemaker provides an electrical stimulus for myocardial contraction.

EDUCATING THE PUBLIC

Nurses not only should acquire a basic knowledge of CPR, but also be able to perform CPR skillfully whenever necessary. To do this, nurses need familiarity with the current guidelines and standards of practice. Nurses also can prepare as teachers of CPR. By doing so, they can teach not only other nurses, physicians, and allied health workers basic life support techniques, but can also reach many persons within their communities who can learn these skills. "The goal should be to train the general public, starting with school children in eighth grade"(4).

Educating the public about major health problems is a nursing responsibility. However, it does no good to acquaint people with the symptoms of myocardial infarction if no provisions are made for quick access into an emergency medical system. Most communities can establish stratified systems of coronary care as outlined below, and nurses can lead in implementing them. A stratified system consists of three levels:

      I. Emergency Life Support Units
          A. Life Support Units
            1. Basic
            2. Advanced

B. Mobile Life Support Units
1. Basic
2. Advanced
II. Coronary Care Units
Intermediate Care Units
III. Regional Reference Centers

Most communities can establish facilities on levels I and II, or they can cooperate with nearby communities to provide such services.

The future delivery of emergency care will depend on advances made in the basic sciences, technology, medicine, and nursing. Inevitably, alterations in standards and guidelines will be necessary. Good practice today may not be good practice tomorrow. Everyone who practices nursing must keep pace with changes as they emerge so he can deliver thoughtful, learned, and compassionate emergency care.

REFERENCES

1. SMITH, B. J. *Fundamentals of Anesthesia Care.* St. Louis, C. V. Mosby Co., 1972, p. 9.
2. AMERICAN HEART ASSOCIATION, CARDIO-PULMONARY RESUSCITATION AND EMERGENCY CARDIAC CARE COMMITTEE AND NATIONAL ACADEMY OF SCIENCES—NATIONAL RESEARCH COUNCIL, MEDICAL SCIENCES DIVISION, EMERGENCY MEDICAL SERVICES COMMITTEE. Standards for cardiopulmonary resuscitation (CPR) and emergency cardiac care (ECC): Part 3. Advanced life support. *JAMA* 2227:853-854, Feb. 18, 1974.
3. ADELHARDT, DIANA, AND OTHERS. Every nurse's station is a life-support station. (editorial) *Heart Lung* 2:832-833, Nov.-Dec. 1973.
4. AMERICAN HEART ASSOCIATION, *op. cit.*, p. 850.

From the *American Journal of Nursing* 75:586-591, Apr. 1975.

Temporary Cardiac Pacemakers

ELIZABETH HAHN WINSLOW • LYNNE BROOKS MARINO

Indications for temporary pacing have broadened considerably in recent years. Temporary pacing is used for the pre- and intraoperative management of patients who require permanent pacemakers, for post-operative care of cardiac surgery patients, for diagnostic studies such as stress tests in which pacing rather than exercise is used to increase the heart rate, for correction of short-term conduction defects and slow impulse formation, and for overdrive suppression of tachyarrhythmias.

A temporary pacemaker consists of a pulse generator and an electrode catheter. Circuitry and batteries within the generator produce pacing impulses and regulate their timing. The catheter carries these impulses to the heart to stimulate electrical excitation and contraction. Portable cardiac monitoring equipment such as telemetry units should not be mistaken for a temporary pacemaker.

The pacemaker may be completely external or partially implanted (transthoracic, epicardial, endocardial). Completely external temporary pacing, historically the first method used, delivers shocks to the heart through electrode plates taped to the chest. This technique, though quickly and easily instituted, is rarely used today because of its unpredictable effectiveness and because the large amount of electrical current required to deliver impulses through the chest wall causes local pain, skeletal muscle contractions, and skin burns.

The major advantage of transthoracic pacing is the rapidity with which it can be initated. A thin wire electrode is inserted directly into the myocardium through a needle in the chest wall. The needle is withdrawn,

MS. WINSLOW, R.N., M.S., *is a clinical specialist in cardiovascular nursing, Hospital of the University of Pennsylvania, Philadelphia.*
MS. MARINO, R.N., *is a staff nurse in the coronary care unit, Saint Francis Hospital, Trenton, N.J. She was head nurse of the medical intensive care unit at Hospital of the University of Pennsylvania at the time this article was written.*

leaving the pacing wire in place. This technique is used only in emergencies because of the risks associated with blind catheter introduction, such as coronary artery trauma and pericardial tamponade.

Temporary epicardial pacing is routinely used after cardiac sugery. Three tiny wires—one sewn loosely to the atrial epicardium, another on the ventricular epicardium, and a third, a subcutaneous, indifferent lead —come out through the chest wall and can be attached to the pulse generator. The origin of each wire is shown by its different length, by labeled adhesive tabs, or by some other method. Ventricular or atrial pacing can be used to provide optimal antiarrhythmic and hemodynamic benefits. The wires are easily pulled out through the skin in a few days or weeks when they are no longer needed.

Transvenous endocardial pacing is the most common method of temporary pacing. The catheter is inserted percutaneously or by cutdown into a vein. The antecubital, femoral, jugular, or subclavian vein may be used. Each approach has advantages and disadvantages. Ordinarily, the antecubital and femoral are used so that the jugular and subclavian veins remain available if permanent pacing is required. Antecubital insertion can be performed with electrographic or fluoroscopic control. Femoral insertion requires guidance by fluoroscopy and, in some institutions, necessitates moving the patient from the intensive care unit to another unit with x-ray facilities. The large femoral vein is less likely to become phlebitic than the smaller antecubital vein.

For ventricular transvenous pacing, the catheter tip is securely wedged between the trabeculae of the right ventricular apex. Achievement of stable atrial transvenous pacing is difficult. The catheter is lodged in the atrial appendage or coronary sinus. A special curved catheter has been helpful in maintaining position stability.

A unipolar (one electrode) or bipolar (two electrodes) catheter may be used. The unipolar catheter must be connected to a ground electrode, a small subcutaneous, metal needle which is connected to the positive pacemaker terminal. The indwelling cardiac electrode is connected to the negative terminal.

The bipolar catheter is more commonly used because it does not require a skin electrode, and its two electrodes permit better contact with the cardiac tissue. Also, if one electrode fails, the bipolar catheter can be converted to a unipolar system by adding a skin electrode. Bipolar lead systems may exhibit different threshold values depending on how the leads are connected to the terminals. Usually threshold is lowest when the distal electrode tip is connected to the negative terminal. The external lead system usually is coded to show which is the distal electrode.

The stimulation threshold is the minimal intensity of the pacing stimulus that maintains continuous capture of the heart. Stimulation threshold measurement is used to verify adequate electrode placement after the catheter is positioned. The output current is gradually decreased until capture is lost and then increased until a QRS complex follows each pacing impulse. The amount of current used when 1:1 capture first occurs is the stimulation threshold. If it exceeds 1.5 milliamperes (mA), the lead is in an unsatisfactory position and must be repositioned.

The threshold may increase or decrease after catheter placement, due to fibrosis around the catheter, infection, drugs, electrolyte changes, and numerous other factors. To compensate for these threshold fluctuations and to maintain constant capture, the impulse strength is set two to three times the threshold value. Consistent pacing may generally be effected by impulses of two to five mA. Because fibrillation threshold generally ranges from 10 to 30 times the stimulation threshold, the impulse strength should not be set too high.

After the stimulation threshold has been determined, the sensitivity threshold should be measured to confirm adequate sensing of intrinsic cardiac activity if demand pacing is used. The rate dial is turned below the patient's heart rate. The sensitivity dial is turned to its most sensitive demand position, fully clockwise in the Medtronic 5880A model. The Sense/Pace indicator should deflect toward Sense. Then, the sensitivity dial is gradually turned to the middle of the sensitivity range, three o'clock on the Medtronic model. An acceptable sensitivity threshold is present if the pacemaker can still accurately sense R waves; if not, the lead should be repositioned. Determination of sensitivity threshold may be difficult or impossible in patients who have rates below 50/min., the lowest pacemaker setting.

Fixed-rated (asynchronous, competitive) and demand (non-competitive) pacemakers are the most common types used. A fixed-rate pacemaker stimulates the heart at its present rate, uninfluenced by the intrinsic electrical activity of the heart. If it is set at 60 it will fire at 60, even if the patient's heart block disappears and he resumes normal sinus rhythm. Competition between paced and spontaneous beats ordinarily does not cause problems even though the pacemaker may fire during the vulnerable period of the cardiac cycle, the T wave, because a significant safety factor exists between the energy needed to pace and the energy needed to produce ventricular fibrillation. However, if the ventricular fibrillation threshold is lowered by myocardial infarction, electrolyte imbalance, or other factors, a pacemaker stimulus firing on the T wave may initiate ventricular tachycardia or ventricular fibrillation. This danger, though exaggerated in the past, is very real and makes the use of demand pacemakers more acceptable than fixed-rate pacemakers.

A demand pacemaker avoids competition by stimulating the heart at a preset rate *only if* the patient's rate falls below a predetermined rate. It is designed to fire when a certain time period elapses without intrinsic cardiac activity. For example, a pacemaker set at 60 will fire if one second elapses without a spontaneous heart beat. The demand pacemaker is inhibited when the intrinsic cardiac rate is adequate. The sensitivity dial must be set correctly to enable proper sensing and pacing.

NURSING IMPLICATIONS

A temporary pacemaker is usually inserted as an emergency or semi-emergency measure. It is rarely inserted on a leisurely, elective basis. The nurse must prepare the patient and his family quickly, yet adequately. The information given depends on the time available, what the patient knows, what he wants to know, and what he needs to know. Good preparation for temporary pacing enhances patient cooperation during pacemaker insertion, assists the patient to cope with the inconveniences which follow the procedure, and fosters an improved attitude toward permanent pacing should it be required.

Patients like Mr. H., who arrived at the hospital with his Merck Manual under one arm and his PDR under the other and recited his medical history like a physician rather than a retired businessman, will want detailed information—including a thorough explanation of the electronic circuitry. After his temporary pacemaker was inserted, formal teaching was done with pictures, diagrams, and booklets. All subsequent procedures were thoroughly explained. Other patients, like Ms. M., feel "ignorance is bliss" and do not want to be told anything. These patients do require and respond well to basic, simple information about the pacemaker and its insertion. Teaching is best done in small amounts, informally, and in response to questions. For example, when Ms. M. asked, "Why won't you let me use this arm?" the possibility of catheter displacement was explained briefly.

All patients should understand the purpose of the pacemaker. They should realize that transvenous, endocardial pacemaker insertion is not similar to open heart surgery—a common, frightening misconception. A diagram showing the catheter following a vein into the heart is often helpful. The patient should know where the insertion procedure will take place, that it will take about an hour, that he will be awake because local anesthesia is used, and that the major discomfort will be having to lie relatively still on his back during the procedure. If possible, the patient should be told the site of the pacemaker insertion—arm, groin, or neck. This is especially important if the neck is used because some patients have a "cut-throat phobia" and need time to ventilate their fears and control their anxiety. If possible, the usual postinsertion routines should be explained briefly. After the pacemaker has been inserted and the patient's condition has stabilized, the nurse can reinforce previous information and give additional information.

Following temporary pacemaker insertion, the nurse checks vital signs, dressings, and monitor pattern, administers analgesics, and makes the patient comfortable. She records on the Kardex the date and site of pacemaker insertion and the following pacemaker settings: rate, mA, fixed rate or demand, on or off. These settings must be changed on the record when they are changed on the pacemaker.

The pacemaker dials should be protected so the patient or health personnel do not inadvertently alter them. Shortly after Mr. S., a confused elderly gentleman, had his pacemaker inserted, the nurse noticed a chaotic, variable pacemaker pattern on his monitor. She found Mr. S. totally frustrated and exasperated—no matter how he turned the dials his television would not go on! Some pacemaker models have plastic shields that protect the control settings; otherwise, transparent tape will fix the settings. An extension pacemaker cable may be useful for patients who persistently tamper with the pacemaker and for those who are bothered by its weight, about ¾ pound. The extension cable permits placement of the pacemaker box near but not on the patient.

The nurse should understand the pacemaker settings and when to alter them. For example, the nurse might be instructed to gradually increase the mA to five if capture is lost. She should know how and when to turn the pacemaker on and off. Some models have a safety lock on the on/off switch that requires two hands to operate. The nurse might be instructed to turn on a fixed-rate pacemaker if the patient's rate drops below 60. If the pacemaker rarely needs to pace, the nurse may be asked to check pacemaker function routinely to ascertain that it will work properly if required. For example, for the patient with a demand pacemaker but an adequate spontaneous rate of 80, she would turn the rate from its setting at 60 to 85, observe and document proper pacemaker function, and then reset the rate at 60. If pacing is to be stopped or interrupted, this should be done gradually or with cardiac stimulating drugs. Abrupt cessation of pacing may be followed by a period of asystole before the idioventricular pacemaker resumes activity because this subsidiary pacemaker has been suppressed by the artificial pacemaker. In general, the higher the pacing rate, the longer the asystole following pacing interruption. The nurse should know how the pacemaker demonstrates pacing or sensing. Most models have a needle or light which indicates pacing and sensing. In some older models an electrocardiogram must be taken to ascertain pacemaker function.

The nurse must understand how the pacemaker demonstrates battery failure and how to obtain and load new batteries. Most pacemakers lose sensing function with early battery depletion; later, pacing function is lost. In some models the Sense/Pace indicator stops functioning before any pacemaker action is altered significantly. The pacemaker artifact may suggest battery depletion by a decrease in amplitude. To detect this alteration, monitor strips must be taken at regular intervals and compared to previous strips.

Pacemakers are powered by mercury transistor batteries that last two to four months. Loading procedure varies with different models but in general is relatively simple and similar to loading flashlight batteries. Some models feature a storage capacitor that provides about 10 seconds of continuous operation while the battery is being changed. All hospital units housing patients with temporary pacemakers should have fresh batteries and extra pacemakers readily available.

The pacemaker box must be properly maintained. It should not be autoclaved or immersed in liquids. Gas autoclaving may be used, if necessary; otherwise, occasional sponging with water or alcohol is all that is required.

It is also important to understand the care of the catheter site and extremity, complications associated with temporary pacing, and additional resuscitative measures indicated if a patient with a temporary pacemaker arrests.

INSERTION SITES

The catheter site and surrounding skin should be inspected regularly for signs of inflammation or infection. If present, these are reported to the physician. When a transvenous, endocardial catheter is present, the dressing is changed every other day. Extreme care must be used to prevent catheter displacement, especially if the catheter is not sutured to the skin. The skin around the catheter is cleansed with an antiseptic solution. Antibiotic ointment and a dry, sterile dressing are applied to the insertion site. The date of the dressing change is written on the dressing, and the dressing change and appearance of the site are recorded in the nurses' notes.

In post-thoracotomy patients with temporary epicardial pacemaker catheters, the sites where the wires exit through the skin usually do not require dressings or special care unless drainage or infection is present. Then, a procedure similar to that described above is used, or the wires are removed.

If the patient has an antecubital pacemaker, an armboard and pillows are used to prevent all but minimal arm movement. It is especially important to prevent extremity abduction when atrial pacing is used because wire displacement is a common problem. In patients with endocardial atrial wires a pillow is placed between the arm and the bedrail while the patient is in bed; before he gets out of bed, his arm is secured to his side with Kling or Ace bandages. Analgesics are administered to allay the resulting arm stiffness and pain. Range of motion exercises are begun as soon as the pacemaker is removed.

We do not yet permit our patients with femoral temporary pacemakers to walk although some institutions do, without significant problems with pacemaker wire dislodgement. We allow chair privileges, but we are careful to prevent marked hip flexion when positioning the patient. Most patients seem to prefer femoral pacemakers to antecubital pacemakers because the femoral site does not entail extremity immobilization and discomfort.

ELECTRICAL HAZARDS

Temporary external pacemakers are more sensitive to electrical interference than permanent implanted pacemakers. The health team must be aware of the possible hazards and conscientiously protect the patient from them.

The pacemaker catheter itself is insulated and electrically safe. However, the catheter's metal tips, which are inserted into the pacemaker box terminals, can be electrical hazards. The metal tips are safe if they are embedded in the insulated pacemaker terminals on the newer model pacemakers. The metal tips are not safe if they are stuck through the terminal holes on the older model pacemakers, or if they are disconnected from the pacemaker and flapping loosely. In a freak accident several years ago a patient's rosary beads and crucifix hit the exposed metal pacemaker tips and short circuited the pacemaker. Exposed metal catheter tips can provide a low-resistance pathway for otherwise harmless current leakage directly to the patient's heart. Therefore, exposed tips must be covered with a rubber glove or dressing. If they are diconnected from the pacemaker box they should be taped to the patient.

All demand pacemakers must be sensitive to intrinsic cardiac activity. This capacity makes them inherently sensitive to external electrical fields as well. Better shielding and filtering devices make newer pacemakers less sensitive to external signals, but the danger still exists. The electrical interference may suppress pacemaker output or stimulate asynchronous operation, depending on the type of interference and the pacemaker.

Electrocautery and electrocoagulating equipment, diathermy, and microwave ovens, well-known sources of strong pacemaker interference, should be avoided or used cautiously. Some apparently innocuous, everyday, electric devices, such as electric razors, may also produce pacemaker dysfunction. All electrical equipment used on patients with temporary pacemakers must be properly grounded. Personnel should be careful not to have physical contact with the patient while operating an electrical device. In our hospital patients with temporary pacemakers are not permitted to use the electric bed control, the television control, an electric razor, or similar electrical equipment.

OTHER COMPLICATIONS

The most common problem associated with temporary pacing is electro-mechanical failure of the pacemaker-catheter system. If the pacemaker is not working properly, the nurse must rapidly determine and alleviate the cause of the failure. She should first note the presence of absence of the EKG pacing artifact. If pacing has stopped and the artifact is absent but the pacemaker box continues to discharge, she should check the connections between the box and the catheter. If the box is not discharging, the batteries or the box need to be replaced. If a pacing spike is present but capture is absent or intermittent, the catheter may be malpositioned, the pacing threshold increased, or an electrode may have failed. This problem is usually solved by repositioning the catheter, increasing the pacemaker output, or converting a bipolar system to a unipolar system. Until the physician arrives the nurse should reposition the patient—helping him lie on his right or left side often establishes better pacemaker contact and capture—or increase the output one or two milliamperes, or as instructed.

Aberrant pacemaker stimulation may occur. The pacemaker may cause chest wall twitching or it may stimulate the phrenic nerve. Mr. J. shouted frantically for help several hours after his pacemaker was inserted. He was hiccoughing each time the pacemaker fired—80 times a minute—and was extremely uncomfortable. The nurse helped him roll onto his side. This position change temporarily controlled his hiccoughs until his physician could reposition the wire.

Demand pacemakers are subject to specific sensing problems. Catheter repositioning is usually needed if the pacemaker does not accurately sense intrinsic cardiac activity. Sometimes the pacemaker will sense a

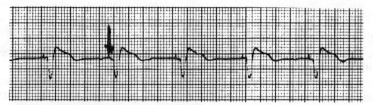

Normal ventricular pacing: *arrow points to artifact preceding QRS.*

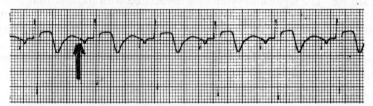

Normal atrial pacing: *arrow points to artifact preceding P wave.*

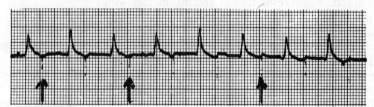

Pacer malfunction: *pacer is firing below stimulation threshold.*

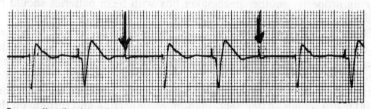

Pacer malfunction: *intermittent non-capture (arrows); other impulses stimulate ventricle.*

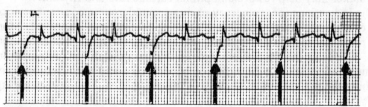

Pacer malfunction: *pacer (arrows) not sensing, not capturing; first impulse appears on the T wave.*

large T wave as a ventricular depolarization. Decreasing the pacemaker sensitivity usually corrects this problem.

Arrhythmias, septicemia, pulmonary embolization, venous thrombosis, and myocardial perforation are other complications associated with temporary pacing. These complications, fortunately infrequent, should be watched for. The signs and symptoms associated with the first four complications are well known. Myocardial perforation is usually benign, causing aberrant pacemaker stimulation like hiccoughs. It is treated by wire repositioning. Occasionally myocardial perforation causes cardiac tamponade, and emergency measures are required to correct the resulting decrease in cardiac output.

CARDIAC ARREST

If a patient with a temporary pacemaker is found in cardiac arrest, the nurse should begin resuscitation and do the following:
• Turn the pacemaker on if it is off.
• Increase the mA, for example, from three to five, because the patient's threshold may have increased and made his heart unresponsive to the present pacing stimulus.
• Increase the rate to 60 if it is below 60 because the patient may need a faster rate to maintain an adequate cardiac output.
• Observe for pacemaker function by looking at the pacemaker box indicator, and EKG, and by palpating a pulse. If the pacemaker is not working properly, another pacemaker box with fresh batteries should be obtained and hooked up immediately.

If the patient requires defibrillation, the pacemaker should be turned off, and, if time allows, both wires should be disconnected from the pacemaker terminals. These actions will prevent diverting the current from its cardiac pathway and will also prevent possible pacemaker damage even though most pacemakers are made to withstand shocks up to 400 watt seconds. After defibrillation, reconnecting and turning on the pacemaker may help restore an optimal cardiac rate and rhythm.

The indications for temporary pacing are undergoing constant revision and extension. Pacemaker design is being altered and improved. More and more people have temporary pacemakers for more and more reasons. Knowing the indications, goals, and complications of temporary pacing; understanding the types of pacemakers and their settings; and teaching the patient and his family facilitate successful temporary pacing.

BIBLIOGRAPHY

ANDREOLI, K. G., AND OTHERS, *Comprehensive Cardiac Care*. 2d ed. St. Louis, C. V. Mosby Co., 1971.

BELLET, SAMUEL. *Essentials of Cariac Arrhythmias*. Philadelphia, W. B. Saunders Co., 1972.

CAGIN, N. A., AND OTHERS. Unipolar subclavian and bipolar femoral catheter electrodes to pace heart: comparison of effectiveness. *NY State J.Med.* 72:1037-1040, May 1, 1972.

CHENG, T. O. Percutaneous transfemoral venous cardiac pacing. *Chest* 60:73-78, July 1971.

CRYSTAL, R. G., AND OTHERS. Inhibition of discharge of an external demand pacemaker by an electric razor. *Am.J.Cardiol.* 27:695-697, June 1971.

ESCHER, D. J., AND OTHERS. Transvenous emergency cardiac pacing. *Ann.NY Acad. Sci.* 167:582-596, Oct. 1969.

HODAM, R. P., AND STARR, ALBERT. Temporary postoperative epicardial pacing electrodes: their value and management after open-heart surgery. *Ann.Thorac. Surg.* 8:506-510, Dec. 1969.

MEDTRONIC, INC. *Model 5880A External Demand Pacemaker*. Minneapolis, Minn., Medtronic, Inc., 1972.

MELTZER, L. E., AND OTHERS. *Intensive Coronary Care*. rev. ed. Philadelphia, Charles Press, 1970.

ROSENTHAL, J. E., AND COHEN, L. S. Temporary pacemaking: indications and results. *Conn.Med.* 35:736-743, Dec. 1971.

SPANDAU, M. M. Insertion of temporary cardiac pacemakers without fluoroscopy. *Am.J.Nurs.* 70:1011-1013, May 1970.

From the American Journal of Nursing 75:52-55, Jan. 1975.

The Intra-aortic Balloon Pump

KATHLEEN SCESA DORR

The sheer complexity of this new, lifesaving procedure may be overwhelming. Care must be taken to meet the emotional and physical needs of the patient behind the machines.

The development of cardiogenic shock after an acute myocardial infarction is an ominous sign. High mortality rates indicate that present medical therapy is inadequate. The intra-aortic balloon pump, a mechanical aid to the circulatory function of the failing heart, is being used more and more frequently[1].

Intra-aortic balloon pumping presents a multitude of problems for patients, nurses, and physicians. Based on our experiences with 20 persons who have required the balloon pump we have evolved some recommendations for their nursing care. These patients have clinical signs and symptoms of hypotension, tachycardia, narrowing pulse pressure, changes in sensorium, oliguria or anuria, and a generally poor response to medical management following myocardial infarction[2]. The pump may also be used when cardiopulmonary bypass cannot be terminated successfully after open heart surgery[3].

Intra-aortic balloon pumping temporarily assists left ventricular function on the principle of counterpulsation. The balloon is passed into the descending thoracic aorta via a femoral artery. The balloon is inflated with helium during diastole, and deflated just before systole[4]. Inflation and deflation are automatically correlated with the ECG by a computer in the pump machine.

The experienced critical care nurse is noted for her flexibility and creativity in problem solving. She must adapt to an environment that changes in a matter of seconds. The challenge of caring for patients on the balloon pump lies in the great need for flexibility due to everchanging problems.

The patient who requires intra-aortic balloon pumping is critically ill and needs quick, expert care if he is to survive. At any one time during the initial phase of balloon insertion several physicians may be doing separate procedures on each of the patient's extremities. The balloon must be inserted, as well as an arterial line, a Swan-Ganz catheter to measure pulmonary artery and wedge pressures and sample mixed venous blood, a central venous pressure line, and a peripheral intravenous line. At our hospital the surgical service provides the special instruments and assistance for the femoral cutdown and balloon insertion. But when the multiple procedures are done in an ICU for the first time, frustration and critical time loss can occur due to lack of vital equipment and unfamiliarity with the technique.

To alleviate problems, inservice education should provide each ICU nurse with the experience of simulated balloon pump operation, troubleshooting, and maintenance requirements. The medical and nursing staffs must agree about the type and amount of equipment needed for the patient. A procedure should be written for obtaining and setting up equipment. Staffing patterns should be altered to allow at least three nurses to assist the physicians when balloon pumping is started. Even with the best planning, however, there is great stress and apprehension the first time the balloon pump is used. Its very complexity almost ensures that this procedure will not go perfectly the first time.

MULTIPLE LINES AND TUBES

The patient will have a line to the pump, an arterial line, a pulmonary artery line, a CVP line, and Foley catheter. There may also be a nasogastric tube, an endotracheal tube to assist ventilation, and, of course, ECG leads. The mere presence of so many tubes and lines to and from a patient may be overwhelming to inexperienced nurses.

To organize and record information from invasive lines, we maintain a continuous patient flow sheet of vital signs, pressure measurements, fluid intake and output, and laboratory results. If the transducers to readout equipment for arterial lines and pulmonary artery lines are kept calibrated and in working order, pressure measurements are simple, mechanical, and quickly obtained. Improperly functioning monitors have been

MS. DORR (*B.S., Chico State College, Chico, Calif.; M.S., University of California Medical Center, San Francisco) was assistant head nurse and inservice coordinator in the intensive care unit, Samuel Merritt Hospital, Oakland, Calif., when this article was written. She is an instructor at Tacoma General Hospital School of Nursing, Tacoma, Wash.*

one of our greatest irritations. Time spent fixing and calibrating machines draws the nurse away from her patient.

The sites of invasive-line insertions require daily care. Cleansing the area of insertion for the urinary catheter and checking intravenous insertion sites are readily accepted practices. Central venous pressure, Swan-Ganz, and arterial line sites also require care. The sites are less apt to become pathways for infection if they are cleansed every day with acetone, followed by Betadine, and then a small amount of antibiotic ointment applied with a sterile, occlusive dressing.

We use a heparin flush system to keep the arterial, CVP, and Swan-Ganz lines patent. A plastic pouch of 500 cc. 5% dextrose and 0.2% sodium chloride with 1,000 units heparin is used with a pressure bag and in-line intraflow valve to deliver as little as 3 cc. per hour through each line.

Insertion of the balloon via a femoral artery cutdown has significant implications for nursing care. After the balloon has been inserted, a chest x-ray is taken to check balloon location. Does one elevate the head of the bed to a high Fowler's position for this? Will a kink at the femoral site occur and occlude passage of helium to the balloon?

The answer to both these questions is no. Sitting the patient up does not block helium passage, but it does allow the balloon to move higher in the thoracic aorta and possibly cause trauma by rubbing against the aortic wall or protruding into the left subclavian artery. Also, the x-ray may show the balloon in a higher position than when it was inserted with the patient lying flat. For these reasons, the patient must be kept flat or elevated no more than 15 or 30 degrees.

Balloon insertion may also lead to vascular insufficiency in the leg with the cutdown. Most of our patients had diminished perfusion, and the involved leg was cooler to the touch and had weaker pulses than the other leg. Two patients required femoral bypass operations to correct circulatory impairment. Therefore, frequent monitoring of leg perfusion is necessary.

The large femoral incision to accommodate insertion of the balloon requires the same care as any surgical incision, with special measures to preserve the line's position.

Unfortunately, foot drop developed on the cannulated leg in two of our early patients. In our preoccupation with maintaining lines, regulating fluids, dealing with the patient and his family, and operating several machines we neglected range-of-motion exercises to all extremities. Although the list of priorities seems long, exercising the extremities, without flexing the hip joint of the cannulated leg, is a must. If the patient cannot cooperate the nurse must do it for him. A foot board is also essential for dorsal and plantar flexion.

Control of balloon action is based on the ECG signal. The R—R interval is used as a base to determine timing for inflation and deflation of the balloon. A clear ECG pattern is vital, and the nurse must constantly watch for interference with the pattern. Problems may occur when respiratory equipment is used, when the patient is moved and turned, or when improperly grounded equipment is brought into the area. We have found that chest leads rather than limb leads produce the stronger ECG signal necessary for balloon pumping.

The balloon pump patient, like any patient, must be turned frequently to prevent the development of bedsores. He can be turned from side to side every hour and the ECG maintained if close attention is paid to the many lines.

TROUBLESHOOTING

Our most frequent problems with the operation of the balloon pump have been high PVC rate, high leak rate, and inability to keep the patient on the automatic cycle. Due to machine malfunction, we also had complete helium loss on one occasion. In any event, because the nurse is with the patient constantly she must be prepared for problems as they arise. The instruction booklet for the particular machine being used should be read carefully. It presents clear steps to follow when any abnormal conditions occur.

The AVCO Intra-Aortic Balloon Pump (Roche Medical Electronics Division, Hoffmann-La Roche Inc.) has a status monitor with a panel of diagnostic indicators that light when abnormal conditions arise. However, this panel does not warn of volume leaks if the patient is on manual control rather than automatic cycle. Manual control allows the machine to pump in the presence of atrial fibrillation or frequent atrial or ventricular ectopic beats.

The line of the balloon must be purged with helium before resuming pumping if the pump has been turned off or on standby for any reason. The sleeve vent used for purging must be kept open for a full minute(5). The system must also be purged with helium after the cold tray used to collect condensation has been drained(5). Failure to empty the cold tray and cleanse the blower filter daily are often forgotten maintenance procedures. If the cold tray is not emptied, the accumulated condensation will back up into the helium line and may decrease helium flow. If the filter gets blocked, the pump may overheat.

Obtaining blood samples can be confusing and time consuming to the novice. The arterial line can be used for the routine samples and blood gases, but getting blood to determine co-oximeter CO_2 and O_2 content requires more than one person and close coordination with the laboratory doing the analysis. Errors and patient expense can be reduced if a definite procedure is established by nursing and laboratory personnel that outlines what is expected of the nurse making the blood collection.

A discrepancy can also develop when blood O_2 contents are ordered taken with the patient "on" and "off" the pump. Theoretically, the patient is "off" the pump if it is set on a 1:8 pumping cycle (one counterpulsation per eight cardiac beats) rather than the 1:1 pumping cycle. Some physicians believe, however, that placing the pump on standby for 10 minutes will not cause clotting around the balloon and will produce a more accurate "off pump" blood sample. It is wise to check the preference of the doctor writing the order.

Our patients usually are intubated initially and placed on a volume respirator. Standard, sterile, oral-pharyngeal and tracheal suctioning maintains tracheal toilet. Suctioning alone cannot prevent atelectasis. Frequent turning from side to side along with cupping and vibration are necessary. Auscultation of the lungs informs the nurse of the progress of respiratory care. Repeated experience is necessary to distinguish the sound of the balloon's inflation and deflation from breath sounds when auscultating the posterior and anterior lung fields.

As the patient's condition stabilizes, he may be extubated. Blow bottles or intermittent positive pressure breathing treatments are begun on an hourly or less frequent basis. Any tracheal suctioning now becomes more difficult, and the patient finds coughing, deep breathing, and frequent position changes less tolerable. Timely use of medication to alleviate any pain, planned rest periods, and clear explanations of why such things have to be done seem to be the only aids one can offer.

EMOTIONAL PROBLEMS

The patient knows he is very sick. He feels alone, exhausted, and frightened. He is surrounded by strange, noisy machines. He craves peace and rest. He sees and hears many physicians and nurses talking about him in jargon he doesn't comprehend.

How does the nurse help this patient? First, she must provide him with a means of communication, especially if he is intubated. Some patients find mouthing words and hand gestures adequate. Writing notes may be more effective. Once communication is established, the nurse endeavors to keep the patient oriented to date, time, and place, and explains the what, why, and who of everything that is happening to him. She tries to grant any requests that do not conflict with his treatment.

While medical and nursing skill is saving the patient's life, outside the ICU his family waits in fear, disbelief, or perhaps guilt. All the concern and busyness around the patient may leave little time for the family. But time must be found for them, for they are an important part of the critical care environment. They assist nursing care with the gentle touch and supportive words they provide the patient. Their attention and concern may be all that sustains the patient's will to live. Yet families, too, need explanations and support. They often see little hope and already may have begun the grieving process. They may ask nurses questions "too trivial" to ask doctors. Although the nurse caring for the patient usually cannot leave his bedside to speak with the family in the initial period, arrangements can be made with fellow staff members to help them.

Once the patient is stabilized, a cardiac catheterization may be ordered to learn whether the underlying problems can be remedied by surgical intervention. The thought of transporting a patient dependent on counterpulsation in an elevator may seem impossible, but it can be done. Some models of the balloon pump have a second source of power provided by batteries that permit mobility. Before transportation is initiated, one must determine whether the patient's bed will pass through all corridor and elevator doors or if transfer to a stretcher is necessary. Will pump and patient both fit in the elevator? Will the patient need ventilatory assistance during transport and in the special procedures laboratory? What is to be done with the lines and transducers? How many people are needed for the transfer? All this can be accomplished through careful planning and communication.

Once the patient arrives at the destination point, the power source must be switched from battery to electricity. Plugging in the machine without switching the power source causes dead batteries and machine shutdown in 45 minutes.

When a patient on the balloon pump has a cardiac arrest, standard cardiopulmonary resuscitation is begun. Pump support is ineffective when the patient is in ventricular fibrillation or standstill, so measures must be taken to reestablish some sort of ECG pattern. If the pump is switched to standby for defibrillation, the balloon line is disconnected from the pump and 30 to 50 cc. of air are inserted with a syringe to inflate and deflate the balloon several times every 10 minutes. The pump should remain on standby for only a maximum of 30 minutes(5). This prevents blood from becoming trapped in the folds of the deflated balloon and the development of thrombi.

The patient in cardiogenic shock may be maintained on intravenous vasopressors or peripheral vascular dilators before and during balloon pumping. Efforts are made to reduce the use of these medications so that the patient eventually can be weaned off both the pump and drugs. Patients differ, obviously, but frequent laboratory blood tests are a guide to the medications each person requires. Antibiotics are given if the patient's history and condition require them.

During cardiac assist, with the balloon inflating on a 1:1 ratio with each R-R interval on the ECG, baseline pressures, cardiac output, and blood oxygen levels are determined. These are used to guide the weaning of the patient from the 1:1 pumping cycle through 1:2, 1:4, and 1:8 cycles. If there is no indication of circulatory failure and the patient remains in satisfactory condition on the 1:8 cycle, usually for 24 hours, the balloon is removed by the surgical team.

Following balloon removal, the patient is still monitored closely. Respiratory care continues. Depending on the patient's progress, he is soon assisted in getting out of bed. Our patients have been depressed, confused, and fearful after the balloon was removed. They require constant encouragement and emotional support as well as physical care until they have recuperated from both the procedure and the myocardial infarction.

REFERENCES

1. SCHEIDT, S., AND OTHERS. Intra-aortic balloon counterpulsation in cardiogenic shock. *N.Engl.J.Med.* 288-980, May 10, 1973.
2. CLARK, N. F. Pump failure. *Nurs.Clin.North Am.* 7:529-539, Sept. 1972.
3. HOUSEMAN, L. B., AND OTHERS. Counterpulsation for intraoperative cardiogenic shock. *JAMA* 244:1131-1133, May 21, 1973.
4. SANDERS, C. A., AND OTHERS. Mechanical circulatory assistance: current status. *N.Engl.J.Med.* 285:348-350, Aug. 5, 1971.
5. *Operator's Manual*, AVCO Intra-aortic balloon pump, Model IABP-7, Cranbury, N.J., Roche Medical Electronic Division, Hoffmann-LaRoche, Inc.

From the *American Journal of Nursing* 75:967-970, June 1975.

External Counterpulsation for Cardiogenic Shock

LINDA A. BEGLEY

This noninvasive technique for treating severe cardiac failure reduces myocardial work while it promotes myocardial perfusion.

Despite rigorous medical management, the mortality associated with cardiogenic shock remains 85 to 90 percent. Whenever the underlying cause of the circulatory shock is correctable, circulatory assist techniques may be employed to maintain perfusion of vital organs and tissues until the cardiovascular system is capable of resuming its function(1).

Clinical applications of an external counterpulsation device (ECP) have successfully reversed the deleterious efferts of cardiogenic shock. This mechanical means of assisting the circulation is becoming the treatment of choice for cardiogenic shock. Effective nursing care for patients on ECP therapy requires that nurses understand its concepts and principles.

Cardiogenic shock is usually a complication of acute myocardial infarction and occurs when left ventricular cardiac output is reduced markedly. Peripheral vasoconstriction and tachycardia result when the body attempts to increase peripheral resistance to compensate for the falling cardiac output and to maintain blood pressure. When its coronary blood supply is reduced during the course of cardiogenic shock, the heart tends to undergo progressive damage. Shock reduces the coronary blood supply, weakening the heart and further decreasing cardiac output(2).

LINDA BEGLEY, R.N., M.S., *is a staff nurse at Nassau Hospital, Mineola, N.Y. At the time this paper was written, she was working with Mr. Birtwell and Dr. Soroff at Boston University in the experimental testing of external counterpulsation techniques.*

Ideally, the treatment for cardiogenic shock is to help the heart pump more blood with less effort. Increased flow with perfusion of vital organs is of prime importance but it must be done without overloading the weakened left ventricle. Assisted circulation has as its goal the support of the failing circulation. This is accomplished in two ways. First, by raising the *diastolic* pressure, myocardial and coronary perfusion is increased. This process improves myocardial oxygenation, improves perfusion of vital organs, and by itself aids in reversing the tendency toward lowered pumping capacity. Second, the work of the heart is reduced by taking the pressure off the impaired left ventricle, thereby enabling the heart to increase its stroke volume. This further increases the systemic blood flow. This is achieved by decreasing the *systolic* pressure.

The physiological rationale for counterpulsation includes two concepts. The most effective perfusion of the myocardium with arterial blood occurs during diastole, because the pressure exerted by the heart's contraction during systole decreases the volume of its own vasculature. By increasing diastolic pressure, counterpulsation markedly increases coronary perfusion.

The amount of work the left ventricle must do and the degree of myocardial oxygen consumption are both more closely related to the systolic pressure than to the volume of blood pumped, because it is the systolic pressure which the ventricle works against. Therefore, to the extent that counterpulsation reduces systolic pressure, it reduces the work of the heart(3).

HOW IT WORKS

Counterpulsation raises the diastolic pressure and lowers the systolic pressure to assist circulation. It accomplishes this by synchronizing its pumping action with the heart's own action. However, as the name implies, the pumping pressure is exerted in an opposite way: the pump pressure peaks during diastole and bottoms out during systole. Diastolic pressure is increased; systolic pressure tends to fall.

In external counterpulsation, the patient's legs are used as pumping chambers. Two tapered, rigid cylinders enclose the legs from ankle to thigh, with the feet sticking out of the narrow ends. A water-filled bag completely fills the space between the leg and cylinder, making the device adaptable to a wide variety of anatomic configurations. Water is pumped in and out of the bag through a connecting tube, and exerts a uniform pressure over the entire surface of the legs and on their veins and arteries. By controlling these external pressures through the alternate infusion and removal of water, vascular pressures and system hemodynamics are altered. The pump is controlled by the electrocardiogram and is provided with delay and duration electronic circuits that permit proper phasing of the pump with cardiac action(3).

The normal capacity of the vascular bed is a function of the difference between the internal pressure of the vessels and the pressure that surrounds them. The extravascular pressure is normally that of atmospheric pressure (assumed to be zero), with some variations caused by muscular activity. Similarly, the coronary vascular system is affected by myocardial contractions. If the external pressure is made positive, the capacity of the vascular bed will decrease. Applied when the heart is in diastole, positive pressure forces increase myocardial perfusion, increase coronary vessel perfusion and development, increase systemic perfusion of vital organs, and return venous blood to the right heart.

If the external pressure on the vascular system is made negative, the capacity of the vascular bed will increase. This is accomplished during cardiac systole and reduces the pressure against which the left ventricle must eject its volume by reducing resistance in the aorta. The negative pressure effect "aspirates" blood out of the heart. Reverse flow in the veins is prevented by natural venous valves.

In addition to the effects produced by alternating the pressure within

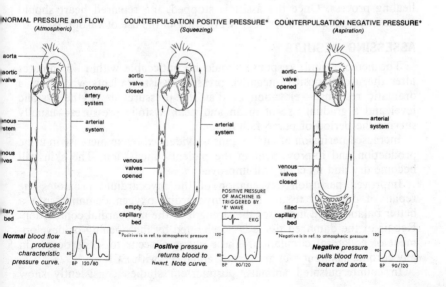

NORMAL PRESSURE and FLOW
(Atmospheric)

aorta
aortic valve
coronary artery system
nous stem
arterial system
nous ves
llary bed

Normal blood flow produces characteristic pressure curve.

BP 120/80

COUNTERPULSATION POSITIVE PRESSURE*
(Squeezing)

aortic valve closed
arterial system
venous valves opened
empty capillary bed

POSITIVE PRESSURE OF MACHINE IS TRIGGERED BY 'R' WAVE

EKG

*Positive is in ref. to atmospheric pressure

Positive pressure returns blood to heart. Note curve.

BP 80/120

COUNTERPULSATION NEGATIVE PRESSURE*
(Aspiration)

aortic valve opened
arterial system
venous valves closed
filled capillary bed

*Negative is in ref. to atmospheric pressure

Negative pressure pulls blood from heart and aorta.

BP 90/120

the water-filled seals, the negative pressure phase may be enhanced by a negative pressure vacuum. The airtight seal surrounding the patient's legs and fitting tightly around the waist allows a vacuum air pressure to be exerted during the negative pressure phase (cardiac systole, pump diastole). Extravascular pressure is reduced even further, decreasing aortic resistance to a much greater degree, and allowing the weakened heart to pump more blood.

Hemodynamically, the results of ECP are striking. When positive-negative pressure is applied to the vascular system arterial pressure measurements are affected. Negative pressure, the aspiration phase, reduces the systolic pressure of the heart. The systolic pressure measurement falls from 120 mm. Hg to 80 mm. Hg. Positive pressure applied during the diastolic squeezing phase greatly increases the blood flow and pressure, and a diastolic reading of 120 mm. Hg is noted. The resulting blood pressure would be read as 80/120.

Regional arterial pressures not only increase arterial flow but also promote venous return and blood volume distribution. Thus, the heart is assisted from both directions. During the cardiogenic shock state, this alternation of blood pressures allows the weakened heart time to repair itself: it is no longer pumping blood against increased resistance. The heart is resting and the increased perfusion state during diastole should be of benefit in increasing the oxygen supply and thus accelerating the healing process. Once the assist is stopped, the repaired heart should maintain an adequate arterial pressure without the use of vasopressors.

ASSESSING RESULTS

The hemodynamic response should be noticeable within 45 minutes after the use of positive-negative pressure assist. Patients who show a dramatic response—elevation of diastolic pressure above the systolic level and a gradual rise of mean and peak systolic pressures—usually survive the period of pump failure.

Increased perfusion of vital organs is evidenced by an increase in urine production and improvement in the patient's mentation. The skin will become dry and its color will improve.

Improved perfusion oxygenation of the myocardium promotes the repair of damaged tissue, brings myocardial oxygen demands into a better balance, and increases the strength of the myocardial contraction. Repair of the damaged tissue is accelerated by the opening or development of collateral circulation. These changes occur to some degree in any coronary patient, but are greatly enhanced with ECP.

In counterpulsated animals, postmortem studies consistently show clear evidence of more and larger collaterals. Collateral channel development in the myocardium produced by the counterpulsation process represents part of the explanation for the improved survival rate of patients. Apparently, counterpulsation produces a sustained change in the coronary vascular structure(4).

External counterpulsation is a noninvasive procedure and can be performed at the bedside. There is no evidence of impairment of peripheral circulation or aggravation hemolysis and no reason to anticipate thromboembolism. The only contraindication for its use is in patients with aortic insufficiency.

The actual pressure used is quite modest; a maximum of 200 mm. Hg, which is roughly equivalent to diving to the bottom of a six-foot pool.

THE NURSE'S ROLE

The nurse assumes a crucial role in assessing the patient's physiological status and in appraising the need for prompt counterpulsation. Her constant presence at the patient's bedside provides her with the opportunity and obligation to observe the patient critically and to evaluate change. The nurse's ability to integrate information into a meaningful evaluation of the patient's status determines the value of these data to the physician in instituting therapy and ultimately helping the patient(5).

Early signs of impending shock include the following: muscular weakness and profound fatigue due to reduced transport of oxygen and nutrients to the muscles; reduced cardiac output, as evidenced by cool, clammy skin caused by sympathetic stimulation and decreased metabolic rate; tachycardia as a compensatory mechanism; and restlessness and a slowing of the mental processes due to inadequate cerebral circulation.

Urine output is an important guide for evaluating circulatory status. Decreased blood flow through the kidneys results in a low urine output. Reduction of urine flow below 30 cc./hr. is a strong indication of shock.

A low systolic blood pressure (80 mm. Hg or less) is a clinical criterion for the diagnosis of cardiogenic shock. However, hypotension is not a reliable index of shock from myocardial inefficiency. The intense vasoconstriction resulting from the release of catecholamines or the intravenous infusion of vasopressors makes it possible for a patient in shock to have a normal blood pressure reading. More accurate measurements of blood pressures are obtained by direct intravascular monitoring.

Measurement of central venous pressure reflects right heart efficiency and can be an important guide for regulation of intravenous therapy. CVP is an indirect measurement of the functioning of the left ventricle.

A pulmonary artery catheter is inserted for measurement of pulmonary pressures and cardiac output. This directly determines left ventricular function.

Specifically, the nurse must become familiar with the measurements obtained from the ECP console itself, particularly the appropriate systolic and diastolic measurements. Arterial pressure and EKG tracings also are displayed.

The average treatment time for the patient is three hours. As his condition begins to improve and stabilize, it is important to provide reassurance for the patient and respond to him with human concern. He is faced at once with specific fears of the procedure itself and fears concerning the heart attack. Continued explanation that ECP is helping his heart by allowing it to rest and heal helps the patient to understand the treatment.

Clinical experience with ECP has been encouraging. In one study 20 patients in cardiogenic shock following myocardial infarction were treated with ECP. Eleven patients died during or soon after treatment. One patient survived for three days and another for three weeks; both died in the hospital of complications apparently unrelated to counterpulsation. Seven patients were discharged from the hospital and remained well. The 45-percent survival rate, which included the two short-term survivors, is a significant improvement over the usual 15-percent survival rate in cases of cardiogenic shock(6).

Eventually, assisted circulation will be an important tool in the prevention of myocardial infarctions and treatment of angina pectoris. The opening of coronary collateral channels and relief of left ventricular myocardial strain are the principles underlying this treatment. Increased use of ECP in many aspects of coronary care will demand that nurses acquire new knowledge and new competence in working with medical technology.

REFERENCES

1. BIRTWELL, W. C., AND OTHERS. Synchronous pressure assist-counterpulsation. *Progr.Cardiovasc.Dis.* 11:323-337, Jan. 1969.
2. GUYTON, A. C., *Textbook of Medical Physiology.* 4th ed. Philadelphia, W. B. Saunders Co., 1971, p. 343.
3. SOROFF, H. S., AND BIRTWELL, W. C. Assisted circulation: a progress report. *Hosp.Practice* 6:139-140, Apr. 1971.
4. SOROFF, H. S., AND OTHERS. Physiological support of heart action. *N.Engl.J.Med.* 280-694, Mar. 1969.
5. MORRIS, D. G. The patient in cardiogenic shock. *Cardiovasc.Nurs.* 5:15-17, July-Aug. 1969.
6. SOROFF, H. S., AND OTHERS. External counterpulsation; management of cardiogenic shock after myocardial infarction. *JAMA* 229:1441-1450, Sept. 9, 1974.

From the *American Journal of Nursing* 72:705-709, Apr. 1972.

Socioemotional Component
of Coronary Care

MARCELLA Z. DAVIS

Although techniques to save lives of those who suffer heart attacks have vastly improved, there is growing evidence to suggest that significant numbers of patients whose lives have been saved suffer psychologic traúma which seriously affects all aspects of their lves.

To my knowledge, there has been no systematic research which has attempted to relate specific events and interactions occurring in the coronary care unit with posthospital patient behavior. Nonetheless, there is mounting evidence of socioemotional difficulties of patients who have had heart attacks and are admitted to CCUs for intensive monitoring and care[1,2]. Some studies suggest that what occurs in the CCU has an impact on posthospital attitudes and behavior[3,4].

SOCIOEMOTIONAL STRESS POINTS

Basically, there are four elements in the coronary patient's situation influencing his socioemotional safety: (*a*) his entry into and exit from the CCU, (*b*) the nature of the CCU environment, (*c*) the nature of his illness, and (*d*) his interaction with the staff. These elements are common to hospital situations and patients in general: however, in the context of the CCU, they are greatly accentuated.

CCU ENTRY AND EXIT The two points of transition, entry into and exit from the CCU, are characterized by a disjuncture with the familiar and a

DR. DAVIS *currently is studying, lecturing, and writing in England on the social-psychologic aspects of illness. She was graduated from the Englewood Hospital School of Nursing in N.J. She received her B.S. in nursing from New York University in N.Y., her M.S. from Teacher's College, Columbia University in New York City, and her D.N.S. from the University of California School of Nursing, San Francisco.*

confrontation with the unfamiliar and strange. Both are stress-generating conditions.

Particularly in the beginning phases of any major serious illness, the patient and his significant others are cast into a crisis situation. As it is used here, crisis is seen as ". . . a sudden and unanticipated disruption of extensive and protracted significance in the everyday activities, understandings and expectations of a social unit, in this instance the family"(5). The pacing of events in a crisis depend on any number of factors, including the nature of the illness. For instance, in some illnesses, such as multiple sclerosis, realization of what is occurring may emerge slowly for the patient and his significant others over a period of weeks, months, or even years(6).

For patients admitted to the CCU, the unfolding of events typically is compressed in time. Even for those who initially misread their symptoms as "heartburn" or "indigestion," and thereby delay their entry into the CCU, the movement of events may take place over only a few hours(7). For these patients, therefore, there is an abrupt disjuncture in their normal flow of events and taken-for-granted routines. Continuity with respect to relationships with others, perceptions of self, expectations and understandings about themselves and their subjective world are dramatically threatened and altered. Not only is the familiar and immediate present in jeopardy, but what lies ahead is unknown and, at best, ambiguous for the patient in a CCU.

These circumstances become compounded for the patient and his others when he enters the unfamiliar environment of a CCU. Even though he is now a patient in a hospital, the major part of his identity is still socially anchored.

When a patient enters a CCU, the needs of his socioemotional self are dramatically pushed into the background as attention to the physiologic takes precedent. However, even when the crisis may be over, there generally is not a redress in the balance of forces. Most often, the socioemotional component is attended to *if* there is time, *if* one remembers, and *if* the staff understands this to be an area of need for patients.

Exit from the CCU may also occur with abruptness. For example, patients may be transferred to a general ward with no prior notice, even in the middle of the night. Adapting to a hospital environment and trying to locate familiar landmarks is difficult under the best of circumstances. Middle-of-the-night transfers, which may be for administrative convenience, increase the stress for patients. One patient aptly remarked that in the dimness of the night, the appearance of "rows of white lumps lying still on the bed" was surpassed in its bizarre imagery only by the equally strange quality of the coronary care unit itself.

Also, by the time a patient is transferred to the general ward the staff's perception of him has usually shifted from seeing him as a critically ill patient to one who is recovering and getting better. The patient, on the other hand, may still perceive his situation to be highly precarious and in effect, still think of himself as "on the brink of death." One patient remarked, "The whole time I was lying there (CCU) I wondered, how close to God am I now?" When such discrepant perceptions are held and the staff have not identified and clarified signs of improvement for the patient while he is in the CCU, the patient is left to his own devices to fathom the unknown with all its frightening ambiguities.

Finally, it is not uncommon for patients who have survived their heart attack to imbue the staff and the equipment in the CCU not only with lifesaving potential, but, more omnipotently, with the capacity to bring the dead back to life. An exit from this life-restoring, lifesaving situation is, therefore, a tremendous threat to the patient, particularly if he does not share the staff's view of him as someone who is making progress. It is no wonder, then, some patients succumb to a second heart attack at the point of exit.

CCU ENVIRONMENT Any hospital environment, to be sure, differs markedly from that of one's home, but the CCU differs in many important respects from even a typical hospital environment. So different are conditions, that even nurses and physicians who were new to the situation frequently comment on the time it took for them to become accustomed to what seemed strange or threatening on initial encounter. While it is desirable for the staff to feel comfortable within the CCU, familiarity, all too frequently, allows them to forget how strange the setting once did appear. It may prevent the staff from recognizing how strange the environment appears to a newly admitted patient and his family.

Coronary care units were devised to increase lifesaving potential by facilitating the work of the professional staff. However, the emphasis on equipment seems, at times, to obscure the staff's recognition of other than physiologic factors in the lifesaving drama. For example, such environmental features as the continuously lit, intense bright lights, while facilitating around-the-clock work by staff, may cause patients to lose all sense of time. The array of complex machinery, the plastic tubing emanating from and into the patient and machines, and the monotonous patterns of buzzing, humming, and clicking sounds from the various machines are also thought to contribute to the patient's sense of confusion and general disorientation.

Hooked up to a combination of machines and tubes, a patient finds his bodily movements markedly restricted. As a result, he usually avoids the little movement he is able to make for fear of causing something to go awry. Consequently, patients frequently comment about feeling trapped(8).

It is interesting to note that these sensations, common to patients in the CCU, have been found to occur among people in other situations, for example, the patient on a respirator, a lonely isloated explorer, a prisoner subjected to brainwashing techniques, and so forth(9). While these situations are different in their social context, they share certain common environmental features. These are environments which are spatially confined and narrowly circumscribed, allow for only limited body movement, and have a restriction of stimuli—all of which contribute to disorientation and confusion of time and place. It is not surprising, then, that the visual and auditory strangeness of the CCU can confirm, in a highly dramatic manner for the patient, that he has experienced a profound alteration of drastic and lasting significance.

NATURE OF ILLNESS Heart disease, like stroke, cancer, and, at one time, polio, is one of those serious illnesses about which most persons in our society have some knowledge from either direct contact with the illness through a relative or friend or exposure to such public media as T.V., radio, and newspapers. The informal, commonsense beliefs acquired in these ways guide the patient and those close to him in their thinking about and actions toward the illness.

The commonly held perception of most lay persons about a heart attack is either that of instant death or of the victim's having been pulled from the brink of death. In either case, the view persists that a heart attack is a disability requiring profound alterations in one's total lifestyle and concept of self.

With the number of deaths from coronary heart disease approaching a peak of 500,000 annually, it is understandable why the public holds these views(10). The impressive advances in lifesaving measures—including both the development of mechanical equipment and improved skills of physicians and nurses—which now save lives that once were lost, have not, in and of themselves, dispelled the commonly held expectation of death or disability from a heart attack.

Equally important as the imagery and commonsense beliefs with which the coronary patient comes to the hospital is his experience in the hospital. Few illnesses require as swift and total onslaught on the patient by the professional staff as a heart attack. The split-second actions of the

CCU staff, particularly on admission, leave little doubt in the patient's mind of the critical nature of his status. Moreover, the very nature of the illness requires that all, or nearly all, bodily functions and care be assigned to others. It requires little imagination to appreciate that when a patient is suddenly and completely divested of control of his body, he may experience this as a fundamental threat to his ego, even when he "knows" that it is being done to help him.

INTERACTION WITH STAFF To believe oneself to be on the brink of death; to vacillate in quick order between not knowing what to expect from one's body and yet, expecting the worst; and to interpret such ordinary utterances as, "Lie still and you'll be all right," as obtuse and filled with ill forebodings, reflect the predicament of the patient in the CCU as he tries to cope with uncertainty in an unfamiliar setting.

Unfortunately, the patient's search for understanding about himself is often not furthered by his interaction with staff. In a study of the environment of the ICU, De Meyer, for example, reports that patients believed "people (staff) talked about them in the conversation"(11). This style of interaction, so common in hospitals, occurs too often in the CCU as well. One patient in a CCU observed, "The docs just want to get that heart goin' . . . they think that everything else will take care of itself, but it doesn't."

Also, the hustle and bustle of the staff create a general air of crisis, which only reinforces the fears the patient already has about himself and what may happen to him. Consequently, when the staff fail to communicate with the patient or are excessively guarded in communication with him, the ambiguities of his situation are aggravated. He is left to such ineffective devices as reading expressions or catching a word here and there to fathom what is occurring to him. Wynn comments that "failure to give a simple and adequate explanation to the patient . . . often leads to his formulating his own . . . which are both bizarre and extremely frightening" (12,13).

It is of interest to note the sharp contrast between the paucity of information offered the patient and the tremendous amount gathered from him. Nurses and physicians are continuously gathering new data and reinterpreting old signs in order to guide their behavior toward the patient. He is pricked, probed, and palpated. Even those functions he assumed to be aspects of his most private self are now open to scrutiny by many others (strangers in effect) for still further information.

The continuous, massive intake of information by staff about the patient guides their behavior toward him. But what information does the patient have to guide *his* behavior? Admittedly, the amount and type of information needed by a patient and by staff members are different. However, a basic requirement remains: information for both must be sufficient to facilitate correct interpretations and appropriate behavior.

NURSE INTERVENTIONS

Disjuncture, discontinuity, ambiguity, and unpredictability are features which characterize the experience of patients in the CCU and, to a lesser extent, their family and close friends. Since these circumstances are highly problematic, nursing interventions are suggested which are designed to ameliorate the situation by (*a*) reducing the patient's perceived threat to self, (*b*) managing the physical environment, and (*c*) lessening discontinuity in "significant other" relationships.

TO REDUCE PATIENT'S PERCEIVED THREAT TO SELF Much of what the patient sees and experiences is unclear, confusing, and threatening. Under such conditions, patients who are not offered explanations on an ongoing basis will misinterpret benign aspects of their situations and ascribe meanings to them that can have dire and threatening consequences for themselves. For example, the small red light on the monitor indicates that the machine is in working order. However, one patient interpreted this to signify that he was continually in danger. Also, when patients do not know that static registered on the monitor can be due to the smallest arm and body movements, they may understandably assume it to be an indication of cardiac malfunctioning.

In addition, some procedures, while routine and simple in and of themselves, are viewed by some patients as having life-threatening consequences. For example, Cassem reports that some patients viewed the taking of vital signs every 15 minutes as a means of keeping them alive. One patient reasoned, ". . . I knew they (staff) were trying to keep me awake because if I went to sleep, I would die"(14).

Earlier, it was suggested that transfer from the CCU to the general ward is often a stressful transition. To more adequately prepare a patient for this transition, the staff should, from the moment of the patient's entry onto the CCU, offer explanations that help him understand and interpret the meaning of particular signs. For example, "Your heart beat is slower now, Mr. Jones. That is a good sign." When the patient receives information on an ongoing basis, he then is able to formulate a more accurate concept of his condition than if he is left to his own resources.

Prior to transfer out of the CCU, a patient should know the signs which legitimately mark the progress he had made. Alone, statements such as "you are getting better" tell the patient very little. He needs to know the signs which indicate he is getting better and know, too, how he can recognize them. For example, as supportive equipment is gradually removed, a patient should know explicitly that this means he is progressing.

My intention here is not to establish a list of every possible misinterpretation and concern and how each might be corrected. Rather, it is to emphasize that only through monitoring *both* physiologic and psychologic signs that questions, concerns, and fears can be identified, alleviated, and, in some instances, prevented. A nurse can be said to be psychologically monitoring a patient when, in the process of caring for him, she elicits information on how he is perceiving his environment, his physical condition, and the procedures and routines performed on him. This information may be elicited in such a specific statement as, "Mr. Jones, I notice you keep staring at that light. Does something about it trouble you?" or in as prosaic a question as, "How are things going for you this morning, Mrs. Smith?"

TO MANAGE THE PHYSICAL ENVIRONMENT Several features of the CCU environment have been described as producing stress. Some of these are amenable to therapeutic nurse intervention. For example, since it is common for patients in the CCU to experience disruption in their time orientation, a clock and a calendar with the exact day clearly circled and the preceding day clearly crossed out can be placed within view of the patient. However, DeMeyer cautions that since lights are usually on continuously, the hands of a clock pointing to 2:00 will not always tell the patient whether it is 2:00 A.M. or 2:00 P.M.(15). Additional information may have to be provided by the nurse if the patient, for example, is not to feel disappointment or anxiety when his wife seemingly fails to keep her 2:00 P.M. visit when, in fact, it is 2:00 A.M.

Still other interventions are possible for coping with the patient's disorientation to time and space. For some, placing a small bedside radio near him or permitting him to control the operation of a T.V. set by a remote control switch, for instance, can do much toward furthering his sense of reality.

TO LESSEN DISCONTINUITY IN "SIGNIFICANT OTHER" RELATIONSHIPS The central focus in the CCU is, of course, the patient, and the staff's efforts are directed mainly toward him. However, we also know that a patient's identity is intricately enmeshed in his associations and relationships with such significant others as family members and close friends. Nurse interventions, therefore, should also be directed toward alleviating some of the stress from the abrupt disruption in "significant other" relationships brought on by the acute coronary illness.

Baden reports that when nurses in a CCU telephone patients' families on a daily basis to relay information about the patients, "patients and their families quickly learn to trust the staff"(16). Equally important was the reduction in the number of incoming calls, which can be a disruptive element in a tightly organized and busy unit.

Patients, too, wish to maintain communications with their families and close friends. Assurance by the nurse that they will receive messages from those close to them can do much toward reducing the stress from discontinuity in social relationships. Inasmuch as messages can also give rise to anxiety, admittedly this is an area around which there are certain differences of opinion among professionals. If there is a conflict and the nurse, on information at her disposal, believes it is important for the patient to receive messages from those close to him, it is her responsibility to discuss this point with the patient's physician.

The patient's family and those close to him also require information about the patient's condition on an ongoing basis. Such information as what specific signs mean or what the patient and his family may expect can help to establish shared understandings among the patient, his family, and the staff. Pinneo suggests that a room near the CCU be established specifically for family and close friends(17). This might well facilitate communicating with the family. The establishment of an open and trusting relationship between the patient's family and the staff have important implications for how much the family may later cooperate in the long-term work of rehabilitating the patient.

To minimize the socioemotional disruption in the transfer of the patient from the CCU, whenever possible, the ward nurse should be introduced to the patient and his family while he is still in the CCU. This would provide an opportunity for the nurse from the general ward to explain to the patient and his family what the atmosphere and routines on her ward are like. Another device for easing the transition from the CCU to the general ward is the establishment of a small room immediately adjacent to and in view of the "parent" CCU. This is commonly known as a postcoronary unit; if strategically employed, this unit can serve as a kind of psychologic "halfway house" for easing the stresses attendant to a patient's release from the CCU.

The weight of clinical evidence to date suggests that an explicit focus on the socioemotional component of patient care in the CCU might do much to further the welfare of cardiac patients and their families. A focus on the interpersonal and environmental components of patient care offers nurses opportunities to further health and reduce stress.

REFERENCES

1. WISHNIE, H. A. Psychological hazards of convalescence following myocardial infarction. *JAMA* 215:1292-1296, Feb. 22, 1971.
2. WYNN, ALLAN. Unwarranted emotional distress in men with ischaemic heart disease (IHD). *Med.J.Aust.* 2:847-851, Nov. 4, 1967.
3. WISHNIE, *op. cit.*
4. DREW, JACQUELINE A. *Evaluation of Needs of Patients Who Have Had Heart Attack or Stroke,* prepared by Applied Health Research Corporation for San Francisco Heart Association, July 1970. (Unpublished manuscript)
5. DAVIS, FRED. *Passage Through Crises: Polio Victims and Their Families.* Indianapolis, Bobbs-Merrill Co., 1963, p. 17.
6. DAVIS, MARCELLA Z. *Transition to a Devalued Status; the Case of Multiple Sclerosis.* San Francisco. School of Nursing, University of California, 1970. (Unpublished doctoral dissertation)
7. DREW, *op. cit.*
8. DE MEYER, JOANNA. Environment of the intensive care unit. *Nurs.Forum* 6:262-272, Summer 1967.
9. SOLOMON, PHILIP, AND OTHERS. Sensory deprivation; a review. *Am.J.Psychiatry* 114:357-363, Oct. 1957.
10. INTER-SOCIETY COMMISSION FOR HEART DISEASE RESOURCES. Resources for the optimal care of patients with acute myocardial infarction. *Circulation* May 1971, P. A-171.
11. DE MEYER, *op. cit.*
12. WYNN, *op. cit.*, p. 849.
13. MILLER, G. M., AND BREWER, JEAN. Factors influencing the rehabilitation of the patient with ischaemic heart disease. *Med.J.Aust.* 3:413, Feb. 22, 1969.
14. CASSEUM, N. H., AND OTHERS. Reaction of coronary patients to the CCU nurse. *Am.J.Nurs.* 70:323, Feb. 1970.
15. DE MEYER, *op. cit.*, p. 268.
16. BADEN, CATHERINE. Pointers coronary patients have given me for improving their care. *Consultant* 9:45-48, July-Aug. 1969.
17. PINNEO, ROSE. Nursing in a coronary care unit. *Cardiovasc.Nurs.* 3:1-4, Jan.-Feb. 1967.

From the *American Journal of Nursing* 72:1812-1816, Oct. 1972.

Cardiac Rest: Bed or Chair?

DEBORAH KUTTIN GOLDSTROM

The goal in bed rest following a myocardial infarction is to rest the heart. Yet, studies indicate that the heart actually works harder during bed rest than chair rest.

The "arm chair treatment" as a means of therapy for the patient who has had a myocardial infarction was instituted by Dr. Samuel A. Levine in the 1930's and has been challenged by cardiac authorities ever since. Yet, evidence has been presented that patients do well, if not better, when allowed to sit in a chair instead of lying in a bed. Coe, for example, has reported evidence from catheterization studies that the heart does less work in the erect sitting position than in the supine position(1).

HAZARDS OF BED REST

A variety of major hazards associated with bedrest have been identified. Obviously such hazards as increased work load on the heart through an increase in cardiac output, reduction of cardiac reserve, increased use of Valsalva maneuver during movement in bed, increased possibility of thrombosis formation, and so forth have particular relevance for the cardiac patient.

INCREASED WORK LOAD ON HEART The average heart rate per minute in the standing position is 89; in the sitting position, 79; and in the prone position, 69. Although the cardiac rate decreases in a lying down position, the cardiac output increases due to greater venous return. Holmgren and Ovenfors measured the blood volume of the heart and found that in a standing position, the volume was 771 ml.; in a sitting position, 819

MS. GOLDSTROM *is a staff nurse at North Shore Hospital in Manhasset, New York. She received her B.S. degree from the American University Lucy Webb Hayes School of Nursing in Washington, D.C.*

ml.; and in a lying position, 995 ml.(2). The rise in heart volume due to increased venous return produces an enlargement of the heart and causes an increase in stroke volume. This means that the cardiac muscle must do more work per contraction.

With an increase in stroke volume, cardiac output increases. Cardiac output usually varies between four and seven liters per minute in the erect position and between five and nine liters per minute in the supine position(3). Though the work performed by the heart is increased and the cardiac output is greater, with the vasodilation that occurs with the change in gravity, the blood pressure remains unchanged or drops slightly in the supine position(3).

REDUCTION OF CARDIAC RESERVE Though there is an initial decrease in heart rate during bed rest, this is not a sustained decrease. Taylor, in a study of essentially normal adults, found that after three weeks of bed rest the heart rate during moderate work increased by 40 beats per minute over the pre-bed rest rate. These subjects required 5 to 10 weeks of reconditioning before their heart rates, during work, returned to their pre-bed rest levels. Also, since tachycardia reduces diastolic filling time and causes heart muscle to fatigue quickly, Taylor's subjects had a decrease in cardiac reserve which was demonstrated by a 75 percent decrease in their ability to walk 3.5 miles an hour on a 10 percent incline after their period of bed rest(4). One advantage of the armchair treatment, then, is the prevention of a reduction in cardiac reserve.

ORTHOSTATIC HYPOTENSION Lying in bed affects the whole circulatory system: the effects of gravity are reduced and there is a generalized vasodilatation accompanied by increased venous return, cardiac output, and central blood volume(5). When a patient stands up after lying in bed for only a few days, he may experience orthostatic hypotension. Blood suddenly flows from central areas to the lower extremities which decreases the circulating volume, venous return, and cardiac output. Blood pressure drops, causing the patient to feel shaky, dizzy, and faint(6). In Taylor's study, subjects required more than five weeks to compensate for these effects after three weeks of bed rest(4).

INCREASED USE OF VALSALVA MANEUVER Another factor affecting the workload of the heart during bed rest is the Valsalva maneuver. While lying in bed, patients frequently use their arms to aid in moving. Most often when they do this, they hold their breath and keep their chest fixed. In straining during this movement, air is pushed against the closed glottis which raises the intrathoracic pressure and produces an involuntary Valsalva maneuver. The increased intrathoracic pressure, at first, reduces the venous return and the filling pressure of the heart. When air is exhaled, the intrathoracic pressure falls. A sudden increase in venous return to the heart occurs which results in tachycardia and may even produce cardiac arrest in an already failing heart. It has been estimated that patients on bed rest use this maneuver between 10 and 20 times per hour(7).

This involuntary Valsalva maneuver also occurs when patients get on and off a bed pan and when straining to have a bowel movement. Dock found that changes in pulse and blood pressure when a bed pan is used are greater than those which result from rising slowly and moving to and from the commode(8).

If the patient is to remain in bed, these effects can be prevented by instructing the patient to breathe through his mouth while moving around. Valsalvian effects can also be partially avoided through the use of a bedside commode instead of a bed pan and rest in a chair rather than a bed.

THROMBUS FORMATION Thrombus formation is another hazard of bedrest. Muscular contractions which ordinarily promote venous return from the extremities are usually significantly decreased during bed rest. This change in activity predisposes to thromboembolic complications by contributing to venous stasis in the extremities, particularly the legs.

There are a number of theories on factors ultimately resulting in the formation of thrombi during bed rest—generally each can be directly related to consequences of immobility.

Osteoblastic cells, which build up the matrix of bone, are stimulated by stresses of weight bearing on bones during mobility. During bed rest, when these stresses are reduced, activity of osteoblastic cells is decreased while cells which destroy bone matrix continue their activity, causing demineralizaton of bone and release of such minerals as calcium into the blood stream. It is believed that this addition of calcium may combine with material from platelets to activate prothrombin which forms thrombin—thus activating the chain of clot formation(7).

In another theory, external pressure on the blood vessels is considered the prime factor in thrombus formation. Pressure reduces circulatory flow and damages the intima of the vessels. Platelets tend to collect over the damaged area, and it is believed this platelet conglomerate may be the basis for a clot. Whatever the cause, the incidence of thrombosis is directly proportional to the number of days in bed(7).

ELECTROLYTE AND MINERAL CHANGES The relationship of immobility to demineralization of the bones and the possible thromboembolic complications which can occur have already been described. While calcium plays a role in blood coagulation, additional calcium in the blood can have other consequences. Kidney and bladder stones may result from calcium which enters the blood stream and is filtered out through the kidneys, where it may be deposited as calcium salts. But, for the cardiac patient, a particularly dangerous possibility is that the elevated calcium level in the blood may increase cardiac irritability.

It has been demonstrated that in the supine position there is a decrease in the secretion of adrenal mineralcorticoids, which normally affect sodium and potassium balance. Surprisingly, the effect of this on urinary excretion of sodium and potassium during bed rest has not been shown to be significant(9). Still, any factor which can affect electrolyte balance should be considered, for a significant imbalance of electrolytes, particularly potassium, affects cardiac conduction and rhythm.

CONSTIPATION Constipation may be due to a generalized decrease in activity and lowered metabolism associated with bed rest. However, it is complicated by the use of the bed pan.

In using a bed pan, the patient is forced into an unnatural position for defecation in which he must lean back to support himself and keep his legs extended instead of flexed at the knees. Such an unnatural posture interferes with normal defecation reflexes and mechanisms. In addition to the difficult and precarious position a patient must assume, the embarrassment of sitting in the middle of a bed partially separated from other patients by only a filmsy curtain or screen to defecate would probably make a patient deny any urge as long as possible(10).

When the patient does use the bed pan to move his bowels, the activity used in getting on the pan and the strain of trying to defecate a hard and bulky stool causes the Valsalva maneuver and puts a dangerous load on the already damaged heart(10).

RESPIRATORY CHANGES Changes in the shape and movement of the chest which reduce its maximum capacity occur in the supine position. Wade, in a study of 10 patients, found that, because of extension of the thoracic vertebrae and the position of the ribs, the chest circumference increased in the supine position. But the chest expansion during tidal respiration and the chest elevation during deep inspiration decreased(11).

Furthermore, the increased volume of blood in the thorax due to increased venous return and cardiac output, as described previously, reduces the area for lung expansion within the chest. As a result of these two factors, the vital capacity on lying down is reduced by 4 percent or 300 to 400 cm.(12).

The rate and depth of ventilation also decrease when lying down. Browse found the average ventilation rate to be 19 breaths per minute when a person is erect and 16 breaths per minute after he has been in bed one hour. Because both the tidal volume and ventilation rates decrease when a person assumes the supine position, the minute volume usually falls(12). Svanberg has noted a minute volume decrease from 10.8 liters per minute in a sitting position to 9.4 liters per minute in the supine position(13).

McIlroy, measuring the work of breathing, found that the effort required to breathe in a supine position was double that required in an erect position(14). And, because a patient must work harder to breathe, he takes fewer deep breaths and alveoli tend to collapse decreasing aerating surface. Thus, a patient on bed rest must expend more energy to get less air.

In addition to the decrease in vital capacity, decreased respiratory rate, and decreased tidal volume, the diameter of the bronchioles is also decreased in the supine position. The diameter of the bronchioles is normally maintained by the negative intrapleural pressure. However, elevation of the diaphragm and increase in intrathoracic blood volume in the supine position reduce the negative pressure, and the bronchioles are partially compressed from these pressure changes. The clearance of secretions from the bronchial tree is then reduced and the patient can develop either a bronchiole obstruction from a mucus plug or such infections as bronchitis or hypostatic pneumonia as a result of stasis of secretions(12).

EFFECTS ON ACID-BASE BALANCE The decrease in respiratory movement and in the movement of secretions results in a limited exchange of carbon dioxide and oxygen. Hypoxemia leading to tissue hypoxia occurs with the decrease in inspired oxygen, and carbon dioxide build up in the blood develops with the limited gas exchange. Because of increased arterial and venous concentrations of carbon dioxide, the patient may eventually go into respiratory acidosis or carbon dioxide narcosis. This can result in respiratory or cardiac failure(7).

Respiratory complications from bed rest can be reduced by a high Fowler's position, but they are better handled by getting the patient up in a chair to increase the ease of respirations and to facilitate the depth of respirations.

Most of the hazards of bed rest described here can directly produce adverse cardiac effects. In addition, there are a number of other complications which may not directly affect the heart, but can complicate a patient's general condition. Included are such problems are difficulty in voiding, decubitus ulcers, and diminished motor function. But, is chair rest really any better or might it result in even more serious complications than those associated with bed rest?

In 1952, Levine and Lown reported a study of armchair treatment of 81 patients with acute coronary thrombosis(15). Most patients were placed on chair rest within the first two days following their acute episode. By the end of the first week, all patients in the study were on chair rest. They were carefully positioned in comfortable chairs so that no pressure was exerted by the chair on the popliteal spaces. They were allowed to remain in the chair until they began to feel tired, which was usually about one to two hours. By the end of the first week, they were spending most of the day in a chair. No patients who remained in shock, had marked debility, or had concomitant cerebrovascular accidents were placed on chair rest.

While on chair rest, the patients fed themselves and either used a bedside commode or the bathroom. Most were allowed to take a few steps by the end of the third week and the average hospitalization period for these patients was about four weeks.

Of the 81 patients, eight died: four in the first week and four in the second. The average age of the patients who died was 73 years. Four of them had had a previous coronary occlusion. On admission, seven of these patients had pulmonary edema and paroxysmal tachycardia, and three were in shock.

Of the surviving 73 patients, only six developed complications during chair rest therapy. One had paroxysmal tachycardia on the thirteenth day, another experienced recurrent pain on the twenty-first day. Among the other four patients, one developed hepatitis, two had hematuria, and one had a fever.

Dr. Levine concluded that the incidence of complications was negligible and attributed none to the form of treatment. The absence of pulmonary congestion and edema was as significant as the rarity of complications in general. Patients who were dyspneic or had pulmonary rales on admission rapidly improved on chair rest. Post mortem examinations were done only on four of the patients who had died; but even in these patients, most of whom had been admitted with pulmonary edema, their lungs were remarkably clear(15).

About 26 months after the initial study, Avard M. Mitchell, James B.

Dealy, and Bernard Lown did a follow-up study of these 73 patients. The study revealed that 17 of the patients who had recovered from the acute episode of myocardial infarction had subsequently died, eight within the first 12 months following the acute episode and nine during the second 12 months. In 16 of the 17 patients, death was due to cardiac factors attributed to either intractable congestive heart failure or recurrent episodes of coronary thrombosis(16).

Of the 56 who had survived over the two-year period, 52 were reexamined. Since a major objection to chair rest during the acute phase of an M.I. is the possibility of increasing the stress on the infarcted area, causing weakness and ventricular aneurysm, particular attention was paid to signs of this complication. However, only six of the 52 patients had persistent elevation of the ST segment, suggestive of ventricular aneurysm, and in none of these was an aneurysm confirmed in x-ray and fluoroscopic examinations. Also, the incidence of such other complications as angina, new infarction, and congestive failure which can often follow an acute M.I. was quite low. From these results, the researchers concluded that there were no long-term adverse effects which could be directly attributed to chair rest as opposed to bed rest in the treatment of acute myocardial infarction(16).

Mitchell, Dealy, and Lown also made additional observations of 13 newly admitted patients with M.I.'s being treated with chair rest to determine the presence and significance of any changes in blood pressure, pulse, and respiration when the patient moved from the bed to the chair. No significant changes occurred immediately, and, except for an average 4 mm. Hg drop in blood pressure, there were no significant differences in the average of readings taken in the chair, compared to those in the bed(16).

From their data, the researchers concluded that there was no reason to believe that the work of the heart is increased either as a result of a change from bed to chair or as a result of remaining in the chair. The constancy of the pulse and respiration rates when compared with the slight decrease in the blood pressure suggested to them that the cardiac work load may be decreased by chair treatment, confirming Coe's catheterization studies of heart work. This decrease would then result in a firmer and smaller scar. Though the patients did not ambulate early, these researchers also found that when patients began their convalescence, they progressed more quickly and easily than patients who had been treated with bed rest(16).

As can be seen from various studies, chair rest, at the very least, has not proved to be more harmful than bed rest and, in fact, many of the disadvantages of bed rest were negated through the use of the chair treatment. There were lower mortality rates, minimal incidence of such complications as pulmonary edema and loss of vasomotor reflexes, and a shorter period of convalescence with more rapid rehabilitation and return to work. Patients displayed more optimistic attitudes on chair rest and took an interest in their form of treatment.

According to these studies, there is no reason why the chair treatment cannot be employed one to two days after a myocardial infarction before the debilitating effects of bed rest occur.

CHAIR REST: NURSING CARE

Nursing care of the patient on chair rest does not differ greatly from that of one on bed rest. In her explanation to the patient before getting him into the chair, the nurse must emphasize that he is expected to rest in the chair as he would in the bed. It is also necessary to explain to all who come in contact with the patient, such as lab personnel, dietary, and housekeeping, that the patient is critically ill; otherwise they might take for granted that the patient is well and expect him to do more for himself than he should.

In transferring the patient, from bed to chair, two people should assist him first to dangle on the side of the bed and then to get out of the bed into the chair. The patient's pulse is checked before, after, and during he process of going from bed to chair; a fast pulse is a sign for the nurse to go more gradually. As the patient lowers into the chair, he should be reminded not to hold his breath, which could stimulate the Valsalva maneuver.

The chair should be comfortable, but not so soft that the patient sinks into it. This can cause hip flexion and affect circulation to lower extremities. Also, the back of the chair should be high enough to adequately support the patient's head. Both the positioning of the patient and the design of the chair should be such that no pressure is exerted on the popliteal or femoral spaces.

The ideal chair is one that has a footrest attached and allows for several changes of position so that the back of the chair can be put down and the foot support elevated independently to different degrees. At intervals during the day, the feet should be elevated to encourage venous return from the lower extremities.

Levine and Lown used the patient's feeling of fatigue to determine the length of time out of bed. Generally, within a period of a week, the patients gradually increased their length of chair rest from an initial one to two hours until they were spending most of the day out of bed.

Beckwith and his colleagues, on the other hand, in similar studies set up a schedule for their patients: 30 minutes three times a day for three days, 60 minutes three times a day for the next three, and 90 minutes three times a day for following three days(17).

Whatever the prescribed regimen, the nurse should monitor the patient's vital signs, cardiac rhythm, and so forth as carefully while the patient is in the chair as she would if he were in bed.

Chair rest should not be misconstrued to be early ambulation. A patient is usually allowed to use the bedside commode instead of a bed pan because it is less physically taxing. Also, since it is believed that the slight exertion of self-feeding is balanced by a reduction in anxiety and increase in appetite, the patient can ordinarily feed himself. However, his tray should still be set up—his meat cut, bread buttered, containers opened, and so forth. And, he must still be bathed(15).

CONCLUSION

In the treatment of patients with myocardial infarctions, all physicians agree that therapy should be directed to decreasing the workload of the heart, resulting in an optimal situation for healing of the infarcted area of muscle and the formation of a small firm scar. They do not agree on whether this is achieved through complete bed rest or rest in a chair.

The many disadvantages and hazards of the immobility in complete bed rest indicate that this approach to cardiac therapy does not really rest the heart as much as would be expected or desired. And, for better than 20 years, chair rest for cardiac patients has been studied and found to negate many of the harmful effects of bed rest. Yet, this approach to rest has never really gained popularity.

REFERENCES

1. Coe, W. S. Cardiac work and the chair treatment of acute coronary thrombosis. *Ann.Intern.Med.* 40:47, Jan. 1954.
2. Holmgren, A., and Ovenfors, C. O. Heart volume at rest and during muscular work in the supine and in the sitting position. *Acta Med.Scand.* 167:267-277, July 15, 1960.
3. Browse, N. L. *Physiology and Pathology of Bed Rest.* Springfield, Ill. Charles C Thomas Publisher, 1965, pp. 34-36.
4. Taylor, H. L. Effects of bed rest on cardiovascular function and work performance. *J.Appl.Physiol.* 2:223-239, Nov. 1949.
5. Browse, *op. cit.*, pp. 11-17.
6. *Ibid.*, App. 29-31.

7. OLSON, E. V., ed. The hazards of immobility. *Am.J.Nurs.* 67:780-797, Apr. 1967.
8. DOCK, WILLIAM. The therapeutic use and the hazards of bed rest. *Conn.State Med.J.* 11:607, Sept. 1947.
9. BROWSE, *op. cit.*, pp. 102-103.
10. *Ibid.*, pp. 180-183.
11. WADE, O. L. Movement of thoracic cage and diaphragm in respiration. *J.Physiol.* 124:193-212, May 28, 1954.
12. BROWSE, *op. cit.*, pp. 50-55.
13. SVANBERG, L. Influence of posture on the lung volumes, ventilation and circulation in normals. *Scandinav.J.Clin. and Lab.Invest.*, 9 (Suppl. 25): 1-195, 1957.
14. MC ILROY, M. B., AND OTHERS. The work of breathing in normal subjects. *Clin.Sci.* 13:127, Feb. 1954.
15. LEVINE, S. A., AND LOWN, BERNARD, "Armchair" treatment of acute coronary thrombosis. *JAMA* 148:1366, Apr. 19, 1952.
16. MITCHELL, A. M., AND OTHERS. Further observations on the armchair treatment of acute myocardial infarction. *JAMA* 155:810-814, June 26, 1954.
17. BUCKWITH, JULIAN, AND OTHERS. The management of myocardial infraction with particular reference to the chair treatment. *Ann.Intern.Med.* 41:1195, Dec. 1954.

From the *American Journal of Nursing* 73:1226-1227, July 1973.

Bed Exercises for Acute Cardiac Patients

MARY ANN LAVIN

A patient with acute myocardial infarction needs rest. At the same time, he needs exercise to prevent venous stasis, thrombosis, and embolization. The nurse then must encourage rest and also allow or recommend activities to prevent the complications of enforced rest. To decide which activity to recommend for a patient with an acute myocardial infarction, the nurse needs a rationale, a knowledge of the usual cardiovascular response, and an evaluation of that patient's probable response.

One rationale for activity is based on the energy costs of self-care activities in calories per minute. The calorie is the unit which expresses "the quantity of energy released from different foods or expended by different functional processes of the body(1)." Energy expenditure may also be expressed in liters of oxygen consumed per minute (5 cal./min. = 1 L. O_2/min.). For example, the use of the bedpan requires 4.2 cal./min. while use of the bedside commode requires only 3.6 cal:/min. Since using a commode requires less energy than using a bedpan, bedside commodes are preferred for patients in coronary care units.

Realizing that the patient needs exercise to prevent venous stasis, thrombosis, and embolization, the nurse must decide on specific exercises. Two types, rhythmic (dynamic or isotonic) and isometric (static), are frequently recommended for patients with acute myocardial infarction. Rhythmic exercise involves muscle contraction accompanied by a change in muscle length, such as active and passive flexion of the limbs. Isomet-

MS. LAVIN, *a graduate of St. John's Hospital School of Nursing, St. Louis, Missouri, received her B.S.N. and M.S.N. from St. Louis University, St. Louis, Missouri. She is assistant professor of nursing and director of the cardiovascular nursing graduate major at St. Louis University School of Nursing and Allied Health Professions. This investigation was supported by PHS Training Grant D10 NU 00184-05, National Institutes of Health, Division of Nursing.*

ric exercise involves muscular contraction with both ends of the muscle fixed and no movement in the involved joint, such as holding objects. Clinically, the common isometric exercises are hand-grip, quadriceps-setting, and gluteal-setting. Walking with heavy luggage or lifting weights are combinations of rhythmic and isometric exercise.

The purpose of rhythmic exercise is to increase muscle strength and endurance and to improve cardiopulmonary and peripheral circulatory status(2). Rhythmic exercise is indicated in muscle training, in cardiac rehabilitation, in treating peripheral circulatory disorders like Buerger's disease, and in preventing venous stasis. On the other hand, the purpose of isometric exercise is to improve the strength of a muscle group. Isometric handgrip has been used recently in testing for left ventricular dysfunction(3,4).

In spite of the limited indications for isometric exercise by patients with cardiac disease, nurses sometimes recommend isometric exercise to patients in coronary care units, encouraging "gluteal-setting" or suggesting that a patient "push against the footboard to get some exercise while you're in bed." These suggestions may cause harm.

The patient's cardiovascular responses can be evaluated by assessing heart rhythm, heart rate, blood pressure, respiratory rate and effort, and skin color and temperature. In the normal person, one cardiovascular response to exercise is cardio-acceleration. However, the patient with an ischemic or infarcted heart may develop bradyarrhythmias, tachyarrhythmias, or ectopic beats.

The cardiovascular responses to rhythmic exercise are increased heart rate, increased cardiac output, decreased peripheral vascular resistance, and little or no change in blood pressure. The systolic pressure increases, the diastolic pressure remains the same or decreases, and the mean pressure increases only slightly. There is decreased blood flow through the muscle during contraction with a compensatory high blood flow during relaxation. The cardiovascular effect of sustained isometric contractions at tensions above 15 percent maximum voluntary contraction (MVC) are moderate increase in heart rate and cardiac output, but a marked rise in systolic, diastolic, and mean blood pressure(5). There is increased blood flow to the contracting musculature, but, because the dilated vessels are compressed by the contracted muscle fibers, this flow is insufficient to supply the metabolic demands of the muscle.

One might expect an increased blood flow through other vascular beds due to the increased blood pressure associated with the isometric contraction, but studies indicate that no increased flow occurs in the noncontracting limbs, liver, or kidney. Evidence shows that compensatory vasoconstriction of these vascular beds occurs during isometric contractions(6). In patients with abnormal cardiac function, isometric exercsie results in a marked rise in left ventricular end diastolic pressure, a rise that either evokes or accentuates left ventricular dysfunction(3).

Cardiovascular responses to rhythmic exercise are preferable, then, to the responses to isometric exercise in the cardiac patient. Rhythmic exercise results primarily in increased blood flow associated with a marked augmentation of myocardial contractility and little pressure change (increased flow load). Isometric exercise results in a marked increase in blood pressure with only some increase in flow (increased afterload). Because an increased flow load results in less myocardial oxygen consumption than an increased after-load, the heart tolerates an increased flow load better than it tolerates an increased afterload(2). An increased after-load may endanger the person with a compromised heart(7).

Furthermore, while the Valsalva maneuver, forced expiration against a closed glottis, is not responsible for the pressure effect of isometric exercise(7), the ease with which the Valsalva occurs during isometric exercise increases the danger to patient safety. This maneuver has been associated with both syncope and premature ventricular contractions(2,8). Thus, the danger of isometric exercise for the cardiac patient is compounded.

Nurses may assume that the isometric exercises recommend to patients with cardiovascular disease are not sustained and therefore not harmful, yet the amount of time a patient maintains an isometric contraction is frequently unknown. He may assume that, if intermittent contractions are good, sustained contractions are better. The amount of time involved in rhythmic exercise can be observed and controlled by the nurse. Because isometric exercise is popular today, cardiac patients need to be taught *not* to engage in isometric exercise.

Rhythmic exercise is preferred to isometric exercise in the prevention of venous stasis, thrombosis, and embolization. Rhythmic exercise, such as passive leg exercises, active flexion and extension of the feet, and turning in bed, may be employed at regular intervals in the care of patients with acute myocardial infarction. A footboard is necessary to prevent foot-drop, but the patient should not use it as an exercise board. Each patient's particular response to exercise should be evaluated by assessing his heart rate and rhythm, respiratory rate and rhythm, skin color and temperature, and blood pressure before, during, and after exercise.

REFERENCES

1. GUYTON, A. C. *Textbook of Medical Physiology.* 4ed. Philadelphia, W. B. Saunders Co., 1971, p. 826.
2. ZOHMAN, L. R., AND TOBIAS, J. S. *Cardiac Rehabilitation.* New York, Grune and Stratton, 1970, pp. 150-151.
3. FISHER, MICHAEL, AND OTHERS. Hemodynamic evaluation of isometric exercise testing in cardiac patients (abstract) *Circulation* 44 (Suppl. 3): 169, Oct. 1970.
4. JACOBS, W. E., AND OTHERS. Hemodynamic responses to isometric handgrip in patients with heart disease (abstract) *Circulation* 42 (Suppl. 3): 169, Oct. 1970.
5. LIND, A. R., and MCNICHOL, G. W. Muscular factors which determine the cardiovascular responses to sustained and rhythmic exercise. *Can.Med.Assoc.J.* 96:713, Mar. 25, 1967.
6. *Ibid.,* p. 707.
7. LIND, A. R., AND OTHERS. Circulatory adjustments to sustained (static) muscular activity. IN *Physical Activity in Health and Disease,* proceedings of the International Symposium on Physical Activity in Health and Disease held at Beitostoien, Norway, 1966, ed. by Karl Evang and K. L. Andersen, Oslo, Universitetsforlaget, 1966, p. 60.
8. HARRISON, T. R., AND REEVES, T. J. *Principles and Problems of Ischemic Heart Disease.* Chicago, Year Book Medical Publishers, 1968, p. 415.

From the *American Journal of Nursing* 72:2174-2177, Dec. 1972.

Hospital Program for Cardiac Rehabilitation

ETHEL M. BARRY • **SHIRLEY ANN KNIGHT**
JOSEPH E. ACKER, JR.

Past experience has shown that about 70 to 80 percent of post myocardial infarction patients throughout the world return to work without special help(1-7). Surprisingly, the return-to-work statistics are no higher among patients who have been given a work evaluation with recommendations by a cardiac team(8).

Possibly, most efforts to improve these figures have been less than successful because attempts were made at least three to six months after the initial illness. Acker estimates that the figures could be increased to 85 to 90 percent by early, organized, inhospital intervention using rehabilitation and exercise principles(9).

Based on this premise, a coronary rehabilitation unit (CRU) was opened at St. Mary's Memorial Hospital in December 1968. The program for early cardiac rehabilitation in the unit has, of course, undergone many modifications based on subsequent studies. But even in the beginning of the program, when 114 patients rehabilitated in the CRU were compared to 114 patients treated the previous year on a routine unit, benefits were evident. The average hospital stay of CRU patients was 3.38 days shorter (22.7 to 19.29 days) and the average convalescence before return to work was 21 days shorter (100.93 to 79.82 days). The patients apparently helped most by this program were those under 50 years of age and those whose job status, economic level, and educational background were poorest.

The program stresses continuity of care, prevention of physical deconditioning, early control of activity (reconditioning), and education of the patient and his family.

The CRU includes 17 small private rooms near the coronary care unit in an area relatively free from traffic. Small rooms discourage large numbers of visitors, and private rooms minimize conflicts and emotional trauma among patients.

An EKG telemetary system permits monitoring of patients whether they are in bed or ambulating. A treadmill is used to test patient's responses to walking, as well as to do diagnostic stress electrocardiography and pulmonary function testing. These are done under the the the supervision of the CRU nurse and physician.

Patients are admitted to the unit on the basis of the following order of priorities:

- the patient who has had a myocardial infarction and has received his initial care in an acute care unit;
- any patient with a questionable diagnosis of myocardial infarction on admission;
- a medical patient with heart disease who poses a specific cardiac problem when he is admitted; and
- a patient admitted to the hospital for diagnostic studies for either hypertension or heart disease.

If such patients do not fill the unit and there is a need for beds, general medical patients may be admitted. However, as soon as possible, general medical patients are moved to other areas. And, occasionally, other low priority patients may be moved to permit admission of higher priority patients.

Both for the morale of the CRU nurses and for better, more efficient patient care, adherence to this priority list is vital. This requires the cooperation of admitting office personnel, hospital administrators, staff physicians, supervising nurses, and CCU nurses.

Nurses who work in the CRU go through a special course in the hospital in which exercise physiology, recognition of psychiatric problems, and principles of rehabilitation are stressed. Care in this unit is considered an extension of care in the CCU. Consequently, CRU nurses are rotated through the hospital's CCU or ICU training course. It is as

MS. BARRY *is the head nurse of the unit. She was graduated from Knoxville General Hospital School of Nursing.* MS. KNIGHT *is a staff nurse in the coronary rehabilitation unit and was graduated from the school of nursing there.* DR. ACKER *is a cardiologist in the Knoxville Cardiovascular Group and chief of the cardiac work evaluation clinic at the University of Tennessee Memorial Research Center, and Hospital in Knoxville. He has written a number of articles on cardiac care. Dr. Acker received his M.D. degree from the University of Tennessee School of Medicine, Memphis. The authors were involved in establishing the coronary rehabilitation unit at St. Mary's Memorial Hospital in Knoxville, Tenn.*

important for the CRU nurse to be thoroughly familiar with EKG inter-pretation and cardiopulmonary resuscitation, including early defibrilla-tion, as it is for the CCU nurse.

HOW THE UNIT WORKS

To insure continuity of care, the patient is visited daily by a CRU nurse while he is still in the coronary care unit. This gives the patient and the nurse an opportunity to become acquainted, and the patient can begin to relate to the personnel on the unit to which he will be trans-ferred. Hopefully, this helps to lessen the psychological impact caused by his removal from the CCU nursing staff, EKG monitoring, and the "intravenous lifeline."

During these visits, the CRU nurse also discusses aspects of the patient's acute illness and care with the CCU nurse and the patient's prognosis and treatment with the attending physician. The closeness of the two units promotes an understanding and appreciation of the role each must play if the patient is to recover and return to a normal or near normal life.

The CCU and CRU nurses must begin from the first day of admission to prepare the patient psychologically for rehabilitation. On the initial visit, the CRU nurse may introduce herself and talk informally. During subsequent visits, she may tell the patient about visiting hours and regu-lations in the CRU, describe the activities he will be able to assume, and stress the fact that he will continue to be observed closely. It is ideal when the CRU nurse can assist with the transfer of the patient upon his discharge from the CCU.

Members of the patient's family also are oriented to the purposes of the CRU. They are often reassured when told that the critical period of the patient's illness is believed to be past and that emphasis in this new area will be upon his gaining strength and learning how to care for him-self in the future. The cooperation of the family is essential and their inclusion and assistance in the overall rehabilitation process is of utmost importance.

In the CRU at St. Mary's Hospital, no visitors except the immediate family are allowed. Incoming calls to patients' rooms are blocked to pre-vent undue disturbance of rest and sleep, but calls may be made from the patient's room during selected periods. The family is allowed to make inquiries by phone to the nurses' station concerning the patient's condi-tion or to have messages relayed to the patient. And, if a patient's condi-tion is unstable or if he is overly apprehensive and desires not to be left alone, a family member may remain in the room overnight.

Early emphasis by the nurse and physician on an orderly activity level progression also encourages the patient and family. As soon as the patient is ready, the physician tells the patient and family what his illness is, how long he will be hospitalized, and when he can expect to return to work. An optimistic description of his convalescence, repeated by the doctor or nurse as often as indicated, helps to change the patient who denies, regresses, or has anxiety depression into someone who is able to confront reality.

NURSING CARE

Routine nursing care of the cardiac patient differs from care of the average hospital patient in that periods of work or activity must be interspersed with periods of rest. This helps to prevent over-taxation of the healing heart or the heart in congestive failure and, therefore, decreases the incidence of angina, arthythmias, dyspnea, and so forth.

For example, after the patient has eaten a meal, he must rest approximately one hour before he is bathed or attempts to bathe. After the bath, he must again rest before any other physical activity is undertaken. The work-rest concept continues throughout the day and indeed during the entire hospitalization.

Routine care is unhurried in an attempt to keep the overall atmosphere of the unit as relaxed and leisurely as possible. The location of the unit and limitation of visitors also keeps noise to a minimum.

The usual cardiac diets—sodium restricted, calorie restricted, or fat controlled—are not well accepted by many patients. Explanations help and usually, after a visit by the dietitian who prepares a list of likes and dislikes, a satisfactory meal plan can be worked out.

Good elimination is important for the cardiac patient. Constipation should be prevented, and fecal impaction should never occur. Most physicians order stool softeners, mild laxatives, or enemas to encourage regular elimination.

If the patient is having difficulty sleeping or appears nervous or restless during the day, a sleeping medication or a tranquilizer may be ordered. Otherwise, such medications are not encouraged or administered on a routine basis.

All procedures—lab tests, x-rays, EKG's—are explained to the patient to prevent his assuming that his condition has worsened. He is protected as much as possible during the rehabilitation period from anxiety and stressful situations.

Team nursing and nursing care plans are considered essential in the cardiac rehabilitation unit, for only with effective team nursing and the

GRADED ACTIVITY LEVELS

LEVEL OF ACTIVITY		METS.*	DAILY LIVING ACTIVITIES	METS.*
I.	Complete Bed Rest	1	May turn self	1
			Watch T.V. & Radio	
			Complete bath (when stable)	1
II.	Complete Bed Rest	1	May be shaved	1
			Feed self	1
			Life onto bedside commode	3
			or bedpan	4
			(specfy bedside commode or	
			bedpan on doctor's orders)	
III.	Complete Bed Rest	1	Read newspaper	1
			Wash face and hands	2
			and brush teeth	2
IV.	Dangle feet	1	Shave self	2
	5 minutes—T.I.D.		Make up face	2
			comb hair	2
			Up on bedside commode	3
V.	Dangle feet	1	Same	
	10 minutes—T.I.D.			
VI.	In bedside chair	1	Same	
	10 minutes—T.I.D.			
VII.	Up in chair	1	Begin partial bath	2
	15 minutes—Q.I.D.			
VIII.	Up in chair	1	Progressive bath	2
	15 minutes—Q.I.D.		Bathroom privileges if bathroom	2
	Walk 1-2 minutes in	2	adjoining—if not—bathroom in	
	room each time up		wheelchair	
IX.	Walk in hall	2	Self care	2
	5 minutes each time up		Dressing, undressing, etc.	
X.	Up ad lib	2	Same	

*METS.—Metabolic Equivalent—one Met. is the approximate energy expenditure while sitting quietly in a chair.

involvement and contribution of the entire staff can each patient's total needs be assessed.

A standarized activity level order sheet is placed on each patient's chart on admission to CCU or CRU and the patient's level of activity is marked on the sheet. This permits individualized orderly progression from early complete restriction of activities to routine ambulation and self care before discharge.

The levels and activities included in each are expressed in metabolic equivalents (METS). One MET respresents the basal energy requirement for an individual and equals approximately 1.3 to 1.5 calories per minute. Most CCU activities are less than two METS. The only activity allowed that requires more than 2 METS is the use of bedpan or bedside commode, which is only for short periods. Early resumption of upright posture is encouraged to prevent deconditioning, and selfcare activities and beginning ambulation are increased gradually for early reconditioning.

The increase in activity level depends on the severity of the myocardial infarction and the patient's tolerance. A patient with an uncomplicated recovery may be at activity level IX, walking in the hall, and ready for discharge home about two weeks after his infarction. The more complicated myocardial infarction patient is more likely to remain hospitalized the average three- to four-week period. Even patients who have not progressed beyond the bed rest stage are instructed to do leg and deep breathing exercises and to turn often in bed. And, increasingly, even patients with complicated conditions are ambulated earlier to prevent deconditioning.

The nurse's role in increasing activity for the cardiac is to observe closely for untoward reactions—chest pain, dyspnea, heart rate above 120, significant arrhythmias, or a 20 to 30 mm. Hg drop in blood pressure—any of which may indicate the need to return to a lower level of activity.

An EKG telemetry monitoring system has proved to be an invaluable asset in caring for cardiac patients on activity level progression. The system makes it possible to transmit with high accuracy the patient's EKG via radio frequency carrier to a central console at the nurses' station. EKG telemetry may be used to observe heart action before and during activity, and any ST or T wave changes which may indicate an adverse response to increased activity can be documented.

Telemetry monitoring is not done routinely on all CRU patients, but the physician may order it to (a) document the relationship of arrhythmias to increased activity postinfarction, (b) monitor the heart action after an elective cardioversion, pacemaker insertion, or pacemaker battery change, (c) document EKG changes during chest pain for diagnostic purposes, (d) document EKG changes during such exercise testing as on a treadmill, or (e) continue monitoring a postinfarction patient with a rhythm disturbance.

TEACHING FOR DISCHARGE

Specific patient and family teaching usually is begun during the last week of hospitalization. By that time, the patient is feeling well physically and has formulated many questions.

Detailed diet instructions are given, and written medication instructions including the name, action, and usual side effects of each drug the patient will be taking are explained. A special anticoagulant instruction sheet, identification card, and calendar are given to patients on anticoagulant therapy. Instructions with special reference to the mechanics of and signs of pacemaker malfunction are given to patients with permanent implants. And each patient receives a general outline of activity instructions to be followed at home and an appointment for a return visit with his physician.

American Heart Association pamphlets and other educational materials are always available on the unit for the patient and family. The most commonly used pamphlets are "After a Coronary," "If You Have Angina," and "Heart Disease Caused by Atherosclerosis."

At intervals, patient group conferences are conducted on the unit by various members of the rehabilitation team. For example, diet conferences are conducted by the hospital dietitian. Also, several closed circuit television programs have been prepared for cardiac patients: "Orientation to Actue Care Areas;" "Anatomy: Normal and What an Infarction Is;" "Physiology: Normal, Effect of an Infarction, and Effect of Inactivity;" "Nursing Care;" "Diet;" "Pharmacology;" "Cardiac Monitoring;" "EKG Telemetry;" Rehabilitation;" and "Pacemaker."

Among the many problems the cardiac patient may have is the common one of finances through the home recuperation period. There are various state, community, and city agencies available to help families in need of social or financial assistance. Those most frequently contacted are the state vocational rehabilitation department, Medicaid, American Heart Association, Public Health Service, and community church and civic organizations. The vocational rehabilitation department is usually the most helpful if the patient will not be able to return to his former employment.

Each patient presents a different psychological reaction to illness (10). Those common to the cardiac patient usually stem from fear of death, uncertainty for the future, fear of invalidism, and, for the male provider, fear of losing his manhood and his role as provider for the family. The patient's psychological symptoms may be manifested as overdependency or helplessness; this patient needs much reassurance and encouragement. Or, a patient may react passively or with apparently no concern about his illness; this patient is one of the most resistant to rehabilitation. And occasionally, a patient may present symptoms of denial and tend to minimize the facts of his illness on the grounds that it is a weakness he will not give in to; this patient takes great risks in his unwillingness to follow the limitations imposed by the illness. Persons who, in the past, have encouraged other people to be dependent on them and give the impression of needing no one's help, usually become increasingly controlling and demanding when they suddenly become ill and need help themselves. This reaction is more common in women than men.

One of the most necessary attributes of a CRU nurse is the ability to listen and hear what is really being said. She must be able to recognize, understand, and cope with a myriad of reactions. And, though she will see a number of problems repeated in a variety of patients, her approach to each must be highly individualized.

The CRU program at St. Mary's Hospital is based on implementation of the principles that discharge planning begins on the day of admission and that rehabilitation must be started in the acute phase of an illness. The activity progress program provides better continuity of care, earlier routine ambulation, smoother convalescence at home, a decrease in average hospitalization, and an increase in the number of patients rehabilitated to old jobs or to a happy, meaningful life.

REFERENCES

1. WEIBLATT, E., AND OTHERS. Return to work and work status following first myocardial infarction. *Am.J.Public Health* 56:169-185, Feb. 1966.
2. KELLERMAN, J. J., AND OTHERS. Return to work after myocardial infarction. *Geriatrics* 23:151-156, Mar. 1968.
3. BIORCK, G., AND WEDELIN. E. M. The return to work of patients with myocardial infarction. *Acta Med.Scand.* 175:215-226, Feb. 1964.
4. WINCOTT, E. A. Return to work after myocardial infarction. *Br.Med.J.* 2:1302-1304, Nov. 26, 1966.
5. PELI, S., AND D'ALONZO, C. A. Immediate mortality and five-year survival of employed men with a first myocardial infarction. *N.Engl.J.Med.* 270:915-922, Apr. 30, 1964.
6. BIORCK, G. The return to work of patients with myocardial infarction. (editorial) *J.Chron.Dis.* 17:653-657, July 1964.
7. LUND-JOHANSEN, P. The work and rehabilitation of patients with coronary heart disease from an urban and rural population of Norway. *Acta Med.Scand.* 177:59-62, Jan. 1968.
8. EZRA, J. Educational role of work evaluation units. IN *Proceed-*

ings. Third National Conference on Work Evaluation Units, held at Washington, D.C., Nov. 17-19, 1966. New York. American Heart Association, 1967, p. 138.
9. ACKER, J. E., JR. Role of the nurse in rehabilitation of the myocardial infarction patient. *J.S.C.Med.Assoc.* 65 (Suppl.) 1:65-66, Dec. 1969.
10. MC MAHAN, A. W. Some emotional aspects of rehabilitation in heart disease. Proceedings of a Research Conference Rehabilitation in Cardiac Disease, held at Boston. Tufts University School of Medicine, 1967, pp. 90-98.

BIBLIOGRAPHY

FAREDUDDIN, K., AND ABELMANN, W. H. Impaired orthostatic tolerance after bed rest in patients with myocardial infarction. *N.Engl.J.Med.* 280:345-350, Feb. 13, 1969.
LEVINE, S. A., AND LOWEN, B. "Armchair" treatment of acute coronary thrombosis. *JAMA* 148:1365-1369, Apr. 19, 1952.
WENGER, N. C. The use of exercise in the rehabilitation of patients after myocardial infarction. *J.S.C.Med.Assoc.* 65 (Suppl.) 1:66-68, Dec. 1969.

Section IV Drug Therapy

Nurses' responsibilities in drug administration demand that they have up-to-date and complete knowledge about the ever-increasing number of medications available. Information about each drug's action, effects, administration, toxicity and interaction potentials, and specifics to be included in patient teaching are vital to effective nursing care. Articles in other sections of this book discuss medication therapy in specific situations. The articles in this section focus on specific drugs used in the treatment of various cardiovascular diseases.

From the *American Journal of Nursing* 74:1062-1065, June 1974.

Digitalis

ELIZABETH HAHN WINSLOW

Digitalis is the most valuable and most commonly used medication for the treatment of heart disease. A complex drug, digitalis affects different areas of the heart in different ways, and affects normal and diseased hearts differently. The actions of digitalis are still not clearly understood despite years of study.

The various digitalis preparations are derived from several plants: digitalis leaf and digitoxin come from the foxglove plant, *Digitalis purpurea;* digoxin and lanatoside C from *Digitalis lanata;* and ouabain from *Strophanthus gratus.* Chemically, digitalis is composed of a sugar, a steroid, and a lactone ring. Digitoxin and digoxin, the most frequently used preparations, have identical structures except that digoxin has an extra hydroxyl group. This makes it a polar compound whereas digitoxin is a nonpolar compound. This minor structural difference creates a real metabolic difference: polar substances are absorbed and exchanged more readily in the body. The steroid portion of digitalis is similar to estrogen, and this may explain why male patients on chronic digitalis therapy occasionally develop gynecomastia.

The margin of safety between therapeutic and toxic doses and between toxic and lethal doses is narrow. When the desired therapeutic response is attained, an estimated 60 percent of the toxic dose has been administered; when the patient has toxic symptoms, approximately 50 percent of the lethal dose has been given(1). The margin of safety is narrowed further because determination of the optimal therapeutic dose is based on a poorly defined and sometimes differing physiological end effect. For

MS. WINSLOW *(B.S., Columbia University, New York, N.Y.; M.S., University of Pennsylvania, Philadelphia) is a cardiovascular nursing clinical specialist at the Hospital of the University of Pennsylvania, Philadelphia.*

example, when digitalis is used to treat congestive heart failure optimal digitalization may be recognized by a resolution of symptoms. But if digitalis is used to slow ventricular response in an atrial arrhythmia, optimal digitalization is recognized by a lowered apical pulse rate. In general, larger doses are needed to control heart rate than to increase the force of myocardial contraction.

One in every five patients who receive digitalis in general hospitals develops some degree of digitalis toxicity(2). And the incidence of toxicity is increasing as more potent digitalis preparations and diuretics are used.

ACTIONS

Digitalis has positive inotropic (increased force of contraction), negative chronotropic (decreased rate), and negative dromotropic (slowed conduction) effects.

Administered locally, digitalis causes intense irritation of subcutaneous or intramuscular tissues. Because of this, and because digitalis is irregularly absorbed by subcutaneous or intramuscular routes, these routes should be avoided if others are available.

The positive inotropic effect, one of the most important effects of digitalis, results from a direct action on the heart muscle. Although the exact mechanism is undetermined, digitalis enables cardiac muscle to convert more of its chemical energy into mechanical energy. This may be caused by digitalis action on the contractile protein, actomyosin. Or digitalis may act on the cell membrane to modify the transport of electrolytes. Some studies suggest that digitalis action is related to increased calcium and sodium levels within the cell coupled with a loss of potassium from the cell(3).

The therapeutic benefits of the positive inotropic effect of digitalis include increased cardiac output, decreased heart size, decreased venous pressure, and relief of edema. The inotropic effect enhances renal perfusion and causes diuresis. Digitalis also has a direct, though minor, renal action which inhibits sodium reabsorption(4).

The negative chronotropic and dromotropic effects of digitalis are caused by its direct action on the heart muscle and by its indirect stimulation of the vagus nerve. Digitalis is the drug of choice in the treatment of supraventricular ectopic rhythms with rapid ventricular response, as in atrial fibrillation, because it slows conduction through the atrioventricular node and, consequently, slows the ventricular response rate. By altering the excitability of atrial muscle, digitalis also helps to convert many atrial arrhythmias to normal sinus rhythm.

The combined actions of digitalis have two major uses: to improve the cardiac contractility and efficiency of patients with congestive heart failure, and to treat rapid, supraventricular, ectopic rhythms by slowing the ventricular response and also by helping to convert them to normal rhythms.

METABOLISM

Digitalis is rapidly and reliably absorbed by oral and intravenous routes. Digitoxin is completely absorbed, extensively recycled through the liver and bowel, and closely bound by serum albumin. Most of it is ultimately excreted in the urine as cardio-inactive metabolites(5).Therefore, digitoxin has a relatively long half-life of five to seven days. Because only a small fraction of digitoxin is excreted unchanged in the urine, excretion cannot be related predictably to renal function.

Digoxin is 80 to 90 percent absorbed, very little of it is recycled or bound to protein, and is excreted largely unchanged in the urine(5). Therefore, digoxin has a short half-life of 1½ days, and its excretion can be directly related to renal function. The difference in the polar characteristics of digitoxin and digoxin contributes to the differences in their metabolism. Digitalis preparations should be given cautiously to patients who have liver or renal disease because these conditions might interfere with the drugs' metabolism and excretion and so permit toxic levels to accumulate.

Digoxin and digitoxin are the most commonly used digitalis preparations. There is much controversy over which is better. Their cardiac effects are the same, but their speed and duration of action differ.

Digoxin is a fast-acting preparation and is given when a rapid effect is needed. Many physicians use digoxin almost exclusively. They reason that, if the patient becomes toxic, digoxin activity will be gone in two to six days whereas digitoxin activity will persist for two to three weeks. Some physicians prefer digoxin for patients with liver disease because it is less actively recycled than digitoxin.

Digitoxin may be chosen for the patient with renal disease because its excretion depends so little on the kidney. Some believe that digitoxin permits smoother digitalization with less variability in the optimal therapeutic level in the body. Also, if a patient forgets to take one or two doses of digitoxin, he still retains some beneficial digitalis effect. If he forgets to take digoxin for two days, however, he may be without any beneficial effects and get into trouble. On the other hand, the patient who forgets to take his medicine is often the patient who also forgets that he has taken it. He may take double or triple doses. For this patient, treatment with

ACTION OF DIGITALIS AFTER A SINGLE, FULL DIGITALIZING, INTRAVENOUS DOSE

	Action Begins	Action Maximal	Action Regresses	Action Gone
Digoxin	5-30 min.	1½-5 hrs.	8-10 hrs.	2-6 days
Digitoxin	26-120 min.	4-12 hrs.	2-3 days	2-3 weeks

Adapted from Louis S. Goodman and Alfred Gilman, *The Pharmacological Basis of Therapeutics*, 4th ed., N.Y., Macmillan Company, 1970, p. 699.

digitoxin would certainly carry a higher risk than the use of digoxin.

DOSAGE

Digitalization builds up the patient's digitalis levels to produce an optimal cardiac effect. Digitalization can be completed in less than 12 hours if fast-acting preparations are used, or digitalization can be done over a period of one to seven days. Digitalizing doses may not be necessary in nonacute situations. Rather, the chosen maintenance dose can be administered and the patient's response closely evaluated. Later, the dosage can be altered if necessary. In general, rapid digitalization should be avoided when slow methods suffice, and oral administration is safer than parenteral.

In order to maintain the beneficial effects of digitalis, a maintenance dose is given to replace the digitalis that is destroyed or eliminated from the body. Thirty-three percent of digoxin and 15-20 percent of digitoxin is excreted daily(5). The maintenance dose is highly individual and varies not only from patient to patient but also from time to time in the same person.

APPROXIMATE DOSAGE SCHEDULE FOR DIGOXIN AND DIGITOXIN

	Total Oral Digitalizing Dose	Daily Oral Maintenance Dose
Digoxin	2-3 mg.	0.25-0.5 mg.
Digitoxin	1-1.5 mg	0.05-0.2 mg.

TOXICITY

Many toxic responses to digitalis are extensions of its therapeutic effects. For this reason, all digitalis preparations are potentially toxic. A preparation that will not cause toxicity when given in excess is also one that will not exert any therapeutic effect.

Anorexia, nausea, and vomiting, often the earliest manifestations of toxicity, occur in 50 to 80 percent of patients receiving the drug(6). Diarrhea also may occur, but it is uncommon. The gastrointestinal effects

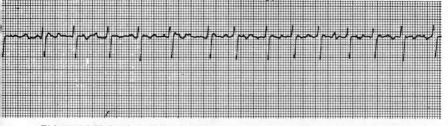

This atrial fibrillation, with a ventricular response of 120/min., was treated with digitalis, which slowed the ventricular response to 60-80/min.

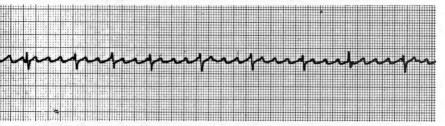

Digitalis was used to slow conduction through the atrioventricular node to lower ventricular response to this atrial flutter (atrial rate 300/min.).

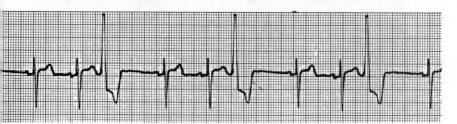

Ventricular premature contractions, seen here in a trigeminal pattern, are often indicative of digitalis toxicity.

are believed to be caused by stimulation of the vomiting center in the medulla rather than by local irritation.

Toxic cardiac effects are common and usually occur early. Cardiac arrhythmias occur in 80 to 90 percent of patients with toxicity(2). Almost every known cardiac arrythmia may be produced. Ventricular premature contractions (VPCs) are the most common but the least specific arrhythmia because there are many other causes of VPCs. Arrhythmias that strongly suggest digitalis toxicity include nonparoxysmal junctional tachycardia, atrial tachycardia with block, marked sinus bradycardia, atrioventricular dissociation with ventricular rate exceeding atrial rate, and coexistence of an ectopic rhythm with depression of conduction. Regularization of *chronic* atrial fibrillation suggests toxicity because it may signal an underlying nonparoxysmal junctional tachycardia(7).

Toxicity can aggravate congestive heart failure. Therefore, all patients with intractable failure should be carefully reevaluated for the possibility of digitalis toxicity.

Visual disturbances occur in 11 to 20 percent of patients with toxicity, usually later than gastrointestinal manifestations or arrhythmias(6). Patients may complain of difficulties in reading, hazy or shimmering vision, halos around dark objects, blind spots, and disturbances of color vision, especially green and yellow. One woman said she saw glittering and moving spots similar to those seen on a television screen before the picture comes on. Patients may not report a visual disturbance unless the nurse inquires specifically about it.

Neurological symptoms, such as headache, drowsiness, insomnia, vertigo, confusion, and delirium also may be present. Easy fatigability and generalized muscle weakness may be especially prominent. One woman described her fatigue as a "most miserable feeling." The neurological manifestations of toxicity are probably related to the direct effects of digitalis on brain cells.

Allergic reactions, such as rash and eosinophilia, are rare with digitalis.

Endocrine alterations, such as gynecomastia may result from the estrogen-like activity of the drug. Some investigators cite this as a toxic effect; others believe it is a side effect because many patients develop it without experiencing any other toxic effects.

Although anorexia, nausea, fatigue, and hazy vision are rather nonspecific and not alarming, they may be the only warning signs of a toxicity that can quickly result in a fatal cardiac arrhythmia.

The treatment of digitalis toxicity is immediate withdrawal of the drug —not just dosage reduction. Most patients with mild toxicity recover completely after digitalis has been discontinued for several days. More active therapy is required if serious cardiac arrhythmias are present.

Potassium is one of the most effective agents used to abolish arrhythmias arising from digitalis toxicity. Potassium is a myocardial depressant and antiarrhythmic and, therefore, has essentially opposite cardiac effects to those of digitalis. Potassium suppresses cardiac excitability, digitalis increases it. The higher the blood level of potassium, the less effective a given dose of digitalis. Conversely, a fall in the serum potassium level enhances the effect of digitalis. The dose of potassium depends on the severity of toxicity, the patient's potassium level, and his response to potassium. Potassium is contraindicated in renal failure and is given cautiously to patients with conduction defects.

Other antiarrhythmic drugs that may be used to treat toxicity include diphenylhydantoin (Dilantin), propranolol (Inderal), lidocaine (Xylocaine), quinidine, and procainamide (Pronestyl). If bradycardia or conduction defects are present, atropine, isoproterenol (Isuprel), or a pacemaker may be used.

In the past 10 years several methods have been developed to determine serum digitalis levels so that toxicity can be diagnosed more accurately. Patients with marked toxicity have significantly higher serum digitalis levels than those who are not toxic. However, substantial overlap exists between toxic and nontoxic levels, and an inadequate level for one patient may be a toxic level for another. Therefore, serum levels are useful only when interpreted in the context of the total clinical picture or when no other information is available about previous digitalization. In general, serum digoxin levels of 2.0 ng./ml. or below and serum digitoxin levels of 20 ng./ml. or below are considered nontoxic(2).

NURSING IMPLICATIONS

If a patient is receiving digitalis for congestive heart failure, the nurse can expect to see a decrease in edema and shortness of breath. If he is taking digitalis for a supraventricular tachycardia, she can expect a slowed heart rate and a decrease in the pulse deficit. A pulse deficit, or radial pulse rate lower than the apical pulse rate, often occurs in patients with atrial fibrillation, as well as other arrhythmias, because the ventricles are stimulated to contract so soon after the previous beat that they do not eject enough blood to produce a palpable peripheral pulse. An apical pulse should be taken in any patient with a pulse deficit. The apical pulse might be 120, indicating a continued need for digitalis and perhaps even an increase in dose, while the radial pulse might inaccurately indicate a controlled rate of 70.

Because digitalis toxicity is both common and serious, the nurse who cares for a patient receiving digitalis must maintain a high index of suspicion and watch for and report any symptoms which might manifest toxicity, no matter how innocuous they seem. An increased pulse rate is just as worrisome as a slow pulse. Irregularities in the cardiac rhythm as well as regularization of a chronic irregular pulse should be recognized as possible indications of toxicity. The nurse should inquire about the presence of non-cardiac symptoms of toxicity. No change is too unimportant to be noted.

Teaching is very important for patients who take this valuable but dangerous drug, and for their families. They should know the name, dosage, and action of the drug. The nurse should point out the importance of not missing a dose (some patients may try to save money by cutting down on the number of pills they take each week), and of not taking extra doses (some patients believe that if one pill is helpful, two must be better, and take extra pills when they do not feel well).

Most patients must take digitalis for the rest of their lives, and some are concerned about becoming "addicted." Therefore, the nurse should assure the person that he need not worry about developing a "drug habit"; chronic digitalis therapy will not harm him if he takes the drug properly.

Written, as well as verbal, medication instructions are helpful. The patient should be asked how he plans to remember to take his pills. If necessary, he can be helped to develop a record-keeping system. Some excellent, inexpensive, commercial products can be recommended to patients.

If the patient must take other drugs, such as diuretics and potassium, he should understand that these medications are in a delicate balance with digitalis. He should not stop taking any medication or alter its dose without consulting his physician.

The patient should know, too, that all drugs, including digitalis, can have adverse side effects. Therefore, he should report any anorexia, nausea, vomiting, visual changes, just not feeling right, or palpitations because these symptoms may indicate that the drug is not working properly.

It is ideal if the patient can take his pulse and recognize abnormal changes in rate or rhythm. However, some patients cannot take an accurate pulse, or become overly concerned about their conditions if they are asked to do so, or are simply uninterested in learning pulse taking. For these patients, learning the common toxic effects of digitalis and a respect for the drug are more important than learning to take their pulse rates. Persons who are willing and able to count their pulses should be taught how to do this and be told what their normal resting pulse rates and rhythms should be. For example, they should be advised to report any resting pulse rate below 60 or above 100 to the doctor and also to report any unusual irregularity or regularity.

Digitalis is valuable for the treatment of congestive heart failure and supraventricular tachycardias. It is dangerous because of the narrow margin between therapeutic and toxic dose levels. A clear understanding and recognition of the therapeutic and toxic actions of digitalis and more time spent teaching patients about digitalis should significantly reduce the high incidence of digitalis toxicity.

REFERENCES

1. FISCH, CHARLES. Digitalis toxicity. (Critical Care Medicine No. 13) *JAMA* 216:1770-1773, June 14, 1971.
2. CHUNG, E. K. The current status of digitalis therapy. *Mod.Treat.* 8:643-714, Aug. 1971.
3. LANGER, GLENN A. The mechanism of action of digitalis. *Hosp.-Practice* 5:55-56, Aug. 1970.
4. GOODMAN, L. S., AND GILMAN, ALFRED *Pharmacological Basis of Therapeutics*, 4th ed. New York, Macmillan Company, 1970, p. 690.
5. DOHERTY, J. E., AND OTHERS. New information regarding digitalis metabolism. *Chest* 59:433-437, Apr. 1971.
6. LELY, A. H., AND VAN ENTER, C. H. J. Noncardiac symptoms of digitalis intoxication. *Am.Heart J.* 83:149-152, Feb. 1972.
7. KASTOR, J. A. Digitalis intoxication in patients with atrial fibrillation. *Circulation* 47:888-896, Apr. 1973.

From the *American Journal of Nursing* 75:1168-1170, July 1975.

Teaching Patients About Nitroglycerin

ELAINE ERICKSON ALLENDORF   •   M. HONOR KEEGAN

Coronary artery disease, accurately dubbed the twentieth century epidemic, is the number one cause of death in the United States, accounting for 660,000 deaths annually.

Angina pectoris, the mildest and often the earliest clinical symptom of coronary artery disease, is considered "the harbinger of sudden death"(1). The Framingham study concluded that one quarter of the males diagnosed as having angina pectoris can expect to sustain a myocardial infarction with five years. This study also demonstrated that there is a 58-percent five-year, postinfarction survival rate among these persons(2). White noted an average survival rate of 9 to 10 years(3).

Angina pectoris is characterized by the paroxysmal occurrence of chest pain, usually in the substernal region. It results from a disparity between myocardial oxygen consumption and supply. When the myocardium is deprived of an adequate blood supply to meet its needs, normal, aerobic metabolism ceases and anaerobic, lactic acid metabolism takes over, resulting in the patient's experience of pain. This pain probably is caused by the irritation of the myocardial neural receptors in response to the presence of the acid byproducts of anerobic metabolism.

Inadequate delivery of oxygenated blood most often is due to degenerative disease of the coronary arteries which feed the heart muscle itself. However, delivery also may be disrupted by aortic valve disease and some forms of anemia. When the body's metabolic requirements increase, as they do with any added stress, the myocardial muscle becomes progressively less able to meet the demand because of inade-

ELAINE ALLENDORF, R.N., M.S., *is a certified nurse practitioner. She works with Dr. Charles Allendorf in Warwick, R.I.* M. HONOR KEEGAN, R.N., M.S., *is an instructor at Massachusetts General Hospital School of Nursing, Boston.*

quate tissue perfusion. At this point, myocardial ischemia occurs and the patient experiences angina.

Anginal pain usually follows exercise, emotional aggravation, stress, or cold. It may radiate to the precordium, upper extremities, neck, jaw, or teeth. The quality of the pain commonly is described as a constriction, tightness, squeezing, or heaviness. The usual duration of the attack is three to five minutes, although it may last up to 15 minutes. Stopping activity and taking nitroglycerin usually produces prompt relief.

Rest, control of risk factors, and appropriate exercise are extremely important in the medical management of persons with angina pectoris. This regimen augments myocardial oxygen consumption and thus relieves pain and prevents or decreases the frequency of attacks. Nitroglycerin is part of this therapy for angina pectoris(4,5).

Nitrates relax smooth muscle. Nitroglycerin alleviates angina in two ways. First, it dilates the walls of the coronary arteries themselves, permitting greater blood flow to the heart muscle. Second, it promotes a generalized systemic vasodilatation which lowers peripheral resistance, lessening the oxygen requirements and workload of the heart. With adequate tissue perfusion, aerobic metabolism is restored and anginal pain is relieved.

The cardiac patient takes his nitroglycerin according to a subjective perception of anginal pain. Therefore, it is his decision and action which will ensure the successful management of his symptoms. It is of paramount importance that the patient be prepared adequately to control his angina.

In light of the person's crucial responsibility for his own care, we attempted to determine patients' existing knowledge about the disease process and to assess the parameters which they use in deciding to take nitroglycerin. An additional goal of our study was to discover what nurses should teach people with angina. Our review of the current literature revealed limited information regarding the nurse's responsibility in preparing people to take nitroglycerin safely and effectively.

WHAT PATIENTS KNEW

Twenty patients with stable angina were selected for the study. These patients were being treated at three large metropolitan hospitals. The study group included both hospitalized patients and those being followed in the clinic. The patients ranged in age from 35 to 62 years, and included 16 men and four women. They had suffered from angina pectoris for two months to 20 years. The study was conducted through a standardized interview.

These 20 persons were generally ill-informed regarding the basic pathophysiology of angina and the prudent use of nitroglycerin. However, although vital knowledge and the action and use of nitroglycerin was lacking, some positive factors were noted. Each of the 20 was able to describe his own symptoms accurately and could identify these as having a cardiac origin rather than involving other body systems.

Patients often are instructed to take nitroglycerin specifically for chest pain. However, because symptoms vary from person to person, the distress of angina may not always manifest itself as pain, but as shortness of breath, constriction, heaviness, or pressure. Therefore, the patient must be aware of his own cardiac symptoms so that he will be alerted to take nitroglycerin appropriately. None of the people interviewed took nitroglycerin for reasons other than angina.

Although they could describe their symptoms, only four could identify the physiological mechanism causing the angina response. Of the remaining patients, most did not know the etiology of their discomfort; others had either inaccurate or inadequate knowledge. "Thin blood," "a cold in the chest," and "collapsed veins" were three reasons cited for angina. These responses indicate that some patients may have a superficial knowledge of their condition. Adequate teaching is necessary if the person is to understand the principle of myocardial oxygen supply and demand as it relates to his symptoms, and thus understand the rationale underlying the prescription of nitroglycerin by the physician.

Even though the majority of patients surveyed lacked sufficient knowledge about the cause of angina, all were able to identify specific circumstances which precipitated attacks. Nineteen ascribed episodes to both physical exertion and emotional stress. Specific activities mentioned were lifting, eating heavy meals, going out into the cold, engaging in sexual intercourse, and smoking.

The patients' ability to identify precipitating factors had little apparent relationship to their use of nitroglycerin prophylactically; only one patient reported using the drug before taking part in angina-producing activities. This implies that they either do not remember to take nitroglycerin before engaging in these activities or, more likely, that they are not taught to do so by health professionals. The person should be instructed to take a tablet three to five minutes before exposure to the aggravating cause; the drug's effect can be expected to last for up to 30 minutes.

Sixteen patients displayed accurate knowledge of nitroglycerin's expected onset of action; four expected the effect to take longer than the normal one to three minutes. All respondents took the drug by the cor-

GUIDELINES FOR TEACHING PATIENTS ABOUT NITROGLYCERIN

Goal: To prepare the patient for the self-administration of nitroglycerin in a safe, therapeutic manner, and to assist him to use good clinical judgment in managing his symptoms.

Before beginning to teach, assess the person's knowledge about his disease and medication. Explore the impact the illness has had on the patient and his family. Determine any fears and questions they may have. Discuss the following material.

Pathophysiology of Angina Pectoris
- Myocardial oxygen supply-and-demand deficit as it relates to pain
- Patient's subjective symptoms
- Precipitating circumstances (physical and emotional)
- Use of rest, in conjunction with medication, to terminate the attack

Nitroglycerin
- Pharmacological action to relieve symptoms
- Drug to be taken when discomfort is not relieved by rest, but patient should not wait for pain to worsen before taking nitroglycerin
- Route of administration: sublingual only; *not* effective if swallowed
- Onset of action: 1-3 minutes; duration of action: 10-30 minutes
- If no relief, take 1-2 tablets at 5 minute intervals, but no more than 3 tablets per attack
- If no relief after 15 minutes, call physician immediately
- Nitroglycerin tablets to be carried by patient at all times
- There is no limit to the number of nitroglycerin tablets which may be taken in a 24-hour period
- Nitroglycerin is not addicting; does not lose its effectiveness in relieving pain even after years of use
- Prophylactic use: take a tablet 3-5 minutes before engaging in activities known to precipitate angina
- Side effects: headache, often pounding in nature; flushing of the skin; dizziness; occasional syncope. Usually subside after drug is taken for an extended period. Avoid standing after taking nitroglycerin
- Store nitroglycerin in a tightly closed, dark, glass container; avoid heat, air, light, and moisture

The drug is potent for up to six months only. Fresh tablets produce a burning sensation in the sublingual mucosa. Nitroglycerin may be kept in the refrigerator to ensure potency.

rect route (sublingual), and 19 were aware that the drug is ineffective if swallowed. However, only five patients knew the medication's mode of action.

The parameters of safety were not well defined in the event that the pain of angina exceeded five minutes. Four patients were not aware that they could take a second tablet should the first one be ineffective after five minutes had elapsed. Due to fear of addiction, five patients took a second tablet only on a rare occasion. Eleven often took a second tablet; of these, six exceeded the limit of three tablets per attack. Lack of knowledge in this particular area is inherently dangerous because excessive use of nitroglycerin increases the predisposition to prolonged hypotention and more severe side effects.

Thirteen patients did not know when to call the physician if nitroglycerin failed to alleviate the anginal pain. The inaccurate knowledge consisted mainly of waiting too long to summon medical assistance. Each patient must be taught never to take more than three tablets per attack or wait longer than 15 minutes to seek medical help if the chest pain does not abate.

A discussion of the drug's side effects and its correct storage is essential. Side effects common to the use of nitroglycerin are flushing, dizziness, weakness, and headache, often manifested as a pounding sensation. In our study, 16 patients had experienced one or more of these side effects. If he is unaware of these possible side effects, the person may become frightened when he experiences them, and avoid using the drug when indicated. If he sits or lies down after taking the first pill, the severity and occurrence of the side effects may be appreciably decreased.

Only seven patients were aware that nitroglycerin loses its potency after six months; five knew how to store the drug. Most of these patients did not realize that nitroglycerin is composed of a volatile substance which is inactivated by exposure to light, heat, air, and moisture. The drug should be kept in a tightly closed, dark, glass container away from heat and light. Fresh tablets are relatively soft, dissolve easily, and produce a mild burning sensation in the sublingual mucosa.

An important, but often overlooked, precaution involves wedging a cotton pledget into the vial to keep the tablets immobile, thus delaying their disintegration. The cotton should not be inserted so tightly that it cannot be easily removed when the person needs nitroglycerin at the onset of an attack.

During the interview patients asked about the storage of nitroglycerin; only two patients asked about angina itself and the effects of cigarette smoking on heart disease. Most patients denied having any questions even though their responses reflected a poor understanding of both angina and nitroglycerin. We hypothesized that these patients didn't ask questions because they had inadequate knowledge on which to base questions, had an overwhelming fear of heart disease and wished to know as little about it as possible, or were denying their heart disease and so believed they did not need the information.

IMPLICATIONS

Although this study was by no means comprehensive, we believe that certain trends can be identified. The 20 study patients were not prepared well enough to assume such a profound responsibility for their own care. On the whole, their knowledge of angina and the use of nitroglycerin were poor, yet this is the key to optimal self care.

Fourteen patients had been taught by a physician, two by a nurse, and four by a physician-nurse team. Those patients who were instructed by the nurse alone or by the physician alone gave more inaccurate responses than the patients who received instruction from a physician-nurse team. Perhaps nurses' reinforcement of physician instruction and the additional information they give have a positive effect on patient learning.

Teaching should be an integral part of nursing intervention in the care of patients with angina pectoris who take nitroglycerin for the relief of symptoms. The informed patient and his family are vital elements of health care. The person must understand what he must do to presrve health, recognize when there is a need of help, and be prepared to take appropriate steps to obtain help.

Certainly, increased knowledge about his condition and its treatment should lead to increased patient compliance with therapy and perhaps to a decreased mortality from heart disease.

REFERENCES

1. FRIEDBERG, C. K. Some comments on reflections on changing interests and new developments in angina pectoris. *Circulation* 46:1039, Dec. 1972.
2. KANNEL, W. B., AND FEINLEIB, MANNING. Natural history of angina pectoris in the Framingham study. *Am.J.Cardiol.* 29:161, Feb. 1972.
3. WHITE, P. D. *Heart Disease.* 4th ed. New York, Macmillan Co., 1951, p. 556.
4. HURST, J. W., AND LOGUE, R. B., EDS. *The Heart, Arteries, and Veins.* 2d ed. New York, Blackiston Division, McGraw-Hill Book Co., 1970. p. 948.
5. KRANTZ, J.C., JR. Action and nomenclature of nitroglycerin and nitrate esters. *AM.J.Cardiol.* 29:436, Mar. 1972.

From the *American Journal of Nursing* 75:620-626, Apr. 1975.

Vasopressor Agents in Shock

JOHN H. MOYER • LEWIS C. MILLS

Shock is often considered synonymous with acute hypotension, but this is a misconception. The physiological changes in shock are both more complex and more variable than those that result from simple reduction in blood pressure. Much of the experimental work in shock has been devoted to the study of physiological changes associated with variations in blood pressure, but the observations made in the laboratory may not apply to the patient in shock. We will consider here some critical hemodynamic changes that are observed with reduction in blood pressure and the use of vasopressor agents as a temporary measure for maintaining arterial pressure so that irreparable tissue damage can be prevented.

The vasopressor drugs we will be most concerned with here are the adrenergic drugs. While they affect many body areas, we shall discuss only their effects on vasculature. Adrenergic drugs resemble the natural neurohormone, norepinephrine, but vary in their tendency to constrict or dilate blood vessels in various parts of the body[1]. Thus, adrenergic drugs produce effects similar to those of the sympathetic nervous system.

Whether vasoconstriction or vasodilation occurs probably depends on the reception sites for these synthetic neurohormones. The alpha receptors tend to produce vasoconstriction and the beta, vasodilation[2].

CEREBRAL CIRCULATION IN SHOCK

Cerebral circulation is not controlled by the sympathetic nervous system but, rather, by the amount of carbon dioxide and the pH of the blood flowing through the brain. Cerebral vessels dilate with a low pH. If

DR. MOYER *is vice-president and director of professional affairs at Conemaugh Valley Memorial Hospital, Johnstown, Pa. Dr. Moyer has done research in renal and cerebral hemodynamics, hypertension, and related pharmacologic studies.* DR. MILLS *is professor of medicine, department of medicine, Hahnemann Medical College and Hospital, Philadelphia, Pa.*

THE EFFECT OF NOREPINEPHRINE
ON BLOOD PRESSURE

	Mean Blood Pressure (mm.Hg)	Cerebral Blood Flow (cc./min.)*
SHOCK (hypotensive level)	58	40
NOREPINEPHRINE (normotensive level)	90	51
AFTER ONE WEEK (post-shock)	86	54

*normal control value = 54 cc./100 Gm. brain/min.

Drug effect is compared in the patient in shock and to normal values in the same patient a week later.

carotid arterial pressure is maintained, cerebral blood flow should be adequate.

Reduction of the mean blood pressure by drugs or hemorrhage also reduces cerebral blood flow. However, unless the blood pressure reduction is marked, cerebral function will not be impaired, because the brain compensates for the slightly lower blood flow by extracting more oxygen from the blood. Obviously if blood pressure is severely depressed, the absolute amount of oxygen available is reduced, cerebral anoxia results, and tissue damage follows.

The point at which ischemia develops is significant. The table (page 182) summarizes a study in which the mean arterial blood pressure is plotted against cerebral blood flow and cerebral oxygen consumption (CMRO$_2$). Initially, as the blood pressure falls, there is little effect on cerebral blood flow. It is not until the blood pressure drops below 60 to 70 mm.Hg that cerebral blood flow begins to decrease. At this point, anoxia has not yet developed because of the brain's ability to extract more oxygen per unit of blood. But when the pressure drops below 50 mm.Hg, cerebral blood flow is severely decreased and sufficient oxygen can no longer be extracted. Anoxia and its related problems develop.

At pressures of 30 mm.Hg, many patients suffer from severe anoxia and have serious manifestations of reduced cerebral metabolism. This is reversed when normal pressure is restored by using a vasopressor agent, which, in turn, increases cerebral blood flow. The critical level for arterial blood pressure, then, is 40 mm.Hg; below that, brain damage may result, depending on the duration of reduced blood flow.

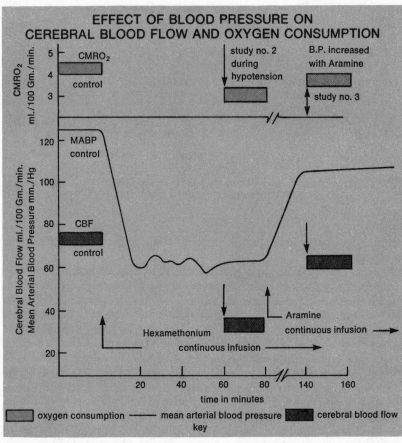

EFFECT OF BLOOD PRESSURE ON CEREBRAL BLOOD FLOW AND OXYGEN CONSUMPTION

Reduction in cerebral blood flow that is associated with a decrease in blood pressure is quickly corrected when the arterial pressure is increased with a vasopressor agent.

The transfusion of blood in hemorrhagic shock produces results similar to the administration of vasopressors. The table shows variation in blood pressure resulting from reduced blood volume. As blood pressure rises to normotensive levels, cerebral blood flow increases. Here, again,

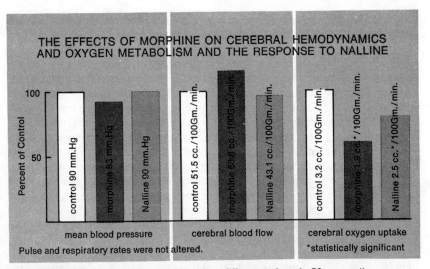

THE EFFECTS OF MORPHINE ON CEREBRAL HEMODYNAMICS
AND OXYGEN METABOLISM AND THE RESPONSE TO NALLINE

Percent of Control

100

50

control 90 mm.Hg

morphine 83 mm.Hg

Nalline 90 mm.Hg

control 51.5 cc./100Gm./min.

morphine 53.8 cc./100Gm./min.

Nalline 43.1 cc./100Gm./min.

control 3.2 cc./100Gm./min.

morphine 1.9 cc.*/100Gm./min.

Nalline 2.5 cc.*/100Gm./min.

mean blood pressure   cerebral blood flow   cerebral oxygen uptake

Pulse and respiratory rates were not altered.   *statistically significant

Marked reduction in arterial-venous oxygen difference (nearly 50 percent)
following administration of morphine indicates a significant decrease in
demand (uptake) of oxygen by the brain or a decrease in cerebral
oxygen requirement. Oxygen requirement rises sharply
after Nalline (nalorphine HCl) is given to block morphine's effects.

this study demonstrates that blood volume itself has little effect on cerebral blood flow as long as the carotid and aortic pressures are adequate to maintain blood flow through the brain.

EFFECTS OF MORPHINE

Morphine has a positive effect on cerebral oxygen consumption, which can be seen in the chart on this page. In this study, morphine was given and then Nalline, which blocks the cerebral effect of morphine. Morphine reduced the brain's oxygen requirement by nearly 50 percent—a particularly beneficial effect in the presence of ischemia or anoxia. Since the oxygen requirement is reduced, the amount of arterial blood flow required to deliver the oxygen is likewise reduced. Thus, in shock, morphine is very efficacious, for it actually protects. If its effects are blocked with Nalline, the cerebral demand for oxygen returns(3).

The critical level at which cerebral circulation becomes definitely inadequate is about 40 mm.Hg (mean arterial blood pressure). Continuing the infusion of a vasopressor until the mean arterial pressure rises above

90 mm.Hg tends to elicit cardiac arrhythmias. It is well to maintain the pressure between 70 and 90 mm.Hg.

WHEN TO USE ADRENERGIC STIMULATORS

SEVERE HYPOTENSIVE EPISODES Even in the early stages, particularly in hemorrhagic or cardiogenic shock, patients can develop such severely reduced cardiac output that the mean blood pressure falls to levels insufficient to sustain flow through vital vascular beds, especially the brain. Cerebral and myocardial function deteriorate rapidly and circulation must be increased to prevent immediate death. Circulation to other organs is of little concern until the brain and heart are adequately perfused. Volume expanders or vasodilators, often the best agents in less acute situations, may act too slowly or they may be contraindicated—for example, large amounts of fluid in cardiogenic shock.

A vasopressor agent, an alpha-beta stimulator such as metaraminol (Aramine) or norepinephrine (Levophed), with or without intravascular volume expansion as indicated, is frequently the initial therapy of choice. Since both Aramine and Levophed cause peripheral vasoconstriction except in the cerebral and small coronary vessels and because the intra-arterial pressure in the arteries supplying these areas is increased by these agents, one would expect the percentage of blood volume to increase in the cerebral and coronary vessels even if there were no increase in total cardiac output. Cardiac output may also be increased by the positive inotropic action of these drugs; thus, cerebral and coronary blood flow would improve. This allows time to take other necessary measures and time for them to become effective. Again, pressure should be raised only to a mean of about 70 to 80 mm.Hg. As other measures become effective, the vasopressors should be discontinued gradually.

HEMORRHAGIC SHOCK Obviously, in hemorrhagic shock, volume replacement and hemostasis are the treatments of choice. Their effectiveness can easily be shown in animal experiments when bleeding can be stopped at will, provided irreversible shock has not been produced. In patients, the bleeding point may not be readily accessible and severe shock may persist in spite of continuous volume replacement. And all solutions used for volume replacement, when given in very large amounts, may have undesirable effects. Administration of an alpha-beta stimulator, such as metaraminol or norepinephrine, will help to maintain essential cerebral and cardiac function by shunting blood to these areas while volume is being replaced or definitive hemostatic procedures are being carried out. Aside from this shunting effect, the venoconstrictor

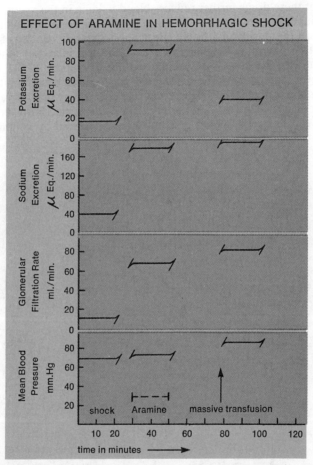

EFFECT OF ARAMINE IN HEMORRHAGIC SHOCK

In hypovolemic shock resulting from a severed artery in a previously normotensive person, the rise in blood pressure produced by Aramine (metaraminol) is accompanied by a rapid increase in renal blood flow and in glomerular filtration rate. A similar response follows blood transfusion. A vasopressor like Aramine may improve renal blood flow by constricting less essential vascular beds without much increase in overall blood pressure.

effect of these drugs further reduces blood volume in the venous vascular bed, shunting more blood centrally and to the arterial vasculature. Coupled with the positive inotropic effect and increased velocity of ejection, circulation time may be shortened. This, in turn, increases tissue perfusion but with the same intravascular volume of blood.

Several factors are to be considered when alpha-beta stimulators are used in hemorrhagic shock. First, the rate of bleeding may increase if the bleeder is a medium or large artery. This may occur, however, if pressure is raised by any means or if viscosity is reduced by volume expan-

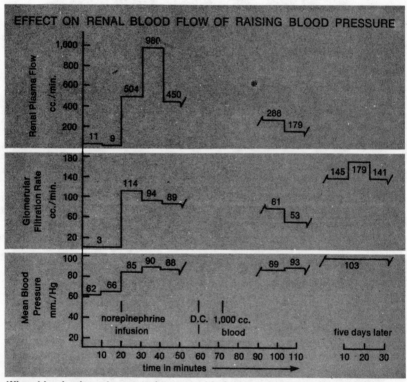

When blood volume is restored to normal in hypovolemic shock, blood flow in all major vascular beds returns toward normal. This is reflected in renal function, although the rate at which improvement occurs varies with the specific vascular bed and with the expander given (whole blood or plasma).

ders. Conversely, if the site is a small vessel or capillary, the vasoconstriction produced by these drugs may reduce bleeding. Pressure should, then, be only moderately elevated.

Next, the effectiveness of alpha-beta stimulators in restoring generalized tissue blood flow is inversely related to the degree of volume deficit. Simultaneous administration of fluid is definitely indicated because these drugs tend to reduce plasma volume and to increase blood viscosity.

Third, elevation of blood pressure does not necessarily indicate comparable increases in cardiac output and tissue blood flow. Other indexes, such as urine flow and skin temperature, should be used. An adequate urine flow usually indicates an intra-arterial pressure great enough to maintain cerebral blood flow.

CARDIOGENIC SHOCK When shock results from narrowing or blockage of the myocardial arterial system, the initial hemodynamic abnormalities are largely related to the loss of functioning cardiac muscle. Pump efficiency is lowered and so is cardiac output. Diastolic arterial pressure falls and the length of diastole may be shortened if tachycardia or arrhythmias are present. Consequently, coronary perfusion may be reduced even further, causing additional myocardial insufficiency. In other types of shock in which the heart is presumed to be normal, compensatory coronary vasodilation protects the heart from moderate reductions in diastolic pressure. In patients with myocardial arterial disease. coronary vasodilation is already at the maximum level. However, perfusion requirements may be somewhat less because blood pressure is low and the work being done by the body is less. Cardiac output falls to a point which varies with the remaining blood supply.

As in any low-flow shock, measures must be instituted to increase tissue blood flow and, ideally, to minimize further cardiac damage by increasing coronary blood flow. One way to do this is by decreasing cardiac work so that the available coronary flow can meet myocardial requirements. Vasodilators may reduce cardiac work by reducing diastolic blood pressure but coronary blood flow will also be reduced, which counteracts the effects of decreasing the cardiac workload.

Conversely, an absolute increase in flow may be produced by raising arterial and, thus, coronary perfusion pressure, unless obstruction is complete. But drugs which raise diastolic blood pressure also increase cardiac work and thereby myocardial oxygen requirements. There is, then, a therapeutic dilemma and each patient's condition requires careful evaluation.

There is no practical way to determine at the bedside whether or not

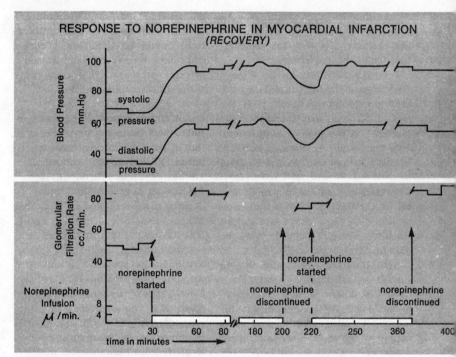

RESPONSE TO NOREPINEPHRINE IN MYOCARDIAL INFARCTION
(RECOVERY)

Renal function was at first moderately depressed in a patient whose blood pressure responded to norephinephrine, but renal blood flow and glomerular filtration rates quickly returned toward normal. Except for a slight decrease when the norepinephrine was discontinued briefly, both blood pressure and renal function were maintained at nearly normal levels and remained stable even after the drug was stopped at the end of six hours.

the effect on flow versus that on myocardial metabolic requirements produced by either type of drug is advantageous. It is difficult to determine readily whether a change in a patient's condition is spontaneous or drug induced. Unfortunately, only a few studies have been done which give sufficient relevant statistics to make therapeutic judgments.

Survival studies in patients, although often not well controlled, suggest that survival rate is increased by such drugs as norepinephrine, metaraminol, and mephentermine (Wyamine)(4). Experimental cardiogenic shock indicates that, at least for short periods in some situations, certain alpha-beta adrenergic stimulators may be beneficial. They may restore to or toward normal the cardiac output, blood pressure, and certain rhythm disturbances. Beta stimulators also appear to increase cardiac output and regional blood flow.

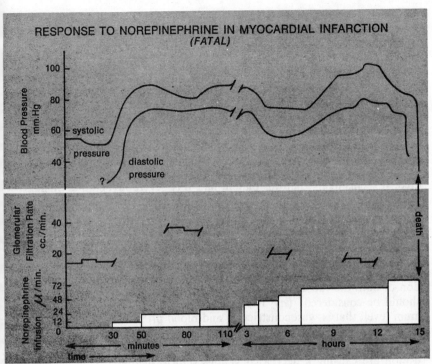

RESPONSE TO NOREPINEPHRINE IN MYOCARDIAL INFARCTION
(FATAL)

A patient in severe shock as a result of an MI had only minimal renal function when norepinephrine was started. Despite fairly good blood pressure response to increasingly large doses of the vasopressor, renal function improved for only a short time and then decreased steadily until death (15 hours post-MI).

When adrenergic stimulators are used for more than a few hours, the response must be evaluated carefully. For example, patient A was admitted with an acute MI and shock. His blood pressure was 70/35; his renal blood flow dropped rapidly from 1,000 ml. to 285 ml./min. Norepinephrine infusion at 6 mcg./min. raised his blood pressure to 96/55, an increase in mean pressure from approximately 47 to 68 mm. Hg. Renal blood flow increased to 650 ml./min. This improvement was maintained, so it was possible to decrease the infusion rate and after six hours to discontinue norepinephrine. No further hypotension occurred and the patient eventually recovered. Of course, the patient might have responded similarly without norepinephrine, but his rapid response to therapy and the absence of any upward trend during three 10-minute control periods suggest that the observed response was true drug effect.

Patient B also was admitted with an MI and shock. His condition was clinically more severe. His blood pressure could be heard at 50 mm. Hg; the pulse pressure was narrow. Renal blood flow was 88 ml./min. After institution of norepinephrine therapy, his blood pressure was 84/72. Renal blood flow increased slightly initially, but only to 190 ml./min. at a time when norepinephrine was being given at 24 mcg./min., a rate four times greater than in patient A. During the succeeding hours, his blood pressure was maintained with increasing amounts of norepinephrine but, as subsequent renal function data showed, at the expense of increasing vasoconstriction and decreasing renal blood flow to levels below the pretreatment shock level. Patient B developed ventricular fibrillation and died. It seems likely that this patient had very severe myocardial damage and that raising his blood pressure, although adequate to maintain cerebral blood flow, was subsequently fruitless because of his deteriorating cardiac status.

Nonetheless, prolonged maintenance of blood pressure at the expense of flow is unwarranted. Finding that ever larger amounts of vasopressors are "required" to maintain blood pressure demands immediate reevaluation of both the therapy and the patient's condition. Several possibilities should be considered: (a) The dosage is excessive and above the optimum level; that is, vasoconstriction and blood pressure have been raised higher than the minimum required levels and are unnecessarily increasing cardiac work. (b) The reduced plasma volume and hemoconcentration are causing a decreased venous return, increased compensatory vasoconstriction, and increased effective peripheral resistance. (c) The blood pH or electrolyte balance or both need to be corrected. (d) The extent of the infarction is so great that recovery is impossible.

The danger of plasma volume depletion and hemoconcentration are real ones in the patient with cardiogenic shock and may be intensified by vasopressors.

ENDOTOXIC SHOCK In this situation, several events occur: There is venular constriction and increased arterial flow to some vascular beds, which result in pooling. Circulating blood volume decreases and, of course, venous return and cardiac output then decrease. Although output produced by some adrenergic stimulators may be of value in elevating perfusion pressure and increasing cardiac output in severe hypotensive episodes while more appropriate therapy is being instituted, the prolonged use of adrenergic stimulators alone does not seem to be of ultimate value and, in some situations, is deleterious(5).

To test this hypothesis further, we gave six dogs metaraminol alone (in minimal amounts of saline) as soon as their blood pressures began to fall. We maintained their blood pressures at about the pre-endotoxin control levels. Initially, cardiac output was maintained better in the treated than in the untreated endotoxin control group. Between three and six hours after administration of metaraminol, the untreated group average declined sharply because three animals died. But after six hours, the average cardiac output in the treated group did not differ significantly from the nontreated group. The respective six-hour mortality rates were 50 percent (treated) and 46 percent (untreated).

CLINICAL USE OF VASOPRESSORS IN SHOCK

HEMORRHAGIC SHOCK If a patient is in severe shock and the basic cause cannot be corrected, it makes no difference what measures are taken to improve the blood pressure because the patient will die.

In hemorrhagic shock, blood flow studies show that in a moderately hypotensive state, a substantial increase in blood pressure may be achieved by giving norepinephrine, which will improve visceral blood flow in general. But the improvement is only temporary; the definitive treatment is to replace the blood as rapidly as possible. Transfusion is specific and much more effective than vasopressors.

As visceral blood flow increases, so do urine and sodium excretion. In fact, urinary output reflects well the rate and adequacy of the renal blood flow. However, a patient suffering from shock due to mercury poisoning, for example, would have renal failure on the basis of renal damage as well as generalized tissue toxicity. Increasing this patient's blood pressure would have little effect on his prognosis.

CARDIOGENIC SHOCK Vasopressor drugs are best used to treat acute hypotension that occurs in myocardial infarction (coronary occlusion). The survival rate following coronary occulusion depends almost completely on the severity of the infarction. Vasopressors are used to keep the blood pressure within normal range, but only as adjunctive thereapy. Mills, in a study of survival after coronary occlusion, compared the response obtained with norepinephrine to that obtained with metaraminol(6). He found the blood pressure response to be the same with both drugs. Metaraminol, however, is apparently less likely to produce arrhythmias. Although it is not as potent as norepinephrine, metaraminol seemed to yield a better survival rate in this particular study.

When a patient becomes hypotensive following an acute MI, the renal blood flow and glomerular filtration rate are reduced below normal. In fact, oliguria or anuria is a rough index of the severity of the circulatory derangement. Renal blood flow may not be severely disturbed in a patient whose lowest blood pressure is 70/38, but it is severely depressed in a patient whose blood pressure is 50/0 or less. In treating such a patient, an increasing amount of norepinephrine is necessary, despite the possibility of harmful effects, if the patient's condition is deteriorating and if irreversible cerebral damage is to be prevented. When some myocardial function returns, chances for recovery improve.

Care is essential in choosing and administering a vasopressor agent, and familiarity with the primary disease being treated is necessary if the correct vasopressor agent is to be used at the correct time. There is little doubt that these agents are helpful and effective, under the right circumstances.

REFERENCES

1. RODMAN, M. J., AND SMITH, D. W. *Pharmacology and Drug Therapy in Nursing.* Philadelphia, J. B. Lippincott Co., 1968, p. 225.
2. *Ibid.,* p. 228.
3. MOYER, J. H., AND OTHERS. Effect of morphine and n-allylnormorphine on cerebral hemodynamics and oxygen metabolism. *Circulation* 15:379-384, Mar. 1957.
4. MILLS, L. C., AND EMKEY, R. D. Pharmacologic properties and comparative efficacy of norepinephrine and metaraminol. IN *Cardiovascular Drug Therapy,* ed. by A. N. Brest and J. H. Moyer. New York, Grune and Stratton, 1965, pp. 110-117.
5. GOURZIS, J. T., AND NICKERSON, M. Intraorgan blood flow distribution in shock. IN *Shock and Hypotension,* ed. by L. J. Mills and J. H. Moyer. New York, Grune and Stratton, 1965, pp. 289-294. *Op. cit.* Mills, pp. 110-117.

From the *American Journal of Nursing* 74:439-443, Mar. 1974.

Anticoagulant Therapy

RUTH MAYER SHAPIRO

Anticoagulants have been prescribed in the treatment of thromboembolic disease for more than 25 years. Heparin and the coumarin derivatives have been widely used and have reduced the mortality and morbidity from diseases such as pulmonary embolism(1). While few experts agree on the best way to give anticoagulants, their goals are the same: to provide effective coagulant therapy, to make administration of the anticoagulant comfortable and acceptable to the patient, and to minimize the incidence of side effects, particularly massive hemorrhage.

One major risk of a vascular disorder is potential occlusion. Blood clots can partially or completely obstruct vessels, either by forming and remaining in a vessel (a thrombus) or by dislodging and moving to another site (and embolus). Any interruption of blood flow in the arterial or venous sytem can precipitate grave sequelae. Treatment is aimed at preventing thrombus formation by decreasing the level of blood coagulability. Anticoagulants are used most commonly to treat venous thrombosis, pulmonary embolism, arterial embolism, disseminated intravascular coagulation, and acute myocardial infarction, as well as for prophylaxis where the risk of thromboembolic disease is high, as in the bedridden, postoperative patient.

There are three types of thrombi. The first is the arterial or white thrombus. This lesion, composed primarily of platelets, forms in areas of rapid blood flow where there is an abnormal or damaged vessel wall, for example, in an artery roughened and thickened by arteriosclerosis. Because anticoagulants have little effect on platelet function, these drugs are of questionable value in the treatment of the white thrombus, except perhaps to prevent clot formation distal to the occlusion. On the other

MS. SHAPIRO *is a clinical research nurse in heparin therapy at Beth Israel Hospital, Boston, Mass. Ms. Shapiro received her B.S.N. from the University of Michigan School of Nursing, Ann Arbor.*

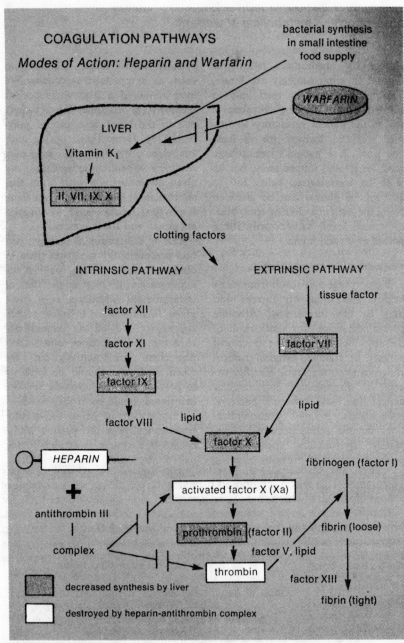

COAGULATION PATHWAYS

Modes of Action: Heparin and Warfarin

bacterial synthesis in small intestine food supply

WARFARIN

LIVER

Vitamin K_1

II, VII, IX, X

clotting factors

INTRINSIC PATHWAY

EXTRINSIC PATHWAY

tissue factor

factor XII

factor XI

factor IX

factor VIII

lipid

factor VII

lipid

factor X

HEPARIN

activated factor X (Xa)

fibrinogen (factor I)

+

antithrombin III

prothrombin (factor II)

fibrin (loose)

complex

factor V, lipid

thrombin

factor XIII

fibrin (tight)

decreased synthesis by liver

destroyed by heparin-antithrombin complex

Heparin acts directly on preformed clotting factors within the coagulation system. Warfarin acts indirectly, decreasing synthesis in the liver.

194

hand, the red thrombus forms typically where blood flows slowly, as in peripheral veins, and may not require an abnormal vessel lining. This thrombus consists primarily of red cells and fibrin. Anticoagulation can be used here to prevent the formation of fibrin.

The third type, referred to as disseminated intravascular coagulation (DIC), occurs when procoagulant material is released into the circulation, as in amniotic fluid embolism, sepsis, metastatic disease, malaria, or incompatible blood transfusions. Systemic clotting begins, depositing fibrin into small vessels throughout the body. Clotting factors are rapidly consumed and the fibrinolytic system is activated so that eventually both massive bleeding and widespread clotting may occur. This catastrophe is also amenable to anticoagulant therapy.

Blood clotting proceeds by two pathways: The intrinsic system, which includes clotting factors XII, XI, and VIII, is stimulated by the activation of factor XII at the surface of an injured vessel. The extrinsic pathway is activated by tissue damage and involves factor VII. Both pathways share factors X, VI, II (prothrombin), and factor I (fibrinogen).

ANTICOAGULANTS

Heparin acts by binding to a plasma co-factor (antithrombin III). This complex rapidly destroys both thrombin and activated factor X (Stuart), which are key clotting factors operative in both the intrinsic and extrinsic pathways of blood clotting. Heparin, therefore, acts immediately and directly to block blood clotting. Heparin does not affect a preformed thrombus other than to prevent its extension and to prevent the accumulation of platelets on the thrombus.

At high concentrations, heparin may also block the thrombin-controlled release of serotonin from platelets. Serotonin causes dyspnea and bronchospasm in patients with pulmonary embolism. Heparin is a strong organic acid which combines with numerous proteins, making its dosage range and possibly its duration of action vary widely in different patients and at different times. In the majority of patients, the half-life of heparin is approximately two hours. Most of the heparin is degraded in the liver, but about 20 percent is excreted through the kidneys. Patients with renal or hepatic disease may therefore build higher blood levels of this drug.

Warfarin acts in a different manner. Vitamin K_1, present in a normal diet and synthesized by bacteria in the small intestine, enables the liver to produce clotting factors II, VII, IX, and X. By interfering with the action of vitamin K, warfarin prevents the synthesis of those clotting factors and thereby affects the intrinsic system (factor IX), the extrinsic system (factor VII), and the common pathway (factors X and II).

HEPARIN	WARFARIN
Mode of action	
directly blocks action of factor Xa and thrombin	indirect; inhibits synthesis of factors II, VII, IX, X
Onset of therapeutic effect	
immediate	at least 3-6 days
Duration of action	
hours; half-life for I.V. heparin is 2 hours; effect gone in 4 to 6 hours	days, depending on dose, liver and renal function, diet
Route of administration	
I.V., SC preferred; IM	PO preferred; IM, I.V.
Reversibility	
immediate; I.V. protamine sulfate or plasma	delayed; vitamin K, IM, I.V., or PO: refractory period to warfarin follows; plasma
Control tests	
whole blood clotting time, partial thromboplastin time, thrombin time	prothrombin time
Appearance across placenta or in milk	
none	occurs

Heparin and warfarin are both potent anticoagulants yet they have substantial and important differences which affect their clinical usefulness.

Unlike heparin, however, warfarin does not immediately affect the coagulation system. Consequently heparin is used to initiate anticoagulation therapy when rapid protection against thrombosis is desired.

ADMINISTERING ANTICOAGULANTS

Heparin is not absorbed from the gastrointestinal tract, so it must be given parenterally. This can be done subcutaneously, or it can be given intravenously by continuous infusion or intermittently through a scalp-vein needle with a special rubber plug (heparin lock). Because muscle tissue is extremely vascular and bleeds easily, the IM route is not recommended. Subcutaneous heparin is often given to prevent thrombus formation in pre- and postoperative patients, usually in doses of 5,000 units every 8 to 12 hours. The advantages of giving heparin subcutaneously are that it is easy to give and requires no special I.V. setups. However, heparin may be inadvertently injected into muscle tissue and cause bleeding. The results of clotting tests are often difficult to interpret, due to the variable absorption rate by both the IM and SC routes.

When given intermittently by the intravenous route, heparin is injected every four to six hours. Its effects are immediate, dissipate quickly when the drug is discontinued, and are readily reversible if necessary. The administration itself is quite painless, once a scalp-vein needle is in place, provided the heparin is injected slowly, at a rate of 1 to 2 cc. per minute. When blood is drawn for clotting tests, it must be drawn at a precise time in relation to the last dose in order for the results of the test to be interpretable.

When heparin is given by continuous I.V. infusion, a constant level of anticoagulation may be maintained, that is, without periods of under anticoagulation or infinite clotting times. Other advantages of this method are that clotting tests may be drawn at any time, multiple injecions are avoided, usually less heparin is needed, and normal hemostasis can be restored in one to two hours after the drug is stopped. The anticoagulation effect can be reversed promptly.

Continuous infusion therapy, however, may be contraindicated in patients with fluid restrictions. Frequent nursing observations are necessary and the flow rate is often difficult to control even with an electric infusion pump. Moreover, the I.V. line may restrict the patient's mobility and can be a problem when other intravenous fluids must be given concurrently. No other medication should be given through the heparin line nor should heparin be piggy-backed into any other line. As a safety measure, a heparin solution, in 5 percent dextrose and water, should be prepared and hung in a quantity no greater than that needed for six hours.

As with any medication, patient response to heparin is extremely variable. Although our study of heparinized patients has disclosed no significant correlation of bleeding complication with age or sex, we suspect that body weight, renal and hepatic function, general state of health, and diet may all affect the heparin dosage required. In addition, individual patient's responses may vary from day to day and necessitate periodic dose changes. An individual's *response* to a given amount, not the amount itself, probably determines, at least to some extent, whether he will be protected from thrombosis or will hemorrhage.

Warfarin may be given IM, although it is generally given orally. Because it can be taken by mouth, it is often used for long-term anticoagulation therapy. Heparin and warfarin may be started at the same time; however, heparin should be continued for 7 to 10 days until the thrombus is firmly adherent to the endothelial wall or until factors predisposing to thrombosis are gone. The prothrombin time (PT), a laboratory measurement of warfarin's activity, must be 1½ to 2½ times greater than normal before it is safe to discontinue the heparin. The PT may rise to the "proper range" in one or two days, but this rise only indicates the fall of factor VII, which has the shortest half-life. This level is not anti-thrombotic and the patient will not be protected until factors IX, X, and II are also depressed, which may take three to six days. This would appear to argue against the "loading dose" theory that larger doses of warfarin should be given the first several days to elevate the PT quickly. In fact, loading doses may predispose the patient to hemorrhage but do not hasten the process that protects him from thrombosis. In our practice, 10 to 15 mg. of warfarin are given every day until the PT comes into the proper range. Thereafter, the dosage is adjusted to maintain that range.

Warfarin is generally given once daily; the dose is adjusted to keep the prothrombin time between 1½ to 2½ times the control time (18 to 30 sec.). The control or normal value must be predetermined in each clinical laboratory where the test is performed, but usually runs between 11 and 14 seconds. With heparin, however, no clinical trial has yet proved that the use of any clotting test will prevent complications, either thrombotic or hemorrhagic. This is probably because a clotting test can represent heparin activity only at a specific moment whereas heparin effect actually varies considerably from moment to moment.

At the Beth Israel Hospital, Boston, we are now conducting a long-term, prospective clinical study to answer some questions about heparin therapy. All consenting patients who are to receive intravenous heparin are randomly enrolled in one of three treatment regimens. One group gets an amount of heparin every four hours that will keep the activated partial thromboplastin time (PTT) within a specified range three hours after the dose of heparin. The second group receives heparin every four hours, but the dose is predetermined on the basis of body weight (75 to 125 units per kilogram per dose) and remains constant throughout the course of therapy. Heparin dosage is expressed in units. One mg. is required to have a biological activity greater than 120 units. But for rough calculations, 1 mg. is considered equivalent to 100 units. The third group receives heparin continuously by an IVAC continuous infusion pump and the dose is adjusted to maintain the PTT within a specified range. Results of each regimen will be analyzed according to a fixed protocol.

Currently in most hospitals, heparin is given every four hours either with or without clotting studies to regulate the dosage. If one employs clotting tests as a guide to therapy, the two most common tests are the Lee-White clotting time, done on whole blood, and the activated partial thromboplastin time, using plasma. In our experience, these tests correlate well with each other; we prefer the PTT because it is easy to perform, can be reproduced, and is accurate. As with PT, the heparin dose is adjusted to keep the PTT between 1½ and 2½ times normal, approximately 50 to 80 seconds in our laboratory.

When heparin and warfarin are given simultaneously, one should be aware that the heparin may affect the PT used to control the dose of warfarin. At low doses of heparin, the effect is minimal; but at high doses of heparin, the PT may be prolonged by several seconds and too low a dose of warfarin may be given.

In an emergency, heparin effect may be reversed by giving protamine sulfate I.V. in a dosage of 1 mg. of protamine sulfate per 100 units of the last dose of heparin. However, if a gross excess of protamine is given, it, too, may delay clotting. Subcutaneous heparin, because of its variable absorption rate, should be neutralized by small doses of protamine at spaced intervals. As an antidote to coumarin derivatives, vitamin K or phytonadione (Aquamephyton) will restore factor synthesis in the liver and is used in cases of induced hypoprothrombinemia. When vitamin K is given IM or I.V., hemostasis returns to normal in approximately six hours. Vitamin K should be used only to combat frank bleeding because it makes the patient refractory to further warfarin therapy for at least one week. If a patient's hemorrhage must be treated immediately, but he is to be warfarinized later, 250 to 500 ml. of plasma can be given to bring the patient's clotting time back to normal levels satisfactorily for a period of several hours.

PRECAUTIONS AND CONTRAINDICATIONS

Hemorrhage may result from many known and unknown factors and may be life threatening. Absolute contraindications for anticoagulant therapy include recent intracranial surgery or trauma, cerebral hemorrhage from stroke, frank bleeding except in disseminated intravascular coagulation, and subacute bacterial endocarditis. Relative contraindications include active duodenal ulcer, platelet dysfunction, thrombocytopenia, a history of previous bleeding on anticoagulation, marked diastolic hypertension, or recent surgery—especially where large, friable areas exist, as in prostatic resections. We have observed a high incidence of hemorrhagic complications, largely due to the injudicious use of polypharmacy. Hemorrhage during anticoagulant therapy is especially common when anticoagulants are given in conjunction with drugs that affect platelet function or when there is physical trauma, such as surgery, accidents, and IM injections.

During anticoagulant therapy, certain precautionary measures must be observed strictly. Large, painful hematomas can develop at the sites of intramuscular injections, *even those given 10 days prior to starting anticoagulants.* We tell our patients not to accept IM injections unless their physicians are actually in the room. Bed rails should be kept up to prevent falls and trauma and the call signal should be in easy reach.

Platelets are of prime importance hemostatically in the patient whose coagulation system is artificially impaired by anticoagulants. Drugs which interfere with the platelet-release reaction are to be avoided. These drugs include antihistamines, phenothiazines, indomethacin, phenylbutazone, glyceryl guaiacolate, and any of the more than 500 aspirin-containing compounds available commercially. In addition, patients on warfarin therapy should not add or delete those drugs known to depress or enhance the action of warfarin, for example, ACTH, adrenocorticosteroids, antibiotics, quinine, and quinidine, as well as various sleeping medications(2).

One should keep in mind, too, that anticoagulants may affect the action of other drugs; for example, warfarin may potentiate the action of tolbutamide and heparin may do the same to insulin(3). One should be alert for any signs of hypoglycemia and recognize that this particular patient's need for antidiabetic agents may fluctuate.

NURSING INTERVENTION

Since preventing complications is better than discovering them, a few more precautions are vital. A nurse should always be aware of any medications ordered for her anticoagulated patient. New medications should be checked with the pharmacy to be sure they do not contain any of the harmful drugs just mentioned. Any questions should be referred immediately to the physician. Intramuscular injection orders should be questioned. At the Beth Israel Hospital, a sign is placed over the patient's bed which states "No IM's, ASA-containing compounds, phenothiazines, or antihistamines." Potentially dangerous situations can be decreased by avoiding arterial and femoral vein punctures and by frequently checking scalp-vein needles and I.V.'s for signs of infiltration. The latter sites should be carefully protected to prevent dislodgement of needles and catheters.

Daily blood studies should all be drawn at one time, if possible, to avoid multiple venipunctures. After removing I.V.'s or drawing blood, one must maintain pressure at the puncture site for at least three minutes, not just until the bleeding stops. Elderly patients, who have decreased venous-wall elasticity, may require a longer time.

When we draw blood for a clotting test, we use a 19- or 21-gauge, scalp-vein needle and two syringes. Two cc. of blood are drawn into the first syringe. The tubing is occluded and a new syringe is added. Then, 4.5 cc. are drawn and added to a Vacutainer citrate tube and gently tilted several times. Care is taken not to bubble the blood when drawing or mixing. The first 2 to 3 cc. of blood are not used for a PT or PTT as they contain thromboplastin which can activate the coagulation pathway, but this blood may be used for any other test. Tissue thromboplastin is released in minute quantities from the vein wall at the time of venipuncture; the first 2 or 3 cc. of blood will flush the needle.

For clotting studies, blood is never drawn from an I.V. line without first copiously flushing it with saline to remove any traces of heparin used to keep the line open. Also, if the same arm is to be used, blood should not be drawn proximal to the heparin administration site. Blood samples should be sent to the laboratory in cups of ice to preserve the clotting factors. Any marked fluctuation from expected values of PT, PTT, or hematocrit should be pointed out immediately to the patient's physician.

Early detection may help to reduce the consequences of bleeding complications. Patients and their families, as well as staff, should be taught to recognize these danger signs: darkened urine or frank hematuria; black, tarry stools; abdominal or flank pain; increased menstrual bleeding (with pad counts if necessary); joint pain or immobility; head pain or change in neurological status; hematomas, especially at IM or I.V. sites; nasal or gum bleeding; and vomiting or coughing blood. For the hospitalized patient, one should also watch for incisional hematomas or bloody drainage, or bleeding from thoracentesis or cutdown sites; all stools should be tested for occult blood. Fecal specimens from menstruating women must be obtained by rectal exam if sanitary pads are used. Urinalysis for red cells should be done routinely. And, of course, vital signs are taken regularly.

When heparin is given intermittently, all schedules should be strictly adhered to because the time between each dose is most important. If a dose is unavoidably delayed by more than 15 minutes, the next dose should be delayed the same time to keep the interval constant. Continuous infusions should not be "caught up" if the infusion has slowed down. The drop rate should be adjusted to restore the proper dose per hour. Many infusion pumps count the drop rate not the drop size. So, if the solution is running in too quickly, the I.V. set may need to be changed to obtain the correct drop size. Heparin doses should never be skipped even if the patient leaves the unit. Coagulation levels could fall dangerously near normal, or even to a hypercoaguable state, and thus expose the patient to the unnecessary risk of a recurrent thromboembolic episode.

When the anticoagulated patient goes home, he may continue on warfarin for a short time or indefinitely. It is imperative that the nurse and physician determine that the patient will continue his anticoagulation in a safe, effective manner. All doctors and dentists who treat the patient should know that he is taking warfarin. Dangerous activities or hobbies may need to be curtailed. Patients who are anticoagulated and their families may be justifiably concerned or frightened about the idea of resuming a normal life because the risks of both rethrombosis or hemorrhage are quite real to them. Explanations about heparin or warfarin should be repeated and reinforced, and learning should be evaluated carefully since anxiety decreases one's receptivity to new information. A reliable family member or friend, therefore, should always be included in these discussions.

The importance of taking warfarin regularly, according to schedule, should be emphasized. A calendar marked with the dose for each day could be checked off each night when the pill is taken. The diet should not have an overabundance or deficiency of foods containing vitamin K. Excessive drinking is to be discouraged. The nurse should caution the patient not to discontinue any present medications or take any new one without first checking with his physician. This includes cold remedies, antacids, sleeping pills, vitamins, or birth control pills. Laxatives and mineral oil may decrease the absorption of vitamin K and warfarin and should be avoided. Again, these patients should know the signs that could indicate bleeding and should have the physician's or hospital's telephone number on hand. We believe strongly that patients are not to be routinely given vitamin K tablets to carry with them if doctors are readily accessible.

Diarrhea, vomiting, or febrile illnesses should be reported promptly because these could affect absorption and metabolism of warfarin. Ideally, an anticoagulated patient at home should be followed by one doctor who is fully familiar with the patient's history and who is concerned enough and able to provide adequate follow-up care. With these precautions, we believe that most patients can take anticoagulants with a minimal risk of bleeding.

REFERENCES

1. BARRITT, D. W., AND JORDAN, S. C. Anticoagulant drugs in the treatment of pulmonary embolism: a controlled trial. *Lancet* 1:1309-1312, June 18, 1960.

2. KOPROWICZ, D. C. Drug interactions with coumarin derivatives. *Am.J.Nurs.* 73:1042-1044, June 1973.
3. TUTTLE, C. B. *Drug interactions. Can.J.Hosp.Pharm.* 22:25-51, May-June 1969.

BIBLIOGRAPHY

DEYKIN, DANIEL. Thrombogenesis. *N.Engl.J.Med.* 276:622-628, Mar. 16, 1967.
————. Current concepts: the use of heparin. *N.Engl.J.Med.* 280:937-938, Apr. 24, 1969.
————. Warfarin therapy. Parts 1 and 2. *N.Engl.J.Med.* 283:691-694, 801-803, Sept. 24, Oct. 8, 1970.
GOODMAN, LOUIS, AND GILMAN, ALFRED EDS. *Pharmacological Basis of Thrapeutics.* 4th ed. New York, Macmillan Co., 1970.
SALZMAN, E. W., AND BRITTEN, ANTHONY. *Hemorrhage and Thrombosis: a Practical Clinical Guide.* Boston, Little, Brown and Co., 1965.
SWANSON, MARGO, AND CACACE, LARRY. Heparin therapy by continuous intravenous infusion. *Am.J.Hosp.Pharm.* 28:792-795, Oct. 1971.

From the *American Journal of Nursing* 73:1042-1044, June 1973.

Drug Interactions with Coumarin Derivatives

DIANNE C. KOPROWICZ

Many people with thromboembolic disorders are being treated with coumarin derivatives on a long-term basis. Many of them have other medical problems which require therapy with additional drugs during coumarin therapy. In recent years, increasing numbers of drugs have become available that interact with coumarin derivatives by potentiating or inhibiting their effects. Potentiating drugs may precipitate hemorrhage; inhibiting drugs may decrease the anticoagulant effects of coumarin derivatives and leave patients liable to thrombus formation.

The coumarin derivatives (acenocoumarol, bishydroxycoumarin, cyclocumarol, ethyl biscoumacetate, phenoprocoumon, sodium warfarin) are absorbed from the gastrointestinal tract. Most of the absorbed coumarin is bound to albumin in the plasma. Coumarins that are bound to plasma proteins are pharmacologically inactive and are not excreted(1). The free coumarin (not bound to plasma protein) is able to exert its pharmacological effect. Free coumarin is metabolized in the liver and its breakdown products are excreted in the urine. As free coumarin is metabolized, the protein-bound coumarin is gradually released and becomes pharmacologically active. The anticoagulant effects of the coumarins last from two to seven days after the last dose, depending on the drug and dose use(2).

The coumarins act by antagonizing vitamin K in the liver. The presence of vitamin K is necessary in the formation of prothrombin. The result of coumarin therapy is a relative hypoprothrombinemia which retards formation of intravascular clots in thromboembolic disorders.

MS. KOPROWICZ *is an assistant professor of nursing at California State University, San Diego. She is a graduate of Jersey City Hospital School of Nursing, Jersey City, N.J. and received her B.A. from Jersey City State College and an M.A. from New York University.*

When a patient is first treated with coumarins, he is usually hospitalized. Initially, his prothrombin time is checked daily and the dosage regulated accordingly. The prothrombin time should be maintained at 1½ to 2 times the normal control time for maximum therapeutic effectiveness(3). The dosages of coumarins given on the first and second days of therapy are generally larger than the maintenance dose because approximately 90 percent of the coumarin is bound to plasma proteins and therefore only a small portion of the dose is free to act(4). The time needed to reach therapeutic levels depends on the drug selected and individual differences among patients(3).

After a patient has been maintained on the same dose of coumarin for several days, he is discharged from the hospital if there are no other problems. His prothrombin time should be monitored frequently: at least once a week for the first month and every two or three weeks thereafter, if the patient appears well controlled.

The chief complication of coumarin therapy is hemorrhage due to marked hypoprothrombinemia. Administering vitamin K, 5 to 10 mg. orally, and omitting one or two doses of coumarin are usually sufficient to control bleeding or shorten an excessively prolonged prothrombin time. In severe hemorrhage, the patient may require a transfusion of whole blood(5).

Drugs which interact with coumarin derivatives fall into the following categories: drugs that affect vitamin K, drugs that compete with coumarins for plasma protein binding, drugs that inhibit or accelerate coumarin metabolism in the liver, and drugs that inhibit or stimulate synthesis of the clotting factor.

Vitamin K is a fat-soluble vitamin that is adequately supplied in most diets. It is also synthesized by intestinal bacteria. Neomycin, chloramphenicol, and chlortetracycline have been shown to reduce bacterial synthesis of vitamin K, thereby reducing the amount of available vitamin K and potentiating the effects of coumarins(6). Cholestyramine resin prevents absorption of vitamin K by trapping bile salts, thereby increasing the effects of coumarins(7). Anabolic steroids, thyroid preparations, and clofibrate decrease serum lipid concentrations and thereby decrease circulating vitamin K and potentiate the effects of coumarins(8). Phenothiazines may induce cholestasis with resulting diminished absorption of vitamin K and potentiation of the effects of coumarins(9).

Drugs that compete with coumarin to bind with plasma proteins displace protein-bound coumarin and increase the amount of free-plasma coumarin, thereby increasing anticoagulation. Chloral hydrate, phenylbutazone, oxyphenbutazone, diazoxide, ethacrynic acid, nalidixic acid, mefanamic acid, sulfinpyrazone, long acting sulfonamides, and indomethacin may all potentiate coumarins by this mechanism(6,10).

Drugs that inhibit metabolism of coumarins in the liver include phenyramidol, allopurinol, methylphenidate, nortriptyline, diphenylhydantoin, disulfiram, tolbutamide, and mercaptopurine. These drugs inhibit the breakdown of coumarins, cause coumarin build-up, and may enhance the action of the coumarins(6,9). Drugs which accelerate coumarin metabolism in the liver may limit the effectiveness of coumarin. These drugs include barbiturates, glutethimide, ethchlorvynol, griseofulvin, and meprobamate(6).

Some drugs stimulate or inhibit clotting factor synthesis. Those that stimulate clotting factor synthesis are adrenocortical hormones and oral contraceptives. These tend to offset coumarin activity. Drugs which inhibit clotting factor synthesis are glucagon, quinidine, and salicylates. These enhance the effects of coumarins(6).

When a patient is being treated with coumarins, it is best if he can avoid taking drugs that are known to interact with the anticoagulant. Since there are so many of these drugs and since patients often have multiple problems requiring treatment with other drugs, this is not always possible. Many drugs that interact with coumarin derivatives can be taken with relative safety along with the coumarins, providing appropriate precautions are observed.

When coumarin therapy is begun, the patient should continue to use those drugs he must take routinely. In this way, his prothrombin time can be stabilized realistically in the presence of other drugs while he is hospitalized. The patient's prothrombin time should be checked frequently and his coumarin dosage adjusted as necessary whenever a drug which interacts with coumarin is added to or eliminated from his regimen.

While the patient is in the hospital, the nurse must be aware of all drugs the patient is taking. All new medication orders must be checked to determine if any of them interact with coumarin. Some drugs that are often used on a p.r.n. basis, such as barbiturates, glutethemide, and salicylates, should not be given at all. Occasionally, more than one physician writes medication orders for a patient. Or the physician may forget that a drug he is ordering interacts with coumarins. When such a drug is ordered, the nurse should discuss the situation with the physician before she gives it. If a drug that interacts with coumarins is added or eliminated, the nurse must be certain the prothrombin time is checked frequently. The physician should be notified if the prothrombin time is less than 1½ times the control or more than double the control time. Either

DRUGS WHICH INTERACT WITH COUMARIN DERIVATIVES

Generic Name or Group	Brand Name	Action on Coumarins
Adrenocortical Steroids	Acthar, Delta-Cortef, Meticortelone, Deltasone, Cortef, others	Inhibits
Allopurinol	Zyloprim	Potentiates
Barbiturates	Amytal, Seconal, Luminal, Nembutal, others	Inhibits
Chloral Hydrate	Noctec, Felsules, Somnos, Hydral, others	Potentiates
Chloramphenicol	Chloromycetin	Potentiates
Cholestyramine resin	Questran, Cuemid	Inhibits
Clofibrate	Atromid-S	Potentiates
Diazoxide	Hyperstat	Potentiates
Diphenylhydantoin	Dilantin, Phenytoin	Potentiates
Disulfiram	Antabuse	Potentiates
Ethacrynic Acid	Edecrin	Potentiates
Ethchlorvynol	Placidyl	Inhibits
Glucagon		Potentiates
Glutethimide	Doriden	Inhibits
Griseofulvin	Fulvicin, Grifulvin	Inhibits
Indomethacin	Indocin	Potentiates
Mefenamic Acid	Ponstel	Potentiates
Mebrobamate	Miltown, Equanil, Meprospan	Inhibits
Mercaptopurine	Purinethol	Potentiates
Methandrostenolone	Dianabol	Potentiates
Methylphenidate	Ritalin	Potentiates
Nalidixic Acid	NegGram	Potentiates
Neomycin	Mycifradin, Neobiotic	Potentiates
Nortriptyline	Aventyl	Potentiates
Oral Contraceptives	Ortho-Novum, Norinyl, Enovid-E, C-Quens, others	Inhibits
Oxphenbutazone	Tandearil	Potentiates
Phenothiazines	Thorazine, Sparine, Compazine, Stelazine, Mellaril, others	Potentiates
Phenylbutazone	Butazolidin	Potentiates
Phenylramidol	Analexin	Potentiates
Quinidine	Cardioquin, Quinaglute	Potentiates
Salicylates	Aspirin, Bufferin, Empirin, APC, Darvon Compound, others	Potentiates
Sulfinpyrazone	Anturane	Potentiates
Sulfonamides (long-acting)	Kynex, Madribon, Madriqid, Levisul, others	Potentiates
Thyroid drugs	Thyroid extract, Proloid, Thyroxin, Cytomel, Synthroid, Choloxin	Potentiates
Tolbutamide	Orinase	Potentiates

development usually indicates that the dosage of coumarin should be altered. Whenever a drug that enhances the effects of coumarin is added to a patient's regimen, the nurse must observe the patient more frequently for signs of internal or external bleeding.

Before leaving the hospital, the patient and his family must learn the actions of coumarins and the precautions required to prevent or minimize complications. The content of the instructions to the patient should be planned by the nurse and physician together to avoid confusion. Teaching should be geared to the patient's needs and capacity to learn.

Before beginning patient teaching, the nurse must evaluate the patient's readiness to retain and use the information. Some patients view taking a medication on a long-term basis as a threat to their independence. Some deny the fact that they are ill and resist taking medication. The nurse will have to identify these feelings and help patients to work them through before they will be ready to learn all details about their medications.

The directions for taking the medication should be reviewed with the patient. It is a good idea to provide tablets of only one strength to eliminate confusion. The patient should be cautioned not to begin or stop *any* medication unless he first checks with the physician responsible for his coumarin therapy. This includes over-the-counter drugs, such as cold preparations, which may contain aspirin, and multivitamins, which may contain vitamin K.

Any abnormal bleeding should be reported to the physician immediately. This includes rectal bleeding, vaginal bleeding, excessive menstrual flow, nasal or skin bleeding, and discolored urine. Some physicians prescribe vitamin K for the patient to carry at all times and use in case of severe bleeding. If this is done, the nurse should review the directions for the use of vitamin K with the patient. The patient should notify his physician if he plans to have minor surgery or tooth extractions. Most physicians discontinue coumarin before these procedures to lessen the risk of hemorrhage. Activities that carry a high risk of injury, such as contact sports, should be avoided.

Patients should avoid excessive use of alcohol and foods which cause diarrhea or vomiting. The superficial gastritis which often results from prolonged drinking can precipitate hemorrhage. Diarrhea or vomiting may inhibit the absorption of coumarins(11).

The patient can obtain a card from the American Heart Association that gives the name and telephone number of his physician and the fact that he is taking anticoagulants. This information is important in the event of accident, severe injury, or bleeding.

The prothrombin time is the most important tool for measuring the effectiveness of the coumarins and protecting the patient from hemorrhage. Therefore, emphasis should be placed on the importance of periodic prothrombin time measurements.

REFERENCES

1. KOCH-WESER, JAN, AND SELLERS, E. M. Drug interactions with coumarin anticoagulants. Part 1. *N.Engl.J.Med.* 285:490, Aug. 26, 1971.
2. AMERICAN MEDICAL ASSOCIATION, COUNCIL ON DRUGS. *American Medical Association Drug Evaluations.* Chicago, The Association, 1971, p. 67.
3. WRIGHT, IRVING Anticoagulant therapy: 1971. *Drug Therapy* 1:13, Jan. 1971.
4. KOCH-WESER, *op.cit.*, p. 489.
5. WRIGHT, *op.cit.*, p. 16.
6. KOCH-WESER, JAN, AND SELLERS, E. M. Drug interactions with coumarin anti-coagulants, Part 2. *N.Engl.J.Med.* 285:549, Sept. 2, 1971
7. DEYKIN, DANIEL. Warfarin interaction. *Drug Therapy* 1:8, Jan. 1974.
8. KOCH-WESER, AND SELLERS E. M. Drug interactions with coumarin anticoagulants, Part 2. *N.Engl.J.Med.* 285:551, Sept. 2, 1971.
9. EIPIE, JOSEPH. Drugs affecting therapy with anticoagulants. *Med.Clin.North Am.* 56:256, Jan. 1972.
10. DEYKIN, *op.cit.*, p. 21.
11. WALDMAN, SAMUEL Anticoagulant therapy: for and against. *Consultant* 6:12, Oct. 1966.

BIBLIOGRAPHY

CECIL, R. L., AND LOEB, R. F. Textbook of Medicine. 13th edition edited by P. B. Beeson and Walsh McDermott. Philadelphia, W. B. Saunders Co., 1971.
GUYTON, A. C. *Textbook of Medical Physiology.* 3rd ed. Philadelphia, W. B. Saunders Co., 1966.
Physicians Desk Reference to Pharmaceutical Specialites and Biologicals. Oradell, N.J., Medical Economics, 1972.
SEAMAN, ARTHUR, AND OTHERS. Long-term anticoagulant prophylaxis after myocardial infarction. *N.Engl.J.Med.* 281:115-119, July 17, 1969.

From the *American Journal of Nursing* 74:1442-1446, Aug. 1974.

Drug Interactions of Common CCU Medications

ARTHUR F. SHINN • **DAVID N. COLLINS**
ELLEN J. HOOPS

The patient who is receiving Isuprel and Inderal may show no therapeutic effects from their use because these drugs antagonize each other.

Most patients receive several different drugs during their hospitalization, many concomitantly. No nurse can afford to ignore the possible physical and pharmacological drug interactions that can and do occur. Many drugs are given intravenously. They are potent agents, and combination therapy is frequent. The nursing staff in our cardiac care unit at William Beaumont Hospital, Royal Oak, Michigan, identified 22 commonly used drugs and asked the hospital's Drug Information Center for data on interactions.

With this information, we formulated two charts that serve as guide-

DR. SHINN *is assistant director of clinical services and clinical education, department of pharmaceutical services, William Beaumont Hospital, Royal Oak, Mich., and adjunct assistant professor of clinical pharmacy, Wayne State University, Detroit, Mich. He received his B.S. degree from Brooklyn College of Pharmacy, Long Island University, Brooklyn, N.Y., and Pharm. D. degree from the University of Michigan, Ann Arbor. MR. COLLINS is a staff pharmacist at William Beaumont Hospital. He received his B.S. degree from Northeastern University College of Pharmacy, Boston, Mass. MS. HOOPS was an instructor, department of nursing education, William Beaumont Hospital, at the time this paper was written. She was responsible for staff development courses concerning critical care and pharmacology. She was graduated from Blodgett Memorial Hospital School of Nursing, Grand Rapids, Mich., and received a B.S.N. degree from Calvin College, Grand Rapids, Mich.*

	aminophylline	ampicillin	atropine	calcium	Coumadin	Demerol	digoxin	Dilantin	glucagon	Heparin	Inderal	Isuprel	Lasix	Levophed	morphine	nitroglycerin	potassium	Pronestyl	Prostaphlin	quinidine	Tensilon	Valium	Xylocaine
aminophylline					X																		
ampicillin					X																		
atropine					X						X	X	X	X				X			X	X	
calcium					X																		
Coumadin	X	X				X	X	X	X			X		X				X	X		X	X	
Demerol			X		X										X							X	X
digoxin and other cardiac glycosides			X	X	X			X			X	X	X	X				X	X	X			
Dilantin			X		X						X		X							X		X	
glucagon					X																		
Heparin			X		X													X					
Inderal			X		X						X	X	X	X	X			X	X				
Isuprel		X			X						X							X					
Lasix		X			X	X					X			X								X	
Levophed		X									X	X			X								
morphine		X	X								X									X	X		
nitroglycerin		X			X						X	X		X									
potassium					X																		
Pronestyl		X			X						X							X	X			X	
Prostaphlin			X		X									X									
quinidine		X	X		X	X		X			X							X		X		X	X
Tensilon		X			X						X							X	X				
Valium		X	X		X			X				X	X										
Xylocaine											X	X											

"X" indicates an interaction between two drugs given concurrently or within the span of action of either.

lines to drug interactions: one identifies physical incompatibilities and the other indicates possible pharmacological interactions. The chart of physical incompatibilities is offered without explanation, except to say that the incompatibilities are demonstrated by such physical means as cloudiness and precipitation.

Drug interaction is the phenomenon that occurs when one drug alters the effect of another drug given with it or during its span of action. A drug effect may be potentiated, antagonized, or otherwise changed by its specific interaction with another drug. These interactions can be detrimental or therapeutic. In fact, many drug regimens prescribed for a patient are based on the expected interaction of the drugs.

There are several mechanisms by which these drug interactions occur in the body: both drugs may have similar or opposite pharmacological

SIGNIFICANT PHYSICAL INCOMPATIBILITIES

	aminophylline	ampicillin	atropine	calcium	Coumadin	Demerol	digoxin and other cardiac glycosides	Dilantin	glucagon	Heparin	Inderal	Isuprel	Lasix	Levophed	morphine	potassium	Pronestyl	Prostaphlin	quinidine	Tensilon	Valium	Xylocaine
aminophylline		X			X	X		X				X		X	X						X	
ampicillin	X		X	X	X	X	X	X	X	X	X	X	X	X	X	X	X	X	X	X	X	X
atropine		X			X			X		X				X				X			X	
calcium		X					X	X													X	
Coumadin	X	X	X					X		X				X							X	
Demerol	X	X						X		X					X						X	
digoxin and other cardiac glycosides		X		X				X													X	
Dilantin	X	X	X	X	X	X	X		X	X	X	X	X	X	X	X	X	X	X	X	X	X
glucagon		X						X													X	
Heparin		X	X		X	X		X						X	X						X	
Inderal		X						X													X	
Isuprel	X	X						X													X	X
Lasix		X						X													X	
Levophed	X	X	X		X			X		X								X			X	X
morphine	X	X				X		X		X											X	
potassium		X						X													X	
Pronestyl		X						X													X	
Prostaphlin		X	X					X						X							X	
quinidine		X						X													X	
Tensilon		X						X													X	
Valium	X	X	X	X	X	X	X	X	X	X	X	X	X	X	X	X	X	X	X	X		X
Xylocaine		X						X				X		X							X	

"X" indicates a physical incompatibility (cloudiness, precipitation, and so forth) as a result of admixture.

effects; a drug may alter the gastrointestinal absorption of another drug; drug metabolism may be changed; excretion may be affected; electrolyte levels may be altered; drugs may act in the same body area, for example, the adrenergic neuron; or they may compete for protein-binding sites. These invisible mechanisms provide the framework for pharmacological drug interactions.

To more fully explain the specific drug interactions, look at each drug listed in the chart, and see which drugs interact with other drugs on the list. Only those drugs that interact are mentioned. To locate a specific interaction, look under both drug headings, in the list that follows.* The interactions are not necessarily discussed in both places.

* MARTIN, E. W. AND OTHERS. *Hazards of Medication*. Philadelphia, J. B. Lippincott Co., 1971, pp. 463, 471, 476-477, 481, 495, 512, 529, 570, 573-574, 579-580, 582, 590, 610-611, 642, 650-651, 653, 670, 686-687, 705, 747, 751-752, 758-759.

AMINOPHYLLINE: Aminophylline and *Coumadin* (warfarin) interact in the body to reduce the effect of Coumadin.

AMPICILLIN: A synergistic antibacterial effect occurs when ampicillin is given with *Prostaphlin* (sodium oxacillin).
Ampicillin enhances the anticoagulant effect of *Coumadin.*

ATROPINE: Atropine, an anticholinergic drug, antagonizes the anticholinesterase effects of *Tensilon* (edrophonium) and is a specific antidote to counteract the muscarinic side effects of Tensilon.
The combination of atropine and *Demerol* (merperidine) produces additive effects, such as dry mucous membranes, flushing, and depressed respirations. This is a hazardous combination in patients with glaucoma.
Conversely, when combined with *morphine*, atropine antagonizes the respiratory depression that commonly occurs. The effect of this combination on the gastrointestinal tract is twofold: atropine contributes to the decrease in intestinal mobility caused by morphine, but antagonizes the smooth muscle spasms often induced by morphine, especially those in the bilary tract.
Organic nitrates and nitrites (*nitroglycerin*) potentiate the side effects of such anticholinergic drugs as atropine. This combination, too, can be hazardous for the patient who has glaucoma.
Additive effects result when atropine and *quinidine* are combined. Quinidine enhances the anticholinergic effects of atropine.
Sympathomimetics such as *Isuprel* (isoproterenol) and *Levophed* (levarterenol) enhance the mydriatic and bronchial-relaxation effect of atropine. This combination could precipitate an acute attack for the patient with narrow-angle glaucoma.

CALCIUM: When serum calcium levels are elevated, the change of *digitalis* toxicity is increased. Calcium is used cautiously in the patient receiving *cardiac glycoside* preparations.
The analgesic effects of *Demerol* and *morphine* are antagonized by intracisternal injection of calcium.

COUMADIN: Antibiotics such as *ampicillin* and *Prostaphlin* interact with Coumadin to increase its anticoagulant effect.
Coumadin and *Dilantin* (diphenylhydantoin) combined increase the effect of each drug. Dilantin displaces Coumadin from plasma-binding sites. This allows a greater amount of free or active Coumadin to be pre-

sent in the serum, resulting in an increased anticoagulant effect. Coumarin derivatives potentiate Dilantin's action in inhibiting its enzymatic breakdown. More active Dilantin remains in the serum, resulting in an increased effect, and can lead to Dilantin toxicity.

The anticoagulant effect of Coumadin can be potentiated by *glucagon*; Coumadin's affinity for glucagon's receptors may be increased. Prolonged use of narcotics, such as *morphine* and *Demerol*, can enhance the anticoagulant effect of Coumadin.

Prothrombin formation in the liver is depressed by *quinidine*, which can potentiate the anticoagulant effects of Coumarin derivatives.

Reports on the interaction between *Valium* (diazepam) and Coumadin are variable and conflicting.

The action of oral anticoagulants is inhibited by *Lasix* (furosemide). Drugs that produce rapid diuresis can encourage the development of vascular thrombosis and emboli and increase the excretion rate of anticoagulants. The activity of the intrinsic clotting system is increased.

The effects of oral anticoagulants may be counteracted by *digitalis* drugs.

DEMEROL: Demerol interacts with *atropine* to increase the atropine effect. *Nitroglycerin* and other nitrates or nitrites enhance the hypotensive effect of Demerol and related narcotics.

DIGOXIN: This drug is described here as an example of cardiac glycosides. Digoxin decreases the anticoagulant effect of *Coumadin*.

Elevated serum calcium levels increase the risk of digitalis toxicity so *calcium* must be used cautiously.

Digoxin and *Dilantin* used concomitantly will intensify the bradycardic effect of digoxin. However, Dilantin has been given to treat the tachyarrhythmias of digitalis toxicity.

Diuretics, such as *Lasix* and thiazides, increase the effect of digitalis by causing hypokalemia. The heart is more sensitive to digitalis and the possibility of digitalis-induced arrhythmias or toxicity is increased in hypokalemia. Diuretics that do not cause loss of potassium (Aldactone, spironolactone, and Dyrenium triamterine) can be given instead or supplemental potassium salts added.

When *potassium* salts produce hyperkalemia, the action of digitalis drugs will be decreased.

For the patient with tachycardia who is taking digitalis drugs, *Isuprel* is contraindicated; it greatly increases the possibility of cardiac arrhythmias.

Additive effects on cardiac function occur when either *Pronestyl* (procainamide) or *quinidine* is used with digoxin. While Pronestyl may be used to treat the digitalis-induced tachyarrhythmias, caution must be taken to avoid over-depression of cardiac function and ventricular fibrillation. Quindine increases the effect of digitalis.

DILANTIN: When used together, Dilantin and *Coumadin* increase the effect of each drug.

Dilantin when used with *digitalis glycosides* will increase the effect of the digitalis preparation. The plasma concentration of the glycoside may be markedly lowered if Dilantin is used continually.

The hypotensive action of diuretics like *Lasix* and antihypertensive drugs can be potentiated when combined with Dilantin.

The combined use of *quinidine* and Dilantin potentiates the effects of quinidine.

GLUCAGON: Glucagon potentiates the effects of oral anticoagulants.

HEPARIN: Both heparin and Coumadin are anticoagulant drugs and thus their combined use produces additive effects. Heparin can be inhibited by *digitalis glycosides.*

INDERAL: Inderal (propanalol HC1) and *morphine* interact in the body to enhance the CNS-depressant effects of Inderal.

Inderal and *Levophed* have antagonistic beta-adrenergic effects: Inderal is a beta-adrenergic blocking agent; Levophed stimulates alpha- and beta-adrenergic activity. Inderal inhibits Levophed's glycogenolytic action and blocks the hyperthermia produced by Levophed. Both these drugs affect beta-adrenergic activity.

A synergistic action can occur with Inderal and cardiac glycosides such as *digoxin*; bradycardia can result. Inderal may cause cardiac arrest in patients with digitalis-induced, partial heart block. Inderal has a place, however, in treating digitalis-induced tachyarrhythmias without heart block.

Inderal's CNS-depressant action is potentiated when *Dilantin* is given.

Inderal potentiates the antihypertensive effects of *Lasix* (also Isordil, isosorbide dinitrate; Ismelin, guanethidine sulfate; Aldomet, methyldopa; and the thiazides).

Antagonistic effects exist when Inderal and *Isuprel* are given together. Both drugs affect beta-adrenergic activity but with opposite pharmacological effects.

There is a synergistic CNS depressant effect when Inderal is given with *morphine*.

The myocardial depressant effects of Inderal and *quinidine* are increased when these drugs are combined. This synergistic action may be beneficial in the treatment of certain cardiac arrhythmias.

ISUPREL: When Isuprel and *digitalis* preparations are given together, puzzling cardiac arrhythmias may develop. If the patient has a tachycardia which resulted from digitalis toxicity, Isuprel is contraindicated.

When Isuprel is used too frequently, a drug interaction between doses can occur. An enzyme (catechol-o-methyl transferase) found in the liver and lung converts the Isuprel to a metabolite (3-methoxyisoproterenol) which is a beta-adrenergic blocking agent. Since Isuprel is a beta-adrenergic drug and this converted metabolite has beta-adrenergic blocking action, the effects are antagonistic.

Isuprel and *Inderal* are antagonistic to each other because of their opposite actions.

When used with *nitroglycerin*, the effects of Isuprel are increased.

LASIX: The anticoagulant effects of *Coumadin* are inhibited by Lasix.

The combination of Lasix and *digitalis* preparations can precipitate digitalis toxicity if Lasix-induced hypokalemia is allowed to occur. The heart is more sensitive to digitalis effect when the patient is hypokalemic. This potential hazard can be avoided if supplemental potassium is given and normal serum potassium levels maintained.

Arterial responsiveness to vasopressor drugs such as *Levophed* have been reported to be decreased when Lasix is given.

LEVOPHED: The arterial response to Levophed can be decreased when diuretics such as *Lasix* are administered.

Levophed can be physiologically antagonized by nitrates and nitrites (*nitroglycerin*) which relax smooth muscle. Muscle response depends on the relative concentrations of each drug and so can vary.

The beta-adrenergic effects of Levophed are blocked by *Inderal*, a beta-adrenergic blocking agent. The myocardium is particularly affected because the myocardial autonomic tissue is characterized by beta-adrenergic receptors and the pharmacological response will depend on the predominating pharmacologically acting drug.

MORPHINE: Morphine and *Inderal* act synergistically to produce CNS depression.

216

Morphine augments the action of *Coumarin* anticoagulants.

NITROGLYCERIN: Nitroglycerin can potentiate some of the side effects of *atropine*. It should be used cautiously in the patient who has glaucoma. The hypotensive effects of *Demerol* and related narcotics may be potentiated by nitroglycerin.

Because nitroglycerin relaxes smooth muscle, it can act as a physiological antagonist to *Levophed*. The actual smooth muscle response to this combination depends on the relative concentrations of each drug.

POTASSIUM: Potassium affects the sensitivity of the heart to *digitalis* preparations. Hypokalemia increases this sensitivity and is a predisposing factor in digitalis toxicity. Conversely, hyperkalemia decreases the effectiveness of digitalis drugs.

PRONESTYL: Pronestyl may increase the effects of the *digitalis glycosides*. The tachyarrhythmias of digitalis toxicity may be treated with Pronestyl but only with caution, to prevent severe depression of cardiac function of ventricular fibrillation.

Pronestyl has anticholinergic properties and, when combined with *atropine*, the anticholinergic effects are increased.

Both Pronestyl and *Xylocaine* (lidocaine) are cardiac-depressant, antiarrhythmic drugs and, when combined, act synergistically on the myocardium and on the central nervous system. Excess cardiac depression, restlessness, and visual hallucinations may result. Cross sensitivity can occur.

The combination of Pronestyl and *quinidine*, both cardiac depressants, increases the action of each in depressing myocardial excitability and conductivity. Lower doses of each drug may be required.

PROSTAPHLIN: Prostaphlin, a penicillin derivative, augments the action of *Coumarin* anticoagulants and inhibits the effect of *heparin*. If intravenous penicillin is withdrawn, severe hemorrhage may result.

QUINIDINE: There are additive anticholinergic effects with the combination of quinidine and *atropine* or any anticholinergic drug. They must, then, be given with caution.

The anticoagulant effect of *Coumadin* can be potentiated by quinidine, which accomplishes this by depression of prothrombin formation or by inhibition of the synthesis of vitamin K-sensitive clotting factors in the liver.

The combination of quinidine and *digoxin* produces an additive digitalis effect and must be used cautiously, for bradycardia is a possible development.

There is an additive effect when *Dilantin* and quinidine are combined. Quinidine has a curare-like action which antagonizes *Tensilon*.

Additive effects result when quinidine and *Pronestyl* are combined, so lower dosages of each drug should be given.

Additive effects also occur when *Inderal* is given with quinidine and bradycardia is possible.

TENSILON: Anticholinergic drugs such as *atropine* antagonize the miotic and other muscarinic effects of an anticholinesterase drug with *Tensilon*.

The anticholinergic activity of *Pronestyl* antagonizes the anticholinesterase effects of Tensilon.

Both *morphine* and *Demerol* can lower intraocular tension and may enhance the reported beneficial effects of Tensilon when used in certain classes of glaucoma.

VALIUM: Reports on the interaction of Valium and *Coumadin* vary and conflict.

The effects of Dilantin are potentiated by Valium and other benzodiazepines, such as Librium and Serax.

The antihypertensive effects of *Lasix* and other diuretics and antihypertensives could be potentiated by Valium. The combination of Valium with *morphine* and *Demerol* can augment the hypotensive effects of the narcotics and the CNS-depressant effects of Valium.

XYLOCAINE: Cross sensitivity between Xylocaine and *quinidine,* and between Xylocaine and *Pronestyl* could take place. A synergistic effect on the CNS as well as on the myocardium may occur when Xylocaine and Pronestyl are given. Depression of cardiac function, restlessness, visual hallucinations, and so forth may occur.

Drug interactions may be therapeutic or detrimental. The presence of a relatively minor undesirable drug interaction does not necessarily preclude the use of that combination in clinical practice.

The complexities of current drug therapy and the expansion of drug knowledge increase the concern for possible drug interactions. The nurse must be alert to possible interactions among the drugs she administers. The drugs mentioned here obviously are not limited to use in a cardiac care unit.

BIBLIOGRAPHY

ADMIXTURE STUDY. rev. ed. Morton Grove, Ill., Baxter Laboratories, Inc., 1967.

GARB, SOLOMON. *Cinical Guide to Undersirable Drug Interaction and Interferences.* New York, Springer Publishing Co., 1971.

HANSTEN, P. D. *Drug Interactions.* 2d ed. Philadelphia, Lea and Febiger, 1973.

HARTSHORN, E. A. *Handbook of Drug Interactions, Part 1.* Cincinnati, Ohio, College of Pharmacy, University of Cincinnati, 1970.

MEYLER, LEOPOLD, AND HERXHEIMER, ANDREW, EDS. *Side Effects of Drugs: a Survey of Unwanted Effects of Drugs Reported in 1965-1967,* Vol. 6. Baltimore, Williams and Wilkins Co., 1969.

MOSER, R. H., ED. *Diseases of Medical Progress: a Study of Iatrogenic Disease.* 3d ed. Springfield, Ill., Charles C. Thomas, Publisher, 1969.

From the *American Journal of Nursing* 74:2176-2180. Dec. 1974.

Aggressive Drug Therapy in Accelerated Hypertension

FRANK A. FINNERTY, JR.

Malignant hypertension may be a reversible disease and survival may be possible if life can be maintained for a reasonable period of time while the arteriolitis heals(1). Patients with malignant hypertension, particularly those with renal insufficiency, frequently die during the early stages of treatment before the benefits of remission can be realized. Therefore, we have adopted the policy of considering all patients in the accelerated phase of hypertension, with or without papilledema, as medical emergencies, and we treat them as vigorously and aggressively as those with hypertensive encephalopathy(2).

In essence, the aim of therapy is to keep the diastolic pressure below 100 mm. Hg (below 90 in patients under 20 years of age and below 80 mm. Hg in children under 10) and the urinary output above two liters per day. These goals can usually be attained by intermittent, repeated intravenous injections of diazoxide (Hyperstat I.V.) and orally administered furosemide (Lasix). Further intravenous diazoxide or hydralazine (Apresoline), a constant infusion of sodium nitroprusside (Nipride), or intermittent, intramuscular injections of hydralazine may be required if the diastolic pressure returns to 100 mm. Hg or above. Repeated injections of diazoxide or hydralazine are continued until a single injection keeps the diastolic pressure under 100 mm. Hg for more than 24 hours.

Diazoxide is available in 20 ml. ampules, 15 mg./ml. The average effective dose is 300 mg., or one ampule. In our experience with over 1,000 treated patients, 95 percent of adult patients respond to this dosage. Children with encephalopathy due to acute nephritis, adults who

DR. FINNERTY (*M.D., Georgetown University School of Medicine, Washington, D.C.*) *is professor of medicine at Georgetown University School of Medicine and chief, cardiovascular research, Georgetown University Medical Division, D.C. General Hospital.*

weigh more than 200 pounds, and patients who do not respond to one ampule of diazoxide may require a dose of diazoxide as high as 5 mg./ kg. The optimum antihypertensive effect of diazoxide is noted in one to two minutes. No individual titration of dosage is necessary. Rather, our studies have demonstrated the need to administer the full dose in a bolus —within 10 seconds—to assure the optimum effect(3).

Nitroprusside is administered by a constant infusion drip of 0.04 to 0.06 mg./ml. The rate of infusion is regulated according to the level of the blood pressure. Nitroprusside's disadvantages include the need to prepare a fresh solution and the need to titrate the dosage, which requires constant monitoring.

Hydralazine can be administered intramuscularly and has a relatively rapid onset of action (30 to 40 minutes), but it is less potent than the other two rapidly acting agents. The frequent occurrence of headache, flushing, and tachycardia further limits its usefulness.

Furosemide is at least 25 times as potent as the thiazide diuretics. Equally important, its potency may be further increased by increasing the dosage(1). Increasing the dose of thiazide diuretics, on the other hand, does not increase their effectiveness. Five grams of chlorothiazide (Diuril) administered twice daily is no more effective than the standard dose of 500 mg. twice daily. The ability to tailor furosemide dosages to the individual situation and furosemide's effectiveness in the face of electrolyte imbalance favor its use in patients with accelerated-phase hypertension. When doses above 160 mg. are needed, we have obtained the best results with once-a-day administration.

An accurate record of urinary output is an absolute necessity for the successful management of these sick patients. When urinary output cannot be maintained above 1,000 ml./day, peritoneal dialysis should be combined with furosemide and repeated as often as necessary. This combination often tides the patient over a critical period and prevents the development of "end stage" renal failure. In our experience, inability to maintain adequate urinary output despite increasing doses of furosemide is the best clinical sign of deteriorating renal function.

When a single injection of diazoxide has kept the diastolic pressure under 100 mm. Hg for more than 24 hours, or preferably a few days sooner, oral antihypertensive agents, such as methyldopa (Aldomet) or hydralazine, are begun. Aldomet is given in multiple doses of 250 mg. four times a day (initial dose 250 mg. once a day); hydralazine in multiple doses of 25 mg. three or four times a day (initial dose 25 mg. twice a day). It is important to initiate therapy with these drugs with small, suboptimal doses in order to avoid side effects. The development of an unpleasant side effect to the first dose of a new drug may stop the patient from continuing therapy for the rest of his life.

Guanethidine (Ismelin) decreases cardiac output, renal blood flow, and the glomerular filtration rate more than the other antihypertensive agents. Therefore, we believe that it is contraindicated for azotemic patients. Rather, furosemide is continued in reduced dosages of 80 to 160 mg. per day.

In the majority of the patients we have followed, several findings adequately attest to the reversibility of the malignant phase of hypertension: the prompt clearing of papilledema and decrease in retinopathy, the significant reduction in serum creatinine three months after diazoxide or other aggressive therapy, and the improvement in renal blood flow and the glomerular filtration rate(2). Such data support the plea for aggressively treating patients in the accelerated phase of hypertension before renal vascular deterioration has proceeded beyond the point of no return. Although such patients should be thoroughly investigated to rule out curable types of hypertension, particularly if a satisfactory therapeutic response is not obtained, therapy should be instituted first and investigations performed after the arterial pressure has been controlled.

RENAL EFFECTS

Aggressive therapy should not be discontinued because of a rise in blood urea nitrogen (BUN) or creatinine, because such rises are usually transitory and caused by a hemodynamic alteration rather than further damage to the kidney. Inulin and PAH (para-aminohippurate) clearance determinations done three months after aggressive therapy usually indicate significant improvement above control values. Serial determinations six and twelve months later have shown continued improvement. Renal biopsies performed in seven patients six months after control of arterial pressure have demonstrated healing of the necrotizing arteriolitis(4). Although it may be argued that gradual rather than acute reduction of arterial pressure might prevent even this transitory worsening of renal function, in our opinion the imminent danger of a cerebral vascular accident in these patients demands emergency treatment. Our experience and that of others has demonstrated that there is a high incidence of cerebral complications when arterial pressure is not under control; that the longer arterial pressure is uncontrolled, the greater the danger of cerebral complications; and that the person's prognosis is grave once these occur(5).

Lowering the arterial pressure with most potent antihypertensive agents, except for the diuretics, is accompanied by a decrease in renal blood flow, glomerular filtration rate, and urinary output, and an increase in sodium retention. Because each of these unfavorable effects on the kidney is greatly enhanced in patients with azotemia, it is readily understandable why reduction of arterial pressure in these patients consistently has aggravated the degree of azotemia, frequently produced congestive heart failure, and hastened the patient's downhill course.

The availability of furosemide and its beneficial effects in high doses, particularly in azotemic patients, suggest that combining it with diazoxide or hydralazine might do away with at least some of the detrimental effects of acute reduction of arterial pressure in hypertensive azotemic patients(6,7). Furosemide by itself has a modest effect on the arterial pressure, a varying effect on the cardiac output, and promotes urinary output and sodium excretion(8). Administering these agents together produces a greater decrease in arterial pressure than that with diazoxide alone, increases cardiac output, and increases urinary sodium excretion and urinary output.

In 1967 Woods and Blythe concluded that the reduction of arterial pressure in patients with malignant hypertension complicated with azotemia did not necessarily result in deterioration of renal function, and might improve survival rates(1). Studies in our laboratory have demonstrated that more aggressive reduction of the arterial pressure while maintaining urinary output and preventing sodium retention improved survival rates in such patients even further(2).

LIMITATIONS

Valuable as it is, the combination of diazoxide and furosemide does have certain limitations.

The alkaline nature of the diazoxide solution makes any extravasation outside the vein painful. Although such extravasation is associated with a severe burning sensation which lasts from one to two hours, no sloughing of tissues has occurred. If there is any extravasation, the immediate injection of saline or procaine (Novocaine) at the site of injection minimizes the discomfort.

The fall of arterial pressure following the administration of diazoxide alone is not associated with postural hypotension, but the addition of furosemide to diazoxide commonly produces postural hypotension by decreasing the plasma volume(9). Therefore, one should instruct the patient to maintain a supine position for three to four hours following the injection.

A transitory hyperglycemia which lasts no more than 12 hours frequently follows the intravenous administration of diazoxide. Wolff *et al.*

and our own studies have demonstrated that pretreatment of patients with tolbutamide (Orinase) will effectively prevent the hyperglycemic effect of diazoxide(1,10). Diazoxide is not contraindicated in patients with diabetes. It would seem, however, that when diazoxide is administered for more than 48 hours, blood sugar levels should be monitored closely. If significant increases in blood sugar occur, tolbutamide can then be given.

The nausea and vomiting which accompany diazoxide therapy are probably related to the drug's muscle-relaxing properties, which include the stomach as well as the uterus. Withholding food two hours before and after the administration of diazoxide has kept the incidence of vomiting to under 10 percent.

We believe that the beneficial results of aggressive treatment of patients with accelerated-phase hypertension are not peculiar to diazoxide or furosemide, but can best be explained by the physiologic hemodynamic effects accompanying the reduction in arterial pressure. That is, cardiac output increases, total peripheral resistance decreases, urinary output increases, and sodium retention is prevented. Although other parenterally administered agents, such as hydralazine or nitroprusside, may be used in combination with furosemide, hydralazine's lack of potency and frequent side effects and the difficulty in preparation and administration of nitroprusside limit their usefulness.

REFERENCES

1. WOODS, J. W., AND BLYTHE, W. B. Management of malignant hypertension complicated by renal insufficiency. *N.Engl.J.Med.* 277:57-61, July 13, 1967.

2. MROCZEK, W. J., AND OTHERS. The value of aggressive therapy in the hypertensive patient with azotemia. *Circulation* 40:893-904, Dec. 1969.

3. ————. The importance of the rapid administration of diazoxide in accelerated hypertension. *N.Eng.J.Med.* 285-603-606, Sept. 9, 1971.

4. FINNERTY, F. A. JR., AND MROCZEK, W. J. (Unpublished data)
5. HARINGTON, M. B., AND KINCAID-SMITH, PRISCILLA. Results of treatment in malignant hypertension: a seven-year experience in 94 cases. *Br.Med.J.* 2:969-980, Nov. 14, 1959.
6. MUTH, R. G. Diuretic properties of furosemide in renal disease. *Ann.Intern.Med.* 69:249-261, Aug. 1968.
7. BERMAN, L. B., AND EBRAHIMI, A. Experiences with furosemide in renal disease. *Proc.Soc.Exp.Biol.Med.* 118:333-336, Feb. 1965.
8. DAVIDOV, M., AND OTHERS. Antihypertensive properties of furosemide. *Circulation* 36:125-135, July 1967.
9. FINNERTY, F. A. JR., AND OTHERS. Clinical evaluation of diazoxide, a new treatment for acute hypertension. *Circulation* 28:203-208, Aug. 1963.
10. WALES, J. K., AND OTHERS. Reversal of diazoxide effects by tolbutamide. Lancet 1:1137-1138, May 27, 1967.

Section V Cardiac Surgery

A discussion of the preoperative, intraoperative, and postoperative nursing care of patients undergoing open heart surgery opens this section. The advent of the pump-oxygenator for cardiopulmonary bypass revolutionized the field of cardiac surgery and made possible the development of the surgical procedures described in other articles in this section. However, unique physical and psychological complications have been associated with open heart surgery, most notably the "indeterminate stimulus experiences" described by Ellis, and these problems challenge nurses to devise nursing interventions for the patients in their care.

From the *American Journal of Nursing* 74:860-867, May 1974.

Cardiopulmonary Bypass

MADELEINE L. LONG • MARY ANN SCHEUHING
JUDITH L. CHRISTIAN

Intricate, life-saving, open heart surgery is possible because of the pump-oxygenator, but the patient depends on more than a machine. The knowledge and skills of those who teach him preoperatively, maintain his physiological functions during surgery, and care for him throughout his postoperative course all contribute to his eventual recovery.

On May 6, 1953, Gibbon performed the world's first successful open heart operation, using total heart-lung bypass, to repair an atrial septal defect in an 18-year-old girl(1). Before the pump-oxygenator was perfected, cardiac surgery was performed by palpation and repair, without direct visualization of the intracardiac defect. Total body hypothermia was usually employed to reduce the body's oxygen consumption.

Cardiopulmonary bypass, or extracorporeal circulation, permits direct visualization of intracardiac defects, and is used during open heart surgical procedures to oxygenate the blood and remove carbon dioxide while

MS. LONG (*St. Agnes Hospital School of Nursing, Philadelphia, Pa.; B.S.Ed., Temple University, Philadelphia, Pa.; M.S., Catholic University, Washington, D.C.*) *is research associate and cardiovascular specialist at Rush-Presbyterian-St. Luke's Medical Center, Chicago, Ill.* DR. SCHEUHING (*Ph.D., Catholic University, Washington, D.C.*) *received an M.S. in nursing at New York Medical College, New York, N.Y., after completing doctoral work in the humanities. She is employed in the emergency room at Burdette Tomlin Memorial Hospital, Cape May Court House, N.J.* M.S. CHRISTIAN (*Memorial Hospital School of Nursing, Springfield, Ill.; B.S., Northwestern University, Chicago, Ill.*) *is supervisor-clinician in the ICU-PCCU at Columbus-Cuneo-Cabrini Medical Center, Chicago, Ill.*

sustaining peripheral blood flow to meet the metabolic needs of the body. An artificial oxygenator must be capable of oxygenating up to five liters of venous blood to 95 percent saturation each minute(2).

To exclude a patient's heart and lungs from his systemic circulation, venous blood is diverted out of the body through the heart-lung machine, oxygenated, and then pumped back to the patient. Whether cardiopulmonary function is provided by the patient's heart and lungs or by artificial devices, body homeostasis must be maintained; if it is not, cellular hypoxia and metabolic acidosis result.

The diagram illustrates the principle that governs cardiopulmonary bypass and the basic components of any heart-lung circuit. Specific system components and the sites of vessel cannulation are selected according to the needs of the patient, the type of cardiac defect, and the preference of the surgeon-perfusionist team.

Before bypass begins, the heart-lung machine is completely filled with

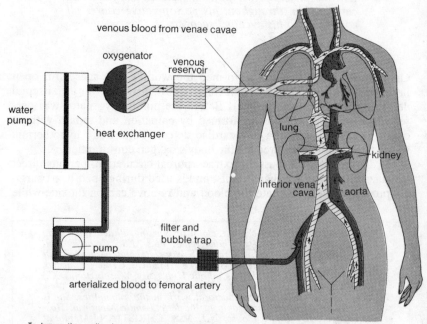

To bypass the cardiopulmonary circulation, catheters are placed in the inferior and superior venae cavae. These divert venous blood to a venous reservoir, heat exchanger, oxygenator, and roller pump. The roller pump propels arterialized blood through the filter and bubble trap. The blood then is returned to the patient through a catheter in the femoral artery.

fluids which will replace the venous blood that is diverted to the heart-lung circuitry. At Rush-Presbyterian-St. Lukes Medical Center, these exchange fluids, called the "prime" or "pump-priming volume," usually include two liters of Ringer's lactate, 44.6 mEq. of sodium bicarbonate, and 500 cc. of 20% osmitrol for an adult patient. This prime dilutes the patient's blood volume by approximately 2,500 cc. When hemodilution exceeds three liters in an adult, it compromises the oxygen-carrying capacity of the blood and is a hypervolemic concern(3).

After the patient has been anticoagulated by the administration of heparin, 3 to 4 mg. per kilogram of body weight, perfusion is begun by diverting the venous blood return from the right heart to the venous reservoir. At the same time, the priming volume is pumped through a catheter in the femoral artery. The venous reservoir is connected to an oxygenator where the venous blood is arterialized. That is, oxygen is taken up and carbon dioxide removed.

The arterialized blood enters a heat exchanger, where its temperature can be maintained at normothermic (98.6° F.) or hypothermic (82° F.) levels. Cooling the circulating blood to moderate hypothermic levels (86° F) decreases the oxygen demands of the tissues by approximately one half the amount needed at normal body temperatures(4). This helps to protect the heart, lungs, and other organ systems from the effects of ischemia and anoxia. If hypothermia is used, rewarming is accomplished toward the end of the procedure by pumping warm water through the heat exchanger.

Having passed through a roller pump, arterialized blood is propelled through a blood filter and bubble trap before it is returned to the patient's circulation via the femoral artery. The filter and bubble trap remove air emboli, tiny clots, fat debris, and other particulate matter from the blood.

Depending on the depth of hypothermia and the patient's body surface area, blood is recirculated through the patient and the heart-lung machine at an approximate rate of 1,000 to 5,000 cc. per minute for an average perfusion time of two hours. While passing through the circuitry, the blood is exposed to substantial trauma by direct contact with oxygen, foreign substances, turbulent flow, mechanical action of the pump, and massive anticoagulation. The most notable physiologic manifestations of trauma are hemolysis or red blood cell damage(5), protein denaturation(6), clotting abnormalities(7), decrease in the number of circulating platelets(8), and platelet aggregation(9). Clinical signs of these plasma and cellular alterations are hemoglobinuria, fat emboli, hemorrhage, and thromboembolism.

INTRAOPERATIVE CASE HISTORY

Mr. T., a 52-year-old foreman, was admitted to our hospital on May 13, 1973. Two months before admission, he experienced exertional and paroxysmal nocturnal dyspnea. His previous medical history included rheumatic fever during childhood and an episode of congestive heart failure with atrial fibrillation, which had been treated successfully with quinidine and digoxin. A cardiac catheterization done in 1964 had shown moderate aortic stenosis.

On May 15, 1973, a second catheterization revealed severe aortic valvular stenosis, left ventricular enlargement, and dilatation of the ascending aorta. Three days later, Mr. T. underwent open heart surgery for an aortic valve replacement. Twelve hours before the operation, a central venous pressure catheter was inserted in the left basilic vein for the administration of preoperative antibiotics and for preoperative monitoring.

After receiving his preoperative medications, Mr. T. was taken to the operating room where he was met by a nurse on the surgical team. She accompanied him into the operating suite and explained that he would be attached to a cardiac monitor and be prepared for anesthesia.

Induction and intubation were accomplished without difficulty, and general anesthesia was begun. A catheter was introduced into the ulnar artery for blood pressure monitoring. The surgeon made a midline sternal-splitting incision, exposing the mediastinum. The pericardium was incised, the heart exposed, and heparin injected into the right atrium.

Before Mr. T. arrived in the operating room the heart-lung machine was prepared by the perfusionist. The priming volume was added and recirculated through the heart-lung circuit to remove all the air bubbles before bypass. After the surgeon cannulated the common femoral artery and both venae cavae, partial bypass was begun and a portion of the venous return was diverted to the heart-lung circuitry. The remaining venous return continued to flow through the patient's heart, lungs, and systemic arteries. Then, cord tapes previously placed around the venae cavae cannulas were tightened to drain all the returning venous blood into the heart-lung machine. The heart was fibrillated and ventilatory assistance discontinued. Mr. T. was now on total cardiopulmonary bypass.

Exposure of the aortic valve revealed marked insufficiency, with shrunken and calcified valve leaflets. The leaflets were excised and a Starr-Edwards aortic valvular prosthesis was implanted. Total cardiopulmonary bypass under normothermia continued at a flow rate of 3,400 to 4,200 cc. per minute. Arterial blood gases and electrolytes were monitored throughout the perfusion to permit correction of metabolic imbalances. Thirty minutes after the bypass was started, Mr. T.'s oxygen tension (pO_2) was 400 mm. Hg; carbon dioxide tension (pCO_2) was 38 mm. Hg; pH was 7.35; oxygen saturation was 100%; serum potassium was 3.9 mEq./L.; and calcium was 7.4 mgm./100 ml. The blood flow rate was 3,400 cc. per minute.

When valve implantation was completed, air bubbles were evacuated from the left ventricle and aorta. Heart conductivity was restored to normal sinus rhythm by direct current defibrillation. Ventilation of the patient was reestablished by respirator while perfusion was gradually decreased to 800 cc. per minute and eventually discontinued. Cardiopulmonary bypass perfusion had lasted 76 minutes.

The arterial and venous cannulas were removed and the remaining incisions sutured. Mr. T. was given 228 mgm. of protamine sulfate I.V. to neutralize the heparin effect. Two chest tubes were left in the mediastinum, and pacing wires were implanted under the wall of the right ventricle. When Mr. T. was transferred to the intensive care unit, he was awake and in satisfactory condition. He recovered fully.

PREOPERATIVE CARE

Preoperative care of all patients undergoing cardiopulmonary bypass involves physiologic and psychologic nursing assessment as well as a significant amount of patient teaching.

The extent of the patient's pathology is determined by cardiac catheterization and angiography. These procedures are explained to the patient and family before they are done. After the decision for surgical intervention is reached, physiologic evaluation of the patient continues, with documentation of his cardiac, pulmonary, renal, neurologic, and hematologic functions. Laboratory studies include electrocardiogram, complete blood count, urinalysis, coagulation profile, determination of blood urea nitrogen, electrolytes, enzymes, and blood type, and cross-matching for 12 units of blood. Radiologic examinations of the thorax delineate heart size and position and identify any intracardiac calcium deposits. Pulmonary disease and left ventricular failure may be detected by pulmonary function tests. This comprehensive evaluation of the patient is necessary to plan surgical therapy and to anticipate potential complications. Skin preparation includes Dial soap showers and the total body application of a depilatory by a surgical technician immediately before surgery. No shaving is done.

In addition to explaining the preoperative examinations and procedures to the patient and his family, the nurse takes a careful history, including specific information about dental problems, medications used, allergies, medical conditions, consumption of alcohol, or cigarette smoking.

Elective cardiac surgery is not performed in the presence of active dental infections, incomplete healing of gums following extractions, or if there is infection elsewhere in the body. These problems predispose the patient to the potentially lethal complication of endocarditis.

Most cardiac patients take medications routinely and some of these can cause life-threatening problems during and after surgery (see chart p. 236). Preexisting health problems, such as gastric ulcers, epilepsy, diabetes, asthma, and any illness necessitating steroid therapy must be noted to ensure prompt recognition of related symptoms and administration of appropriate maintenance medications in the operating room or intensive care unit.

A history of alcoholism is particularly difficult to elicit but highly significant should the patient experience withdrawal symptoms in the immediate postoperative period. These symptoms must be quickly differentiated from the motor and behavioral effects associated with a neurological deficit or impending cardiac failure.

All pertinent information recorded in the nursing history is communicated to the nurses in the operating room, recovery room, and intensive care unit.

While taking the history, the nurse listens to the patient's tone of voice, and manner of speaking, and observes bodily gestures to determine his perceptions of his situation. After taking the history, the nurse gives him an opportunity to explore his feelings about the impending surgery. Verbal reassurances can be particularly supportive at this time. It is well, however, to avoid premature reassurance because this may inhibit the patient's communication of relevant information or negative feelings.

Instructions and explanations are provided before surgery to reduce preoperative stress and postoperative delirium, and enhance his ability to participate in recuperative activities. To limit the incidence and severity of pulmonary complications, for example, the patient is instructed not to smoke, to breathe deeply and cough, and to practice with an intermittent positive pressure apparatus so that he can use it properly in the recovery period. The patient's knowledge and anxiety guide the nurse when she explains his need for surgery, discusses prosthetic valvular devices, incisional sites, and monitoring equipment, and gives general information about the operating room.

Endotracheal intubation and ventilatory assistance are discussed. The patient is told that he will not be able to speak, eat, or drink until the "breathing tube" is removed, usually in about 24 hours. The nurse works with him to develop alternative ways to communicate, such as pointing to his lips to indicate thirst or to his chest to indicate pain.

Patients who wish to visit the intensive care unit before surgery should be permitted to do so. There, they can see monitoring devices, catheters, and chest tubes, and meet a few of the staff members who will care for them postoperatively.

At all times, patient teaching is enhanced by slow, clear enunciation and the avoidance of scientific or technical terms. Some patients ask that all explanations be omitted and such requests should be respected.

CAUSES AND MANIFESTATIONS OF POSTOPERATIVE COMPLICATIONS

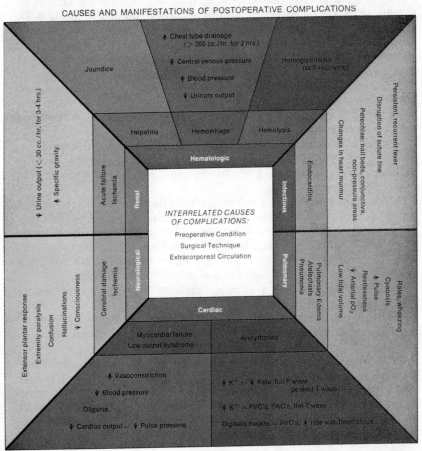

Adapted from material copyrighted by M. Long.

The nurse can reassure the patient and his family that the special equipment and catheters used in the recovery phase are safeguards to ensure a successful postoperative course and should not be interpreted as signs of clinical deterioration. The patient and his family should also be told the estimated length of surgery, the location of waiting areas in the hospital, and the visiting hours in the intensive care unit.

POSTOPERATIVE CARE

Following surgery, the patient is accompanied to the intensive care unit by the surgical-anesthesia team. He may be vasoconstricted and shivering for a brief period if hypothermia was used during cardiopulmonary bypass. The patient is usually responsive on arrival in the ICU, and is asked to move each extremity separately and to squeeze the nurse's hand. Inability to move a limb or inequality in handgrasp strength might indicate cerebral damage due to embolism or hypotension during surgery.

Intensive nursing care during the postoperative period should be geared toward preventing complications. This involves constant assessment of the physiologic parameters which indicate organ system competence or deterioration.

Besides electrocardiographic and central venous pressure monitoring, the nurse observes for adequacy of myocardial functioning, intravascular volume, peripheral perfusion, ventilatory capacity, and for patency of the chest tube drainage system.

Myocardial function and intravascular volume are reflected in the patient's intra-arterial pressure, which is monitored by an oscilloscope. However, the blood pressure is auscultated for comparison. The intra-arterial line is irrigated frequently with heparinized saline to prevent clotting. The dressing at the site is changed daily. If the patient's condition remains stable, the arterial catheter is removed within 72 hours.

Peripheral perfusion is a valuable guide to the patient's circulatory status. Adequacy of perfusion is determined by noting the color, temperature, and pulses of the extremities. Cold extremities and peripheral cyanosis are danger signals and suggest potential cardiopulmonary complications.

It is customary to leave the patient intubated and on controlled ventilatory assistance during the first 24 hours of the postoperative period. Blood gas determinations are made immediately after the patient arrives in the unit and frequently thereafter. The ventilator is adjusted according to the results of these tests. Frequent endotracheal suctioning and position changes are key nursing actions to prevent atelectasis and retention of secretions. Hourly deep breaths are administered with an Ambu bag. An oral airway is left in place for several hours if the patient tends to bite down and obstruct the endotracheal tube.

The patient is usually extubated the morning after surgery if his tidal volume, arterial blood gases, color, and level of consciousness indicate adequate unassisted ventilation. After extubation, his deep breathing and coughing exercises may be enhanced by well-timed analgesic administration.

The patient's chest tubes are connected to a water-sealed drainage system and should be vigorously stripped by the nurse every 30 to 60 minutes to facilitate intrathoracic drainage and prevent clotting. Chest drainage of approximately 50 to 200 cc. an hour is expected during the first two to three hours following surgery. Thereafter, the drainage should decrease to between 50 and 100 cc. per hour. Blood loss is usually replaced by an equal amount of transfused volume. Bright red drainage indicates active bleeding; darker drainage signifies accumulated blood. An operation to renew hemostasis may be necessary if hemorrhage occurs. Chest tubes are removed after 48 hours if the drainage has been less than 15 cc. an hour for six hours.

A continuous electrocardiogram monitors cardiac rate and rhythm. Arrhythmias are not uncommon postoperatively, and acute myocardial infarction is a significant cause of mortality following open heart surgery(10). An increased incidence of ventricular arrhythmias, heart block, and hypotension is associated with ischemic myocardial injury(11). The appearance of frequent premature ventricular beats which interrupt the T wave or are multifocal in origin is a warning of possible ventricular fibrillation(12). A physician should be notified immediately, and anti-arrhythmic therapy instituted.

Serum potassium alterations are common in the postoperative phase and may cause arrhythmias. Measurement of serum electrolytes should be made immediately after the patient is admitted to the unit and frequently thereafter to discover any electrolyte imbalances.

Central venous pressure indicates right heart competence and is used as a guide to fluid administration. A normal CVP ranges between 5 and 15 cm. H_2O. However, multiple factors influence the accuracy of CVP readings and a comprehensive nursing assessment requires the correlation of these readings with other related parameters.

If the CVP is high, for example, the functioning of both ventricles and the pulmonary circulation should be further evaluated. A high CVP reading is a reliable reflection of cardiac failure when it is accompanied by congestive changes in the lungs, such as rales or wheezing, neck vein

DRUGS THAT MAY CAUSE PROBLEMS DURING AND AFTER OPEN HEART SURGERY

DRUGS:	PROBLEMS:
Digitalis Preparations (Discontinued 1-5 days before surgery, depending on preparation.)	Digitalis toxicity in chronically digitalized patients. Cardiopulmonary bypass increases sensitivity to glycosides. CPB causes changes in renal function which decrease dosage needed for maintenance. Give cautiously in postoperative period. Toxicity may be precipitated by hypokalemia.
Antiarrhythmic Agents Diphenylhydantoin (Dilantin) Lidocaine (Xylocaine) Procaine amide (Pronestyl) Quinidine (Discontinued, if possible.)	Myocardial depression. Hypotension.
Anticoagulants Bishydroxycoumarin (Dicumarol) Warfarin (Coumadin) Salicylates (over 3 Gm./day) (Discontinued 3-4 weeks before surgery.)	Bleeding. Possible "rebound effect" on discontinuation.
Antihypertensives Guanethidine	Severe hypotension due to catecholamine depletion.
Methyldopa	Decreased response to vasopressor drugs. Opiates may cause marked hypotension and bradycardia.
Reserpine (Discontinued 10 days before surgery.)	
Diuretics (Discontinued 1-2 days before surgery.)	Hypokalemia, hyponatremia. Dehydration, hypovolemia. Alkalosis.
Beta-Adrenergic Blocking Agents Propranolol (Inderal) (Discontinued 1-2 days before surgery.)	Possible acute heart failure due to depression of myocardial contractility. Decreased response to beta-adrenergic drugs (Isuprel).
Steroids (Continued)	Possible hypotension unless steroids are given. Extreme sensitivity to narcotics and anesthetics.
Antipsychotics Chlorpromazine (Thorazine) (Discontinued 3 days before surgery.)	Hypotension.
Monoamine Oxidase Inhibitors Isocarboxazid (Marplan) Phenelzine (Nardil) Tranylcypromine (Parnate) (Discontinued 3 days before surgery.)	Hypertensive crisis with vasopressors. Coma with hypo- or hypertension. May potentiate the effects of morphine. Prolong the action of barbituates.

distention when the patient is in semi-Fowler's position, sacral edema, narrowing pulse pressure, increased heart rate, and decreased urinary output. A high CVP reading may also indicate excess fluid volume, and neck vein distention may confirm this. Unchecked hypervolemia will result in moist rales, tachycardia, and sacral edema. By the same token, a low CVP reading, which suggests hypovolemia or low effective circulating volume, may be accompanied by decreased urinary output, hypotension, and increased heart rate.

Malpositioned central venous catheters are a source of unreliable measurements and can also cause life-threatening arrhythmias in the immediate postoperative period. Therefore, the nurse observes the manometer fluid for vigorous fluctuations with the heart beat, which indicate right ventricular misplacement. Inordinately elevated CVP readings which are inconsistent with the physical signs of hypervolemia may also indicate that the catheter is in the pulmonary artery. If a chest x-ray confirms misplacement, the catheter is withdrawn to the right atrium.

Two factors related to the patient's surgical experience predispose him to hypervolemia. The previously described pump-priming volume, when composed of non-blood solutions, such as Ringer's lactate, may diffuse into the interstitial space during cardiopulmonary bypass. However, this fluid reenters the systemic circulation postoperatively. In addition, the stress of surgery leads to an elevation of the antidiuretic hormone and aldosterone levels, and this causes salt and water retention.

Therefore, in the postoperative period, a fluid restriction of 1,500 cc. per 24 hours is imposed on the adult patient to prevent hypervolemia or cardiac failure. Once the patient has been extubated, a clear liquid diet is started and intravenous fluids are decreased as oral intake increases. When the patient is able to take 1,250 cc. orally, peripheral intravenous catheters are removed and the remaining fluids are administered through the central venous catheter. If a catheter is left in place for more than 72 hours there is an increased incidence of local infection, thrombophlebitis, and inflammation. These can be detected during daily dressing changes at the insertion site.

Repeated explanations of procedures and therapeutic plans to the patient·and family enhance cooperation and reduce confusion and anxiety. A structured plan for progressive ambulation helps allay the characteristic postoperative depression which may be triggered by the patient's awareness of his weakness and fatigue following surgery.

At this time, the use of a membrane oxygenator during cardiopulmonary bypass has not significantly altered patients' postoperative courses. Clinical use of this technique has been limited. However, one group of investigators has reported that patients who were maintained on the membrane oxygenator exhibited spontaneous ventilation which resulted in early endoctracheal extubation, fewer blood transfusions, and fewer instances of organic brain damage, pneumonia, and atelectasis than patients who underwent cardiopulmonary bypass with a non-membrane oxygenator(13). Also, early results indicate that increased arterial oxygen tensions can be obtained by using a membrane oxygenator. This could alter the degree of ischemia incurred during cardiopulmonary bypass. Although further clinical evaluation will provide more definitive conclusions regarding membrane oxygenation, the fact that there is no direct contact between blood and oxygen appears to permit safer prolonged total cardiopulmonary support.

REFERENCES

1. GIBBON, J. H. Application of a mechanical heart and lung apparatus to cardiac surgery. *Minn.Med.* 37:171-180, 185, Mar. 1954.
2. GALLETTI, P. M. The mechanics of cardiopulmonary bypass. IN *Cardiac Surgery*, ed. by John C. Norman. New York, Appleton-Century-Crofts, 1967, p. 66.
3. NEVILLE, W. E., AND OTHERS. Postperfusion hypervolemia after hemodilution cardiopulmonary bypass. *Arch.Surg.* 93:715-723, Nov. 1966.
4. GALLETTI, P. M., AND BRECHER, G. A. *Heart-Lung Bypass: Principles and Techniques of Extracorporeal Circulation.* New York Grune and Stratton, 1962, p. 294.
5. ANDERSEN, M. N., AND KUCHIBA, K. Blood trauma produced by pump oxygenators: a comparative study of five different units. *J.Thorac.Cardiovasc.Surg.* 57:238-244, Feb. 1969.
6. LEE, W. H., AND OTHERS. Denaturation of plasma proteins as a cause of morbidity and death after intracardiac operations. *Surgery* 50:29-39, July 1961.
7. GRALNICK, H. R., AND FISCHER, R. D. Hemostatic response to open-heart operations. *J.Thorac.Cardiovasc.Surg.* 61:909-915, June 1971.
8. MC KENZIE, F. N., AND OTHERS. Blood platelet behavior during and after open-heart surgery. *Br.Med.J.* 2:795-798, June 28, 1969.
9. DUTTON, R. C., AND EDMUNDS, L. H. Measurement of emboli in extracorporeal perfusion systems. *J.Thorac.Cardiovasc.Surg.* 65:523, April, 1973.
10. ROBERTS, M. C., AND MORROW, A. G. Anatomic studies of hearts containing caged-ball prosthetic valves. *Johns Hopkins Med. J.* 121:271-295, Oct. 1967.
11. LONG, M. L. *Incidence of Myocardial Infarction During and After Open Heart Surgery.* (Unpublished)
12. DHURANDHAR, R. W., AND OTHERS. Primary ventricular fibrillation complicating acute myocardial infarction. *Am.J.Cardiol.* 27:347-351, Apr. 1971.
13. CARLSON, R. G., AND OTHERS. Total cardiopulmonary support with disposable membrane oxygenator during aortocoronary artery-vein graft operations. *Chest* 62:424, 1972.

From the *American Journal of Nursing* 74:862, May 1974.

The Pump and Oxygenator

BARBARA NOBLE

Extracorporeal perfusion is initiated by collecting the patient's venous blood and passing it through an oxygenator. The oxygenated blood is then infused arterially. The normal hemodynamics of blood flow, pressure, and volume are maintained. Total body perfusion occurs when the heart and lungs are completely excluded from the circulation, and the body's vital organs depend totally on two pieces of equipment—the pump and oxygenator.

The heart-lung pump functions as a substitute left ventricle and pushes oxygenated blood through the patient's body. The pump has double rollers. Each roller is directly opposite the other so that each pumps fluid for half a revolution. One roller engages the tubing slightly before the opposite roller completes its stroke. This produces a relatively non-pulsatile blood flow.

During perfusion there is little difference between systolic and diastolic blood pressures. Flow rates are directly proportional to the speed of the pump rotation and the size of the tubing. The rollers do not completely occlude the tubing. Rather, they are carefully adjusted for partial occlusion so that trauma from the crushing effect of the rollers on the blood cells is decreased.

At Strong Memorial Hospital we use only disposable tubing and connectors for the fluid path between the patient and the oxygenator. Disposable equipment eliminates the hazard of using inadequately cleaned equipment.

Several types of oxygenators are available. The bubble, the rotating disc, and the membrane oxygenators are used most commonly.

The membrane oxygenator is the only one that does not permit actual contact between oxygen and blood. The blood and gases flow through

BARBARA NOBLE, R.N., *is an extracorporeal perfusionist, Strong Memorial Hospital, Rochester, N.Y.*

separate compartments; oxygen and carbon dioxide diffuse through a membrane. Elimination of the blood-gas interface is more physiological and less traumatic to blood components than direct contact. Disposable membranes are available, but these are still experimental and relatively expensive.

The rotating disc oxygenator is a horizontal cylinder with a varying number of vertical, rotating discs. Venous blood enters at one end, passes through the cylinder, and is picked up repeatedly by the rotating discs, which direct it to an oxygen-saturated atmosphere. This permanent unit requires meticulous, time-consuming cleaning between procedures.

Several brands of bubble oxygenators are available. They are all similar in terms of disposability, ease of assembly, sterility, and price. Oxygen and carbon dioxide are bubbled through a diffuser into the blood. This creates a blood-gas interface of sufficient duration to permit oxygenation, and sufficient momentum to push inflowing blood into a reservoir.

From the *American Journal of Nursing* 74:868-869, May 1974.

Cardiopulmonary Bypass: Postoperative Complications

ANNE VERDERBER

Some of the significant physiological and psychological complications open heart patients may exhibit are caused by the use of the pump-oxygenator. Others are related to the impact of surgery.

None of the extracorporeal perfusion systems equals the perfection of the human heart and lung. Therefore, physiological changes occur during and after surgery which may affect the patient's postoperative course and treatment.

There are significant changes in the patient's clotting mechanism. This occurs, in part, because the patient is heparinized before he is placed on the pump-oxygenator. Heparinization prevents the clotting of blood in the extracorporeal circuit. Also, fresh, heparinized blood is used to replace blood loss as well as to prime the pump-oxygenator, although many institutions now use non-blood solutions for priming. After surgery is completed, the heparin is neutralized by administration of protamine sulfate. However, heparin is metabolized approximately half as fast as protamine. Therefore, reversal of anticoagulation is often imperfect, resulting in a "heparin rebound" effect which requires the administration of additional protamine(12).

Other changes in the patient's clotting mechanism are due to the

MS. VERDERBER (*B.S.N., Saint John College of Cleveland, Cleveland, Oh.; M.Ed., University of Minnesota, Minneapolis; M.S., University of Wisconsin, Madison) is assistant professor in medical-surgical nursing at San Diego State University.*

mechanical trauma to blood cells by the pump and suction systems. Platelets are damaged and decreased, as are the plasma clotting factors prothrombin and fibrinogen. Hemolysis of red blood cells occurs because of mechanical trauma and the direct exposure of blood to oxygen.

Red blood cells may be hemolyzed more rapidly than the liver and kidneys can metabolize and excrete the damaged cells. If significant hemolysis occurs a mannitol-induced diuresis is usually effective, but "sludging" in the renal tubules may lead to acute tubular necrosis and renal failure.

The patient on a mechanical pump-oxygenator can be compared to a patient in shock, and inadequate perfusion and oxygenation are probably the major causes of postoperative complications. Inadequate or prolonged perfusion can cause tissue anoxia and metabolic acidosis. Therefore, acid-base balance must be monitored during and after open heart surgery. Severe acidosis is treated with sodium bicarbonate or THAM (tromethamine)(3).

Fluid and electrolyte balance must also be monitored carefully during and after surgery. Whenever extracellular fluid volume, blood volume, serum sodium, or cardiac output decreases, the adrenal cortex secretes aldosterone(4). Aldosterone increases renal reabsorption of sodium. This results in water retention and increased excretion of potassium. Furthermore, the hypothalamus stimulates an increase in antidiuretic hormone. ADH causes the distal and collecting tubules of the kidney to reabsorb even more water(4).

It usually takes several days for the patient's fluid balance to return to normal. During that time he is given minimal fluids and must be observed closely for signs of impending congestive heart failure or pulmonary edema. Any potassium loss, which may be accentuated by the use of diuretics, must be replaced. Hypokalemia decreases cardiac contractility, and can result in heart block and other cardiac arrhythmias.

Cerebral edema and brain damage may develop after open heart surgery. Their exact cause has not been determined, but appears to be related to inadequate cerebral perfusion during surgery(5). Air or fat emboli, calcium debris, and microemboli due to damaged red blood cells or inadequately filtered blood have also been implicated. Although cerebral dysfunction is not uncommon following open heart surgery, it is rarely fatal and seldom leaves a permanent deficit(3,5). Improvements in cardiopulmonary bypass techniques have markedly reduced the incidence of emboli. Induced hypothermia, both during and after surgery, reduces the brain's need for oxygen and minimizes cerebral edema and its sequelae.

A more commonly encountered problem is "post-pump psychosis." The patient may experience visual and auditory hallucinations as well as paranoid delusions. These may be caused by preoperative anxiety or by postoperative stress, accentuated by sleep deprivation and increased sensory input. Patients often cease having these experiences as soon as they are transferred out of the intensive care unit. However, psychological disturbances may be caused by cerebral edema or microemboli. Therefore, these patients require a careful neurological assessment.

A frequent complication of cardiopulmonary bypass is respiratory insufficiency. Pulmonary atelectasis, pneumonitis, or both, are frequent complications(6). Many patients have some degree of pulmonary hypertension before surgery, due to congenital or acquired heart disease. Additional damage can develop during the operation. Because the lungs do not function while the patient is on the pump-oxygenator, atelectasis can easily occur unless the patient is hypterventilated intermittently during surgery and in the immediate postoperative period. Also, the bronchial arteries, which perfuse lung tissue during bypass, empty into the left atrium through the pulmonary veins. If the left heart is not sufficiently vented, or drained, it will distend and back pressure on the pulmonary vasculature will cause additional pulmonary damage. Atelectasis can also develop if the patient tends to "splint" his respirations and not cough because of incisional pain.

Post-perfusion lung syndrome, or "pump lung," is the most serious respiratory problem seen in these patients, and is often fatal. Pump lung is characterized by atelectasis, pulmonary edema, and hemorrhage. While its etiology remains unknown, it may be caused by settling of microemboli in small pulmonary vessels, inhibition of surfactant production, or pulmonary hypoperfusion and hypoxia. Hemodilution perfusion (nonblood prime), postoperative ventilatory support, and the shorter duration of total cardiopulmonary perfusion now possible with improved surgical techniques have lowered the incidence of pump lung secondary to open heart surgery(7).

To prevent or minimize respiratory complications, the endotracheal tube is often left in place for one to three days. This facilitates suctioning of the tracheobronchial tree, and also permits ventilatory assistance with a mechanical respirator. If prolonged ventilatory assistance is required, a tracheostomy is usually done.

The shock-like condition which patients may exhibit during cardiopulmonary bypass can persist postoperatively. This is called the "low cardiac output syndrome," and may be caused by metabolic acidosis during cardiopulmonary bypass. Sodium bicarbonate or THAM and adequate mechanical ventilation may correct the metabolic acidosis. Hypoxemia and electrolyte imbalances, such as hypokalemia, hypocalcemia, and hyponatremia, depress cardiac function. These imbalances must be corrected. Occasionally, the only problem is inadequate blood volume replacement. If so, additional blood is all that is needed.

"Low cardiac output syndrome" is seen most often in patients with severe, long-standing heart disease(3). Previously damaged, hypertrophied ventricles which have an inadequate coronary circulation may fail after the insult of surgery. If this happens, extensive therapy, including the use of inotropic drugs, is needed to support the failing heart. Very occasionally, the cause of this syndrome is purely surgical, such as incomplete surgical correction or the implantation of a valve prosthesis which is too large and blocks cardiac blood flow.

Cardiac tamponade must also be ruled out. This is caused by an accumulation of blood and clots within the pericardial sac. Tamponade can usually be determined by the presence of a paradoxical pulse pressure— a drop in the systolic blood pressure of greater than 10 mm.Hg on inspiration. When the patient inhales, accumulated blood compresses the heart and causes a drop in cardiac output. If there is no active bleeding, cardiac tamponade can often be corrected by inserting a drainage tube into the pericardial cavity.

The complications associated with extracorporeal circulation can be serious, and mortality rates for specific kinds of open heart surgery, such as multiple valve replacement, remain relatively high. However, overall mortality rates for open heart surgery have decreased markedly, and many patients with severe disease do remarkably well. Cardioplumonary bypass offers these patients a chance to live completely normal lives.

REFERENCES

1. AMERICAN MEDICAL ASSOCIATION, COUNCIL ON DRUGS. *AMA Drug Evaluations.* Chicago, The Association, 1971.
2. FRIEDBERG, C. K. *Diseases of the Heart.* 3d ed. Philadelphia, W. B. Saunders Co., 1966.
3. SANDERSON, R. G. *The Cardiac Patient, A Comprehensive Approach* (Saunders Monographs in Clinical Nursing, No. 2) Philadelphia, W. B. Saunders Co., 1972, Chaps. 3 and 11.
4. GUYTON, A. C. *Textbook of Medical Physiology.* 4th ed. Philadelphia, W. B. Saunders Co., 1971, Chaps. 24 and 36.
5. JAVID, H., AND OTHERS. Neurological abnormalities following open-heart surgery. *J.Thorac.Cardiovasc.Surg.* 58:502-509, Oct. 1969.
6. GAUERT, W. B., AND OTHERS. Pulmonary complications following extracorporeal circulation. *South.Med.J.* 64:679-686, June 1971.
7. WEEDN, R. J., AND OTHERS. Effects of oxygen and ventilation on pulmonary mechanics and ultrastructure during cardiopulmonary bypass. *Am.J.Surg.* 120:584-590, Nov. 1970.

From the *American Journal of Nursing* 72:469-473, Mar. 1972.

Surgery for Coronary Artery Disease

ETTA RAE BRENER

*Even patients with severe coronary artery disease
can return to work and an active life—free of dyspnea and angina—within six weeks after this surgery.*

In coronary artery disease, atherosclerotic plaques, composed mainly of cholesterol, other lipids, and fibrous tissue, are deposited along the internal wall of a coronary artery. The atherosclerotic plaques are concentrated in the larger sections of the artery and are usually absent in the smaller sections. Thus, typically, the diseased artery has marked narrowing or occlusion in the larger, proximal section, some irregularities in the middle section, and a normal vessel wall in the smaller, distal section(1,2). One or more branches of the right and left coronary arteries may be affected to varying degrees.

These atherosclerotic plaques cause a decrease in the amount of blood delivered to the myocardium. This ischemia results in the familiar symptoms of coronary artery disease—chest pain and decreased exercise tolerance—and usually brings the patient to a physician.

Most commonly, coronary artery disease is treated by such medical measures as diet, exercise, and medication. But, in recent years, surgical methods of treating this disease have been developed. The surgical methods entail constructing new sources of blood supply to the ischemic myocardium.

MS. BRENER *was a part-time staff nurse in the ICU of St. Luke's
Hospital, New York, N.Y. when this article was prepared. She is now
a nursing instructor at Columbia University School of Nursing in
New York City. She received her B.S.N. at Washington University in
St. Louis, Mo. and her M.Ed. at Columbia-Teachers College.*

To treat coronary artery disease surgically, the precise extent of the disease must be defined. This is done primarily by coronary artery cineangiography. The heart is catheterized and radiopaque dye is injected into the coronary arteries. Motion x-ray pictures are taken of these vessels to visualize the precise location and extent of the atherosclerotic lesions.

The degree of disease is determined indirectly by measuring the exercise ability of the patient. The patient walks on a treadmill, the speed and incline of which can be varied. The patient's exercise ability is determined and compared with standard levels for his age. The patient with severe disease will usually have severely decreased exercise ability.

Other tests are also used in diagnosing the disease. The patient with coronary artery disease usually has an electrocardiogram in which the ST segment and T wave are altered. He usually has elevated blood levels of cholesterol (normally 150-250 mg. %) and triglycerides (normally 140 mg. %).

Once the extent of the disease is defined, surgery can be considered. Surgery is considered suitable for the patient who has symptoms of coronary artery disease and has demonstrable, occlusive, atherosclerotic lesions. The surgery consists of bypassing these large, occluding atherosclerotic lesions. The bypasses are constructed with sections of vein or artery which are taken from other portions of the patient's body.

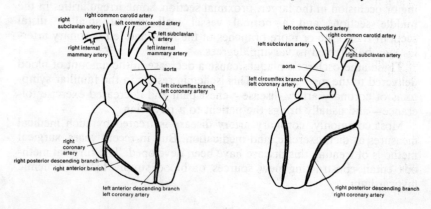

Heart muscle receives its blood supply from the right and left coronary arteries, which are the first arteries to branch off the ascending aorta. The anterior view (left) shows the branching of the right coronary artery and the left coronary artery. The posterior view (right) shows the continuation of the posterior descending branch of the right coronary artery and the circumflex branch of the left coronary artery to the posterior surface of the heart.

SURGERY: VINEBERG PROCEDURE AND VARIATIONS

The first procedure involving bypass grafts was developed by Vineberg in 1946. He implanted the distal end of the internal mammary (also called internal thoracic) artery, which branches from the subclavian artery, into the myocardium near the occluded coronary artery. In three to six months, anastomoses developed between the implanted internal mammary artery and the occluded coronary artery; thus, blood flow to the ischemic myocardium was increased.

In recent years, surgeons have begun making direct anastomoses between the coronary artery and the bypass vessel instead of implanting it in the myocardium and waiting the three to six months for anastomoses to develop.

There are many variations to the direct anastomosis technique, particularly in the use of vessels from different parts of the body for the bypass. For example, in one variation, a section of saphenous vein, about 10 inches long, is removed from its origin in the leg and divided into two

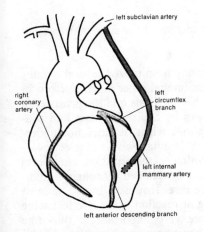

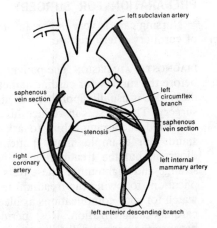

In the early Vineberg procedures, the distal portion of the internal mammary artery was dissected free and anastomosed into the myocardium near the occluded coronary artery. It then took three to six months for an anastomosis to develop between the implanted artery and the occluded artery and for blood flow to area of ischemia to increase.

Variations of the Vineberg procedure may now include direct anastomosis between the internal mammary artery and the occluded coronary artery at a point below the occlusion. Variation shown above was used for a patient with stenosis in three coronary arteries. Saphenous vein sections were used to bypass two of the stenotic areas.

segments. One end is sewn directly into a normal section of the right coronary artery beyond the point of narrowing and disease, and the other end of the section is sewn to the ascending aorta.

One end of the remaining section of saphenous vein is sewn directly to the left circumflex branch beyond the point of disease, and the other end of the section is sewn to the ascending aorta. The distal segment of the left internal mammary artery is dissected free, the proximal end is left attached to the subclavian artery, and the free distal end is sewn directly to the anterior descending branch beyond the point of disease. Thus, the areas of narrowing and diseased wall in the coronary arteries are bypassed, and new sources of blood supply are immediately available to the ischemic myocardium with this direct anastomosis technique.

Some surgeons used a combination of nearby implantation and direct anastomosis.

The surgery is delicate and often requires the use of an operating microscope with 16 magnifications to make these small anastomoses. During surgery, the patient is placed on cardiopulmonary bypass to provide a dry, quiet operating field.

PREPARATION FOR SURGERY

Nursing care is very important in the success of the surgical treatment of coronary artery disease.

DIAGNOSTIC ADMISSION The patient is usually hospitalized several months before the surgery for cardiac catheterization and other diagnostic procedures. He is usually apprehensive about his diagnosis and the prospect of surgery. The nurse can reduce his anxiety by explaining tests and routines and encouraging him to ask questions when he does not understand. For example, many patients are familiar with the electrocardiogram, but the treadmill test and cardiac catheterization may seem strange and frightening. These tests must be explained thoroughly. Complications following the treadmill test are rare. However, the nurse must watch for such complications as bleeding or reaction to the dye following cardiac catheterization. Rest periods are very important at this time because the patient will still experience chest pain and have low exercise ability.

HOME REGIMEN The patient should be given a diet and exercise regimen to follow at home during the waiting period between diagnosis and surgery, and he will require teaching and encouragement concerning them.

His diet may vary, depending on the type of hyperlipidemia he has(3). A representative diet allows 26 percent protein, 38 percent carbohydrate, and 36 percent fat in caloric intake. The ratio of unsaturated to saturated fats allowed is 2:1. And, cholesterol intake is limited to 300 mg. per day. The patient should avoid overindulgence in the five major sources of saturated fat and cholesterol in the American diet: high-fat meats, such as fatty steaks and pork; high-fat dairy products, such as whole milk and cheese; commercial baked goods; spreads, such as butter, the "older" margarines, shortening, and peanut butter; and egg yolks. If the patient is overweight, he should reduce to normal weight(4,5).

Exercise regimens also vary greatly, but they generally follow a pattern of daily, gradually increasing exercise.

SURGICAL ADMISSION When the patient is readmitted for surgery, the nurse helps to prepare him mentally and physically in the preoperative period. She orients the patient to the intensive care unit where he will be immediately after surgery, explains the various pieces of equipment and attachments to be used in his care, and emphasizes the usual ease and rapidity of recovery.

The patient is taught how to use the intermittent positive pressure breathing (IPPB) machine and how to cough effectively. The ICU orientation is best done by the nurse who will be caring for the patient postoperatively; this provides the patient with a familiar face in the unfamiliar environment of the ICU.

The nurse prepares the patient physically in the usual manner—shave, scrub, enema, and preoperative sedation.

POSTOPERATIVE OBSERVATIONS

Following surgery, the patient is brought to the ICU and remains there for about three days. During this period, close observation is essential.

CARDIOVASCULAR The nurse follows the patient's cardiovascular status in several ways. She observes the cardiac monitor carefully for the development of arrythmias. She notes the color and warmth of the skin, the rate and quality of peripheral pulses, and the amount and character of urine output. She frequently measures arterial and venous pressure and specific gravity of the urine. I.V. fluids, I.V. potassium supplements, and blood are ordered and administered on the basis of the patient's cardiovascular fluid and electrolytic status.

RESPIRATORY The patient is intubated and on a respirator until he awakens from anesthesia, which may be several hours. The nurse monitors the patient's respiratory system by observing how the respirator functions in relation to the patient's own breathing efforts and by noting his arterial blood gases. She suctions the patient every hour or more often as needed and notes the quantity and character of his secretions. At least every two hours, she turns the patient. After the patient is extubated, the nurse helps to assure adequate respiratory function by turning the patient, helping him use the IPPB machine, and periodically percussing his back to loosen secretions, encouraging him to cough, and splinting the incision while he is coughing.

CHEST TUBES The patient has chest tubes connected to suction of about 20 cm. water. The nurse milks these chest tubes at intervals, records the amount and type of drainage from them. Initially, the drainage is 10 to 200 cc. per hour and is red in color. After about 24 hours the drainage is minimal and is serosanguinous. The nurse replaces the drainage—cc. for cc.—with either blood or I.V. fluid as ordered.

INFECTION AND PAIN The nurse administers antibiotics which are ordered as a prophylactic measure. She must observe the wound site, chest and urine drainage, and vital signs to determine the effectiveness of the antibiotics. She also administers ordered analgesics to control incisional pain; the patient can easily distinguish between incisional pain and anginal pain, which should no longer be present.

PSYCHOLOGIC SUPPORT The nurse assesses the patient's psychologic status and cares for him in several ways. She assures him of his satisfactory progress and explains any new procedures to him. She helps him to remain oriented to time and place by such techniques as opening the blinds, reminding him of the time and date, and mentioning news outside the hospital. She encourages visiting by immediate family members as permitted by the ICU policy.

POSTOPERATIVE COMPLICATIONS

Some of the more common complications include cardiac arrhythmias, myocardial infarction, bleeding, emboli, pneumonia, and pericarditis. Rarer complications include infection, sternal wound dehiscence, stress ulcers, and renal failure.

ARRHYTHMIAS Cardiac arrhythmias occur. However, they are more rare with this type of surgery than with open heart surgery in which the myocardium is deeply incised and stitched, and ectopic foci are more likely to develop. The most common arrhythmias are those related to ventricular irritability; premature ventricular contractions (PVCs), ventricular tachycardia, and ventricular fibrillation, PVCs are treated with lidocaine; ventricular tachycardia is treated with either lidocaine or countershock; and ventricular fibrillation is treated with countershock. Atrial flutter and atrial fibrillation can also occur; these are treated with digitalis preparations, quinidine, countershock, or a combination of these.

MYOCARDIAL INFARCTION Some patients develop myocardial infarctions which are characterized by EKG changes, cardiac insufficiency, arrhythmias, and anginal pain. The infarction is usually treated by medical measures—rest, medication, diet, and exercise. In very rare instances, the patient is taken back to the operating room, and a new graft, bypassing the new coronary lesion is constructed.

BLEEDING The patient occasionally bleeds excessively from the surgical wound into the chest. To detect this, the nurse observes and records the amount of chest tube drainage hourly and reports excessive bleeding (over 200-300 cc./hour) to the physician. The patient may be taken back to the operating room to have the wound reopened and the bleeders ligated or cauterized.

EMBOLI The patient may develop phlebitis or pulmonary, cerebral, or mesenteric emboli. The nurse helps to prevent this by changing the patient's position frequently and by helping him to ambulate early. Ambulation is usually begun on the second postoperative day. Should emboli develop, they are treated with anticoagulation therapy—heparin and, then, coumadin.

PNEUMONIA Pneumonia is likely to develop in these patients because of ineffective coughing secondary to incisional pain. The nurse plays an important role in preventing pneumonia by administering ordered analgesics and by helping the patient to cough effectively. If pneumonia develops, the nurse continues these measures with increased vigor and administers ordered antibiotics.

PERICARDITIS Pericarditis occurs fairly often. It is caused by an inflammatory reaction of the pericardium which is probably due to the surgical trauma. The pericarditis usually begins with 24 hours after the surgery;

it is characterized by a fever which is often as high as 103°F. Corticosteroids are given, then gradually decreased to control this reaction.

NORMAL POSTOPERATIVE COURSE

Barring the development of complications, recovery is usually surprisingly rapid. On the first postoperative day, the patient dangles and starts on a clear liquid diet. On the second postoperative day, he gets out of bed and eats a regular diet. By the third postoperative day, cardiac monitoring, chest tubes, intravenous lines, and the Foley catheter are discontinued, and the patient is transferred to a regular hospital unit.

The patient remains in the hospital for another 10 days. During this time the nurse encourages him to engage in gradually increasing daily activity. But, she sees that he has frequent rest periods because he still fatigues easily.

Also during this time, the nurse prepares the patient for discharge by reinforcing the diet and exercise instructions which he will need to follow at home. The patient must understand that although the present symptoms are relieved by surgery, the basic mechanism causing atherosclerosis has not been altered. His diet regimen is designed to prevent or slow redevelopment of symptoms of coronary artery disease. The diet is usually the same as the preoperative diet: low in saturated fat and cholesterol. The exercise regimen is also similar to the preoperative one: regular, gradually increasing activity.

The patient usually feels the need to talk about his surgery and to relive the overwhelming experience. The nurse gives him ample opportunity to do so and also explains this need to his family. The patient often has recurrent, unpleasant dreams about the surgery and the nurse can assure him that this is a common experience. She encourages liberal family visiting during this period to enhance psychologic comfort.

The patient is discharged about two weeks after surgery. He recuperates at home for another four weeks and, then, returns to work and full activity. The patient's symptoms of coronary artery disease usually completely disappear, and he gradually reaches higher levels of activity than he was capable of preoperatively.

The results of this surgery are evaluated by the patient's report of his symptoms, and by repeat coronary artery cineangiogram and treadmill test. The success rate of this operation is high: 80 percent of the patients report clinical improvement, and 80 to 90 percent of bypass grafts are demonstrated to be patent. The mortality rate is between 5 and 9.5 percent, as compared to a mortality rate of 25 to 40 percent for acute myocardial infarction(6,7).

CASE HISTORY: MR. S. G.

S. G. is fairly typical of patients who have undergone this type of surgery. For three years, Mr. G. had angina attacks, manifested as a severe burning sensation in his throat, rather than the more common chest pain. Mr. G. was hospitalized twice for observation and rest.

By July 1970, his disease was so severe that he could not walk the three blocks from the subway to his home, nor could he play with his children without experiencing extreme discomfort. Mr. G. was hospitalized for a precise diagnosis at that time. Cineangiography showed complete occlusion of the proximal portion of the right coronal artery with retrograde filling of this artery from the left anterior descending and circumflex branches; stenosis in the proximal portion of the left anterior descending; and stenosis and irregularities in the proximal portion of the left circumflex. He was discharged from the hospital on a preoperative diet and exercise regimen.

Mr. G. reentered the hospital in October 1970 for surgery. Three coronary artery bypass grafts were constructed: the right coronary artery occlusion was bypassed with a saphenous vein section, the left anterior stenosis was bypassed with the left internal mammary artery, and the left circumflex stenosis was bypassed with another section of saphenous vein.

Nursing care for Mr. G. was similar to the general nursing care already described. Mr. G.'s only difficulties were hypotension and a slight pericarditis which occurred within the first 24 hours postoperatively. Large quantities of I.V. fluids and blood, a total of 5,000 c.c., were administered over the first eight hours postoperatively in order to maintain Mr. G.'s blood pressure. And, corticosteroids were administered in decreasing doses to treat the inflammatory reaction and consequent fever which Mr. G. developed the first postoperative night. Mr. G. was rather apprehensive about the development of these complications, and required constant reassurance from the nurse that he really was progressing satisfactorily.

Mr. G. had excellent results from the surgery. His angina disappeared immediately and completely. Six weeks after surgery he was able to walk to and from the subway, work eight hours, play with his children, and, generally, participate fully and actively in life without pain or fear of a heart attack. It is gratifying to see a person who was becoming a cardiac invalid restored to health and vigor.

REFERENCES
1. GREEN, G. E. Microvascular technique in coronary artery surgery. *Am.Heart J.* 79:276-279, Feb. 1970.

2. ———. Direct revascularization: internal mammary artery to left coronary artery anastomosis. *N.Y.State J.Med.* 70:1993-1994, Aug. 1, 1970.
3. LEES, R. S., AND WILSON, D. E. Treatment of hyperlipidemia. *N.Eng.J.Med.* 284:186-195, Jan. 28, 1971.
4. PAGE, I. H., AND STAMLER, J. Diet—and coronary heart disease: Part 1. *Mod.Concepts Cardiovasc.Dis.* 37:119-123, Sept. 1968.
5. PAGE, I. H. Diet—and coronary heart disease. Part 2. *Mod.-Concepts Cardiovasc.Dis.* 37:125-128, Oct. 1968.
6. BREST, A. N., and MOYER, J. H., EDS. *Cardiovascular Disorders.* Philadelphia, F. A. Davis Co., 1968. p. 714.
7. CECIL, R. I., AND LOEB, R. F. *Textbook of Medicine.* 12th edition edited by Paul B. Beeson and Walsh McDermott, Philadelphia, W. B. Saunders Co., 1967, p. 650.

BIBLIOGRAPHY

CLELAND, W. P., AND OTHERS. *Medical and Surgical Cardiology.* Philadelphia, F. A. Davis Co., 1969.

FRIEDBERG, C. K. *Diseases of the Heart.* 3d ed. Philadelphia, W. B. Saunders Co., 1966.

GREEN, G. E., and OTHERS. *Coronary arterial bypass grafts. Am.Thorac.Surg.* 5:443-450, May, 1968.

HATTLER, B. G., JR., AND SABISTON, D. C., JR. Myocardial revascularization. *Surgery 66:* 620-626, Sept. 1969.

JOHNSON, W. D., AND LEPLEY, DERWARD JR. Aggressive surgical approach to coronary disease. *J.Thorac.Cardiovasc.Surg.* 59:128-138, Jan. 1970.

JOHNSON, W. D., AND OTHERS. Extended treatment of severe coronary artery disease: a total surgical approach. *Ann.Surg.* 170:460-470, Sept. 1969.

From the *American Journal of Nursing* 73:2580-2584, Sept. 1973.

Care of a Man with a Partial Artificial Heart

ROBERTA NELSON • JUDY SMITH • RUTH DRUMMOND
HILDE POLLARD • JOYCE BILLINGSLEY
MIRIAM NIKKILA

Techniques in cardiopulmonary bypass for open-heart surgery have stimulated the search for methods to assist a failing heart permanently. One method recently developed uses an implanted auxiliary ventricle—the dynamic aortic patch.

The first patient to receive a dynamic aortic patch was Mr. T., a 63-year-old plant guard from metropolitan Detroit, Michigan(1,2). Mr. T. had severe chronic congestive heart failure and was bedridden with weakness, marked dyspnea, and leg edema. His symptoms were first noted five years earlier, when he complained of difficulty in breathing and a productive, frothy cough. Treatment at that time had consisted of digitalis and diuretics.

His condition had deteriorated during the last several years, and he was transferred to Sinai Hospital of Detroit in July 1971. Prior to his admission, Mr. T. had undergone a series of clinical evaluations. Coronary arteriography and left ventriculography showed more than 70 percent occlusion of three main coronary arteries, and severe left and right ventricular failure. Chest x-rays showed pulmonary vascular congestion in both lung bases. The transverse diameter of the heart had recently increased from 165 mm. to 190 mm.

Laboratory evaluation showed severe liver impairment and reduced renal function, but normal hematologic, endocrine, and gastrointestinal function. The clinical diagnosis at that time included ischemic cardiomyopathy and atherosclerotic heart disease (functional classification of IV-

255

E), diabetes, chronic passive congestion of the liver, probable cardiac cirrhosis, and mild organic brain syndrome.

His response to medication was unsatisfactory. Moreover, it was determined that because of the severity of his cardiac condition, without typical angina symptoms, attempts to surgically repair his coronary circulation would probably be unsuccessful. The partial mechanical heart appeared to offer this patient the best chance for improved functioning.

On August 4, intra-aortic balloon pumping was initiated to determine the patient's response to mechanical cardiac assistance. This pump is a temporary assist device and is a precursor of the dynamic aortic patch(3,4,5,6). The balloon pump consists of a cigar-shaped polyurethane pumping chamber, a catheter, and an external pumping system. The pumping chamber is inserted through the femoral artery and is positioned in the thoracic aorta just below the origin of the left subclavian artery.

The balloon pump operates on the principle of diastolic augmentation. The balloon is inflated during diastole and deflated during systole. This elevates aortic blood pressure immediately after aortic valve closure and increases blood flow to the coronary circulation. The dynamic aortic patch also operates on this principle.

Mr. T. responded satisfactorily to two hours of balloon pumping. His cardiac output increased 16 percent and there were significant decreases in left ventricular end, diastolic, and pulmonary artery pressures.

MS. NELSON, a graduate of Highland Park College of Nursing, Highland Park, Mich., holds an A.B. degree from Highland Park Community College. She was clinical instructor for the Heart Surgery Study Area and surgical ICU at Sinai Hospital of Detroit, Mich., when this article was written. She is now an instructor in practical nursing for the Detroit Board of Education. MS. SMITH, a graduate of Wayne State University School of Nursing, Detroit, Mich., was head nurse of the surgical ICU, Sinai Hospital of Detroit. MS. DRUMMOND, a graduate of the University of Pittsburgh School of Nursing, Pittsburgh, Pa., is home care coordinator, Sinai Hospital of Detroit. MS. POLLARD, a graduate of Holyoke Hospital School of Nursing, Holyoke, Mass., is a staff nurse with the VNA, Roseville, Mich. MS. BILLINGSLEY, a graduate of Wayne State University School of Nursing, is home care coordinator, VNA of Detroit, Inc., Mich. MS. NIKKILA, a graduate of Michael Reese Hospital School of Nursing, Chicago, Ill., holds a B.S. degree in public health nursing from Wayne State University. She is supervisor of the Home Care Program, VNA of Metropolitan Detroit, Inc. The research leading to the development of the patch and the study of the patient were supported in part by USPHS Grant HL-13737.

Because of this favorable response, Mr. T. was considered to be an appropriate candidate for a permanent cardiac assist device.

THE SURGERY

On August 10 the dynamic aortic patch was implanted during total cardiopulmonary bypass. The dynamic aortic patch consists of an ellipsoidial rubber pumping chamber, a gas conduit, and Dacron covering materials. The intravascular surface is Dacron velour, sprayed with a conductive polyurethane. This material has a low thrombogenic potential and permits the growth of a pseudo-intima. The prosthesis was implanted into the lateral surface of the descending thoracic aorta between the origin of the left subclavian artery and the diaphragm.

A gas conduit was then led through a transcutaneous connector in the left hypogastric region to an extracorporeal driving system. EKG leads from the apex of the left ventricle were passed through the connector to the driving unit. The R wave of the electrocardiogram synchronized the external system with the cardiac cycle.

A fixed-rate pacemaker, set at 95 beats per minute, was also implanted in the patient's left chest wall. The pacing electrode was sutured to the left atrium. Following implantation of the patch booster and pacemaker, cardiopulmonary bypass was discontinued and the patch booster was activated immediately. The chest was then closed.

POSTSURGICAL NURSING CARE

Following surgery, Mr. T. was cared for in the Heart Surgery Study Area. His electrocardiogram, arterial and pulmonary artery pressures, and apical heart rate were monitored continuously on a multichannel oscilloscope and digital display.

Respiratory condition, central venous pressure, temperature, urine output, intravenous fluid intake, and chest tube drainage were checked and recorded every 30 minutes. Careful notes were made of the times of intravenous infusions and medications, and results of frequent blood gas and electrolyte determinations were recorded.

We were constantly alert for signs of respiratory complications. The color of Mr. T.'s lips, nail beds, and extremities was observed frequently. We listened to breath sounds to detect accumulated bronchial secretions which might impair oxygen exchange and necessitate deep suctioning.

EKG leads were positioned to leave room for defibrillator paddles, if needed. The electrocardiogram was constantly monitored to detect arrhythmias. Apical and radial pulse rates were frequently compared, and the quality of the radial pulse was noted.

The patient's fluid balance was closely monitored to alert the nurses to any overloading of the circulatory system which would increase the workload of the heart. The patient's chest tubes were connected to suction equipment, and the volume of drainage carefully observed. Since at least 100 ml. of fluid are expected to drain from the chest during the first 60 minutes following lung reexpansion, we watched for any excessive drainage(7).

The specific gravity of the urine was measured every hour to evaluate how well the kidneys were concentrating urine. If urine output was less than 30 ml. per hour, the doctors were notified immediately as this could indicate hypovolemia, hypotension, or renal shutdown.

The external driving unit was placed at the foot of the patient's bed. This instrument was maintained primarily by the engineers, but the nurses were familiar with adjustments needed for changes in heart rate. The skin button, where the gas conduit was externalized, was cleaned with pHisoHex and peroxide. Care was taken not to disturb the tube to the driving unit since tension or kinks in the tube could cause the driving unit to function improperly.

During the first postoperative week, Mr. T. was cooperative even though he was intubated and on a respirator. The psychiatrist on the team suggested we communicate by using a card with all the letters of the alphabet. Mr. T. pointed to the letters of words he wished to say. As his physical condition improved, Mr. T. rebelled against the confinement and restricted activity in the Heart Surgery Study Area and wanted to get up more than the doctors advised.

During the second week. Mr. T. became disoriented and confused. This was thought to reflect the organic brain syndrome diagnosed before surgery. Steps were taken to reinforce his personal identity: his wife was allowed to stay with him for longer periods, she showed him family pictures, told him the time, the day, the place, and discussed his surgery with him. The same nurse cared for Mr. T. each day to provide a frame of reference, and only his wife and sister were permitted to visit. His mental and emotional state progressively improved.

As soon as his condition permitted, Mr. T. was transferred to the Coronary Care Unit, which has a more relaxed atmosphere with homelike furnishing, including pictures, music, and television. He could not see the monitoring equipment, and the wide windows in front of his bed provided a pleasant view. He appeared to be at his emotional best during his stay in the CCU. He was transferred back to the Heart Surgery Study Area on several occasions when his care required it. Because these moves added to his confusion and disorientation, it was necessary to reassure him of his continued improvement. His wife played a major role in providing him with emotional support during this time.

At first Mr. T. was psychologically dependent on the mechanical assist device and this presented a problem. It was not desirable to have the pump on continuously and he often became apprehensive when it was off. Eventually, excursions to the hospital garden in his specially equipped wheelchair provided diversion. A month after surgery, Mr. T.'s tolerance for exercise had improved significantly. He was able to leave his room, walk around.

Mr. T.'s hemodynamic condition had now stabilized. Platelet aggregation and blood coagulation tests were normal, and there was no evidence of hemolysis. The heart size was now essentially normal.

A complete cardiac cathertization, done five weeks after implantation of the patch booster, showed good hemodynamic compensation with a marked increase in cardiac index so we began planning for Mr. T.'s discharge. To make the transition from hospital to home easier for both Mr. T. and his wife, he was transferred back to the CCU, where Ms. T. could stay with him and begin to assume some responsibilities for his care.

HOME CARE

Home care services were coordinated and planned with the Visiting Nurse Association (VNA) and other community agencies serving Mr. T.'s residential area. The VNA, which offers one of the country's first community-based home care programs, serves Detroit and the surrounding tricounty area. Although the agency staff had participated in the home care of artificial kidney patients, much extensive, coordinated planning was required to care for the first patch booster patient.

Planning for home care began with a total team conference, two weeks before Mr. T.'s discharge, attended by surgeons, cardiologists, psychiatrists, nurses, engineers, the home care coordinator, social worker, and hospital administrator. The VNA was represented by the assistant director of nursing services, a medical-surgical consultant, a social work consultant, and the visiting nurse who would be responsible for Mr. T.'s home care. Representatives from the police and fire departments in Mr. T.'s community also participated. Their services were enlisted to prevent intrusions on the patient's privacy and to provide emergency assistance as needed.

The unique circumstances concerning Mr. T. and his assist device were discussed at the conference. The mechanized wheelchair with its self-contained unit, the portable drive unit for the patch booster, and the portable compressed air unit were explained. Initially, Ms. T. would probably need help with Mr. T.'s care around the clock. Therefore, a VNA field nurse would accompany him home and remain there for the first 48 hours. Subsequently, the agency would provide home health aides 24 hours a day. Before the conference ended, Mr. T. and his wife were introduced to the group who would be responsible for his home care.

During the interim before the patient's discharge, the visiting nurse and medical-surgical consultant visited Ms. T. at home to assess her ability to carry out her husband's care and to evaluate the physical setup. The couple lived in a three-bedroom ranch house in a middle-class neighborhood. The visiting nurses felt that Ms. T. was devoted to her husband and sincere in her desire to make the home care plans work.

One week before discharge, the visiting nurse spent a day with Ms. T. and the medical-surgical team at the hospital. Mr. T.'s progress, the operation of the equipment, and the rehabilitation goals were discussed.

On the day Mr. T. was to go home, the visiting nurse arrived early to confer again with the physicians and the psychiatrist, and then she accompanied Mr. and Ms. T. on the 20-mile ride home. Consistent with his pumping regimen in the hospital, the patch booster was disconnected during this time. When they arrived, the neighbors greeted Mr. T. warmly. There was a large "welcome home" sign on the front door. He smiled and, as he entered the house, tears came to his eyes. He said, "I thought I would never make it."

During the first 48 hours at home, Mr. T.'s medical condition remained stable. Engineering technicians visited twice a day to check the equipment and make necessary adjustments. Members of the police and fire departments stopped by often during the first three days. At the beginning, Mr. T. was anxious, and his bed seemed to offer him the most security. He resisted even short walks in or out of doors. He was restless and agitated anywhere but in the bedroom and wanted someone with him most of the time. At times he was mentally confused, especially when the pump had been off for a while. He slept for short intervals, most restfully when someone was in the room with him.

The first few days were also very trying for his wife, who found it difficult to relax and cope with normal activities. The nurse spent a great deal of time talking with her, and gradually she was able to take on more of her husband's care. On the third day, a second visiting nurse arrived with the home health aide. At this time the patch booster was being activated from 12:00 midnight to 7:00 A.M., then two hours on and two hours off throughout the day. The nurse outlined the schedule of duties for the home health aide (see Home Care for Mr. T.). The aide provided opportunities for Ms. T. to have outside activities and rest periods,

---

HOME CARE FOR MR. T.

Vital Signs
Check vital signs, including blood pressure, twice daily.
Observe for shortness of breath, fluid retention, and signs of increased fatigue.

Wound Care
Irrigate, apply prescribed ointment and dry sterile dressing twice daily.
Observe for unusual changes in appearance of wound.

Medication
Instruct wife and home health aide to safely administer medications.
Observe desired and side effects of medication.

Nutrition
Encourage small, frequent meals, high in protein, carbohydrates, and potassium, and low in sodium.
Instruct wife and home health aide in diet modification.
Record and evaluate food intake.
Consult VNA nutritionist regarding problems.

Elimination
Instruct wife and home health aide to test urine daily for sugar and acetone.
Watch for abnormal bowel function, especially constipation.

Activity
Encourage patient to be up and about as tolerated, and as independent as possible.
Increase outdoor walking up to one block daily as tolerated.
Supervise isometric exercises and resistive exercises of the triceps and quadriceps, using 4 lb. weights.
Discuss progress with physical therapy consultant.

Mental and Emotional Behavior
Watch for confusion, disorientation, or erratic behavior.
Encourage patient and wife to verbalize feelings, but attempt to maintain a calm atmosphere.
Limit number of people in home.

Equipment
Instruct patient, wife, and home health aide in use of equipment.
Identify problems and alter as indicated.
Notify engineers, police or fire department in emergency.

---

and assisted with household chores. The nurse continued to visit twice daily to review Mr. T.'s condition, attend to his wound, and supervise the aide.

The home health aide made daily notes about her experience and observations in caring for the patient:

We would get him up and dress him and take walks, first ¼ of a block then ½ block. This he walked without assistance or without a cane. He would see his neighbors and say hello to them; he knew them all. We would take him for rides in the car, which he liked. He was on the pump two hours and off the pump two hours. We would try to do everything possible that he liked. Sometimes he and I would play checkers; he would get a kick when he beat me. He also liked baseball on T.V. I would question him about some of the players for the Tigers so that he would talk about it. When he was on the pump, he liked you to sit with him. Then he would talk about his home in Tennessee, or his guard duty at work, or church, which he liked to talk about most. When he came to the table to eat, he would say a beautiful prayer. I had to see that not more than two visitors came at one time, and that no reporters harassed him. I encouraged him if need be when he was off the pump more than two hours, even if it had to be six hours, that he'd still be all right.

During Mr. T.'s stay at home, VNA specialists, including the nutritionist, physical therapist, and occupational therapist, were consulted on several occasions. The patient's daily living activities were continually reviewed. Muscle strengthening activities, games for diversional activity, and problems concerning food intake were discussed. The engineers moved the pump equipment to the family room to encourage Mr. T. to remain up and about for longer periods of time.

Two weeks after Mr. T.'s discharge from the hospital, he developed a low-grade fever and drainage was noted around the incision and chest button. On October 4, two days later, he was readmitted to the hospital because of anorexia, fever, and malaise. The presence of an empyema was subsequently established. Despite intensive antibiotic treatment, he continued to be lethargic, occasionally confused, and febrile. Severe renal failure developed, and on November 6 peritoneal dialysis begun.

On November 14, following an episode of ventricular fibrillation, Mr. T. died, 96 days after implantation of the dynamic aortic patch. Autopsy revealed extensive thoracic and abdominal infection. The patch booster itself was intact, covered by a firm layer of fibrin, and was not involved in the infectious process. There was no evidence of thromboembolization.

The permanently implanted auxiliary ventricle had provided hemodynamic support to this patient with intractable congestive heart failure. Before surgery, he was bedridden: following surgery, his exercise tolerance improved until he could walk several hundred yards without assistance. Although improved techniques are expected, the equipment and procedures used in the present case appear to be practical for use both in the hospital and at home.

The coordinated efforts of Mr. and Mrs. T., the Visiting Nurse Association, other community resources, and large urban medical center made his discharge and home care possible, after the implantation of a mechanical auxiliary ventricle.

REFERENCES

1. KANTROWITZ, A., AND OTHERS. Current status of intraaortic balloon pump and initial clinical experience with aortic patch mechanical auxiliary ventricle. *Transplant.Proc.* 3:1459-1472, Dec. 1971.
2. ————. Initial clinical experience with a new permanent mechanical auxiliary ventricle: the dynamic aortic patch. *Trans.-Am.Soc.Artif.Intern.Organs* 18:159-167, 1972.
3. ————. Initial clinical experience with intraaortic balloon pumping in cardiogenic shock. *JAMA* 203:113-118, Jan. 8, 1968.
4. SUJANSKY, E., AND OTHERS. A dynamic aortic patch as a permanent mechanical auxiliary ventricle: experimental studies. *Surgery* 66:875-882, Nov. 1969.
5. KANTROWITZ, A., AND OTHERS. Phase-shift balloon pumping in cardiogenic shock. *Progr.Cardiovasc.Dis.* 12:293-301, Nov. 1969.
6. KRAKAUER, J. S., AND OTHERS. Clinical management ancillary to phase-shift balloon pumping in cardiogenic shock. *Am.J.Cardiol.* 27:123-128, Feb. 1971.
7. MARTZ, E. V., AND BEAUMONT, J. D. Computer-based monitoring in an intensive-care unit (ICU): implications for nursing education. *Heart Lung* 1:90-98, Jan.-Feb. 1972.

From the *American Journal of Nursing* 74:240-244, Feb. 1974.

Postoperative Complications: Assessment and Intervention

MICKEY CAMP PARSONS • GWEN J. STEPHENS

Ms. R., a 65-year-old white female, was a patient in the surgical intensive care unit at the University of Colorado Medical Center after undergoing repair of an abdominal aortic aneurysm. Her complicated previous history and numerous postoperative physiologic problems required careful consideration of several biologic parameters which form the bases of nursing assessments and interventions in an acute surgical setting.

In 1953, Ms. R. was found to have hypertension. She was hospitalized several times for this, but her condition worsened, and in 1957 she had several episodes of paroxysmal nocturnal dyspnea, orthopnea, and pulmonary edema with hemoptysis. These signs of progressive left ventricular failure were further complicated by a myocardial infarction later the same year. Eventually her hypertension was adequately controlled with hydrochlorothiazide, and she remained relatively well for several years until low back pain of increasing severity again prompted hospitalization.

A variety of therapeutic measures were tried, including a vagotomy and pyloroplasty. Recovery from this procedure was complicated by thrombophlebitis, pulmonary emboli, and small bowel fistulas. None of these treatments relieved her increasingly severe lower back pain. She was referred to the University of Colorado Medical Center and admitted in August 1972.

MS. PARSONS *is head nurse clinician, surgical intensive therapy unit, University of Colorado Medical Center, Denver. She has an M.N. degree from the University of Washington, Seattle.* MS. STEPHENS *is associate professor at the University of Colorado Medical Center School of Nursing. She has B.S., M.S., and Ph.D. degrees from Northwestern University, Evanston, Ill.*

The examining physicians here discovered a pulsating, lower abdominal mass. Gentle pressure on the mass elicited the back pain she complained of. A diagnosis of abdominal aortic aneurysm was made, and in September she had corrective surgery. The procedure was an aortic-iliac Y graft for correction of the abdominal aortic aneurysm as well as a right iliac aneurysm. In addition, the surgeons resected a length of small bowel for the fistulas which had developed from her previous operation. The operation took nine hours.

A preoperative review of her medical records, consultation with the nursing staff, and a visit with Ms. R. indicated that we had to watch her blood pressure and left ventricular performance closely. The nature of her vascular surgery made it necessary to maintain adequate cardiac output to forestall the possibility of intravascular coagulation in the graft areas. Our knowledge of the circulatory and pulmonary complications she had had before made us more concerned about this possibility.

Because we had seen Ms. R. preoperatively, we were also able to anticipate her emotional needs postoperatively. We had been struck by her courage and stoicism before surgery. She had walked by herself despite her weakness and pain, and was very calm about the surgery and hopeful that it would eliminate her pain. We recognized that any complaint she had should be assessed immediately since Ms. R. did not speak of her discomforts readily. Ms. R. was also alone. She was a widow, she lived out of state, and her daughter would not be able to visit often. Her need for support probably would be greater than she would indicate to us.

When she was transferred to the surgical intensive therapy unit from the recovery room at 8:00 P.M., our initial nursing assessment revealed the following:

Circulatory system: blood pressure 132/90; pulse 76, normal sinus rhythm; central venous pressure (CVP) 12.8 cm. H_2O; pedal pulses palpable; color good; skin warm; wound dressing dry and intact.

Respiratory system: oral endotracheal tube in place; on volume ventilator with 40 percent oxygen; initiating her own respirations at a rate of 18/minute; tidal volume off ventilator 400-600 c.c. with voluntary increase to 800 cc.; minimal clear secretions on suctioning; chest clear to auscultation.

Neurological: awake, alert, responding appropriately to verbal stimuli; moving all extremities on command.

Renal: urine output 40-50 cc./hour; specific gravity 1.016.

Gastrointestinal: abdomen firm, somewhat distended; nasogastric suction tube connected to low intermittent suction, draining light brown fluid.

Emotional: calm, seemed to understand explanations of what was happening to her, assured that she was progressing normally.

According to our assessment, her condition was satisfactory. We discontinued the respirator at 9:15 P.M. and gave her 40 percent oxygen through a neublizer via a T-tube connected to the endotracheal tube. She did well off the respirator. Her arterial blood sample indicated a pO_2 of 119 at 98 percent saturation, pCO_2 35, and a pH of 7.39. At 10:30 P.M. the endotracheal tube was removed without problems. Her blood pressure was 144/100; pulse rate 128 and regular; CVP 14 cm. H_2O; and urinary output for the hour was 95 cc.

PROBLEM 1: HEMORRHAGIC SHOCK

Later that same night, Ms. R.'s pulse rate rose to 144, and her blood pressure fell to 112/84. We notified her physician. When he arrived, a half hour later, her systolic pressure was 108, her CVP measured 9.5 cm. H_2O, and her urinary output had dropped to 24 cc./hour.

Ms. R. was markedly diaphoretic and had cool, pale, clammy skin. She complained of severe abdominal pain. Even with mannitol and plasmanate infusions her blood pressure continued to drop, to 76 systolic, and her abdomen was tender and firm. Her femoral pulses remained satisfactory, but her peripheral pulses were weak. Her CVP had dropped to 3.5 cm. H_2O and her extremities were very cool.

Ms. R.'s anxiety increased as her physiological state worsened. We told her she was receiving treatments to help her improve and a nurse was at her bedside much of the night.

Ms. R. received three units of blood with some temporary moderation of the hypovolemic symptoms, but her respiratory rate increased from 18 at 8 P.M. to 40 by 7 A.M. She was short of breath and complained of abdominal pressure and severe back pain. Her CVP was now increasing: 8.2 cm. H_2O at 7 A.M. and 15 cm. H_2O an hour later. The signs of blood loss coupled with a rising CVP indicated a weakening of left ventricular performance. Her falling urinary output indicated the potential hazard of acute tubular insufficiency secondary to renal ischemia. This, coupled with massive intravenous infusions, posed the problem of pulmonary edema from fluid overload.

Calcium gluconate and digoxin were given to strengthen myocardial contractility, furosemide (Lasix) to stimulate renal tubular function, and metaraminol (Aramine) to raise her blood pressure. By 9 A.M., however, her hematocrit had fallen to 21 percent, compared with an immediate postoperative value of 36 percent. Her abdomen was very distended, and this limited respiratory excursions and so impeded ventilation.

Intra-abdominal bleeding was presumed to be far advanced, and the elevated CVP in combination with hypovolemia and anemia indicated that her cardiac status was precarious.

The most notable physiological change common to all forms of shock is inadequate tissue perfusion, often due to inadequate cardiac output. In hemorrhagic shock, decreased cardiac output is caused by an inadequate venous return.

Several reflex compensatory changes occur in response to inadequate tissue perfusion of the brain and myocardium. There is reflex activation of the sympathetic (adrenergic) division of the autonomic nervous system, and release of catecholamines from the adrenal medulla. These cause an elevation in heart rate, vasoconstriction of vessels in the skin, mucous membranes, and kidneys, and diaphoresis. The catecholamines also stimulate the brain-stem reticular formation to cause anxiety, restlessness, and an enhanced perception of pain.

The compensatory vasoconstriction may be very marked in the kidneys and, in the presence of decreased renal perfusion, the glomerular filtration rate declines markedly. Renal ischemia may lead to acute tubular necrosis.

The hemorrhage-related anemia causes hypoxic stimulation of the respiratory center. This leads to tachypnea. As blood accumulates in the peritoneal cavity it presses on the diaphragm, limiting ventilatory excursions and impeding venous return to the heart. In addition, the presence of blood irritates the peritoneum, causing increased pain and abdominal rigidity, which further restrict breathing movements. Together, these problems cause respiratory insufficiency.

At 10:15 A.M. Ms. R. was returned to the operating room for exploration. She vomited around the nasogastric tube just before she was anesthetized and may have aspirated vomitus at this time. This may have predisposed her to some of the respiratory problems which she later developed.

Ms. R.'s abdomen was filled with clotted blood. During the three-hour exploratory operation the surgeons repaired leaks around the superior aortic graft and the wall of the right iliac artery, and ligated multiple small bleeding points in the aortic bed. At the end of the procedure, Ms. R.'s blood pressure was 145/100 and her hematocrit was 30 percent.

PROBLEM 2: MUCOUS PLUG, MAIN BRONCHUS

Ms. R.'s condition remained stable until the following morning. She was on a volume respirator, which delivered 40 percent oxygen. The respirator was set to deliver a tidal volume of 700 cc. at 30 cm. H_2O

pressure. Ms. R. triggered the respirator at 28 respirations per minute. She soon developed severe tachypnea (44/min.) and 60 cm. H_2O pressure was needed to deliver the same tidal volume. We bag-breathed and suctioned her, which improved her respiratory status. We concluded that a mucous plug had formed in a main bronchus and caused alveolar hypoventilation with rapid hypoxic and hypercapnic stimulation of the respiratory center. If we had not removed the plug, alveolar air beyond the block would be resorbed and the alveoli would collapse, producing atelectasis. Continued perfusion of non-ventilated alveoli will contribute to hypoxia.

As her condition improved, we took Ms. R. off the respirator at intervals. Her tidal volume off the ventilator was adequate this time.

PROBLEM 3: CARDIOPULMONARY ARREST

The following morning the endotracheal tube was removed and the respirator discontinued. We gave Ms. R. six liters of oxygen via nasal prongs and 40 percent oxygen through a neublizer face mask. Her blood pressure remained high (155/100). Three hours later we noted that Ms. R.'s breathing was labored, and shortly thereafter respirations ceased. The cardiac monitor showed no electrical activity. She was cyanotic and unresponsive. Her physician intubated her again and the nurse began cardiac massage. In one minute her heart beat resumed at a slower rate, and within two minutes of the arrest she was in normal sinus rhythm and breathing spontaneously. She was placed on the respirator. She soon was arousable and understood and responded to verbal directions. An hour later she was alert and coherent, so we concluded that there had been no hypoxic brain damage.

Ms. R. was frightened and wrote on a note pad that her chest hurt, and pointed to her sternum. The nurse briefly explained the cardiac massage and told her that, although these procedures were frightening, they were over and she was much improved.

Ms. R.'s respiratory failure, with subsequent cardiac arrest, had probably developed gradually as she became more hypoxic secondary to the increased work of breathing. Mechanical restriction of respiratory excursions caused by pain from her very large abdominal wound and peritoneal irritation from the earlier abdominal bleeding no doubt contributed to the respiratory failure. In addition, reduced alveolar ventitilation secondary to mucous plugs probably had a part in this complication. Ms. R. had had a large mucous plug less than 24 hours earlier, her tidal volume had declined markedly when she was off the respirator, and we had been aspirating large amounts of pulmonary secretions when we suctioned her every half hour. In retrospect, medical and nursing staffs agreed her extubation had been premature.

During the afternoon Ms. R. remained somewhat hypoxic. Her arterial pO_2 was 40, and 40 cm. H_2O pressure was required to deliver a tidal volume of 650 cc., indicating reduced compliance, probably some atelectasis, and perhaps an elevated pulmonary capillary pressure from hypoxic weakening of left ventricular contractions. We increased her inspired oxygen to 70 percent and suctioned her every half hour. Later in the evening the atelectasis appeared to be clearing, her lung compliance was improved, and a pressure of 25 cm. H_2O delivered the same 650 cc. tidal volume.

PROBLEM 4: PREMATURE VENTRICULAR CONTRACTIONS

Toward evening we noted that Ms. R. was having premature ventricular contractions (PVC). We notified the physician and started the lidocaine (Xylocaine) drip which he ordered. Premature ventricular contractions are sometimes caused by digitalis toxicity, hypokalemia, or myocardial hypoxia. However, her serum potassium was 4.4 mEq./L. and her arterial pO_2 was 100 at 98 percent saturation. PVCs may also be a premonitory sign of congestive heart failure and often appear during myocardial ischemia and infarction. There had been a possibility of hypoxic heart damage during the cardiopulmonary arrest or even trauma to the heart from closed chest massage. Whatever its cause, lidocaine controlled this episode of cardiac arrhythmia.

On the fourth postoperative day Ms. R. had a tracheostomy done because of her persistent respiratory insufficiency, and to prevent the complications which may result from prolonged endotracheal intubation, such as tracheal necrosis.

The tracheostomy was particularly disturbing for Ms. R. She wanted to talk. We told her why she needed the tracheostomy and stressed that it was temporary. The fact that it was temporary relieved her the most, and she was able to communicate effectively by writing.

When the tracheostomy was performed, we reduced the inspired oxygen concentration to 55 percent, in order to decrease the risk of oxygen toxicity. The basic mechanism of oxygen toxicity is not known. It may interfere with surfactant and inflame respiratory membranes. As a result, the gaseous diffusion at the alveolar-capillary interface is impeded.

The next day Ms. R. improved enough that we could reduce her inspired oxygen concentration to 45 percent. She dangled for five minutes, but soon became dizzy. The following day we lowered the oxygen concentration further, to 40 percent. That day Ms. R. was able to sit in a chair twice with only moderate elevations in heart and respiratory rates, and mild giddiness.

PROBLEM 5: EARLY LEFT VENTRICULAR FAILURE

On the morning of Ms. R.'s seventh postoperative day, we noted that she had scattered expiratory wheezes accentuated by deep breathing. The physician ordered aminophylline, a drug which acts on the bronchial musculature to dilate the bronchioles. Aminophylline also improves myocardial contractions and has a diuretic effect. Weakening left ventricular performance was causing elevated pulmonary capillary pressure with transudation of capillary fluid into the alveoli. The bronchodilation caused by the aminophylline would enable Ms. R. to expectorate some of this fluid, the diuretic effect would reduce extracellular fluid overload, and the cardiotonic action would lead to improved left ventricular contractility.

The same afternoon we noted an atrial arrhythmia on the monitor. The physican thought that this was caused by the aminophylline and decided to use a diuretic for any further pulmonary wheezing. A diuretic would be less likely to cause arrhythmias and would decrease body fluid volume and lessen the workload of the left ventricle. In addition, we weighed Ms. R. daily to monitor her fluid retention.

With diminished left ventricular performance and consequent decreased cardiac output and inadequate tissue perfusion, compensatory mechanisms improve blood flow. As in shock, there is selective renal vasoconstriction and decreased glomerular filtration. The kidneys' response to decreased perfusion is to secrete renin, which, after a sequence of biochemical reactions, is converted to angiotensin II, a powerful vasoconstrictor. Angiotensin's main action, however, is to stimulate the adrenal cortex to release aldosterone. This mineralocorticoid stimulates the distal renal tubule to resorb elevated amounts of sodium from the glomerular filtrate. Sodium retention increases renal water retention, and the result is an expanded plasma volume. This increases the left ventricle's workload.

The next two days we began weaning Ms. R. from the respirator for half-hour periods. Although she complained of some shortness of breath and had moderately increased heart and respiration rates, her color remained good. She also tolerated being up in a chair three times a day.

PROBLEMS 6: HYPERTENSION

On the tenth day we noted that Ms. R.'s blood pressure, which had been high for several days, was now 200/130. She was given reserpine immediately. This drug depletes catecholamines at the adrenergic terminals, producing vasodilation. However, it also reduces myocardial catecholamines. This decreases myocardial contractility and can cause myocardial failure. Therefore, hydrochlorothiazide was begun the following day. Hydrochlorothiazide decreases the resorption of sodium in the distal renal tubule and lowers body fluid volume. In addition, it may decrease stores of sodium in the blood vessels and decrease their responsiveness to catecholamines.

PROBLEM 7: PLEURAL EFFUSION

The following day, we measured Ms. R.'s tidal volume and found it to be under 350 cc. She was also complaining of difficulty breathing. A chest x-ray showed a left pleural effusion. A thoracentesis yielded 1,300 cc. of serosanguinous fluid. Following this, her tidal volume increased and she breathed more easily. It is likely that the effusion was caused in part by left ventricular failure secondary to hypertension and body fluid overload. An increase in peripheral resistance coupled with an expanded plasma volume lead to discrepancy between left ventricular workload and left ventricular performance. This discrepancy may result in elevated pulmonary capillary pressure and movement of fluid into the pleural space.

On the twelfth postoperative day Ms. R.'s condition had improved so that she was essentially off the volume respirator. We gave her intermittent positive pressure breathing treatments every four hours to expand the alveoli and prevent atelectasis. We also helped her perform bicycling leg exercises. She was out of bed in a chair several times a day.

PROBLEM 8: ARRHYTHMIA

Later that evening the cardiac monitor showed that Ms. R. was having episodes of what appeared to be ventricular tachycardia. Each episode lasted 10 to 15 seconds and converted spontaneously to normal sinus rhythm. Ms. R. had no subjective symptoms during the attack, such as faintness, vertigo, or breathlessness, so we concluded that the tachycardia was not of great hemodynamic significance. That is, her cardiac output appeared not to be markedly diminished during the arrhythmia.

However, because we were not certain that this arrhythmia was not ventricular tachycardia, we started a lidocaine drip. The arrhythmia continued intermittently over the next three days and was not affected by lidocaine. Therefore, the arrrhythmia might be of supraventricular origin caused by digitalis toxicity. This possibility was supported by the appearance of definite premature ventricular contractions and bigeminy. Plasma digoxin and potassium levels were 2.0 nanograms/ml., and 4.1 mEq/L. respectively. Since 1.5 nanograms/ml. is considered a maximal therapeutic blood level of digitalis, and 2.0 may be toxic, the digitalis was discontinued and Ms. R. was given propanolol, a beta-adrenergic blocker. This stabilized her heart rhythm and did not appear to decrease myocardial contractility.

PROBLEM 9: PULMONARY EMBOLUS

On the sixteenth postoperative day, Ms. R. was having some chest discomfort and shortness of breath. A lung scan showed a right upper lobe defect. This was assumed to be a pulmonary embolus and anticoagulant therapy was started.

Over the next two days Ms. R.'s general condition improved gradually. She took fluids well and was passing stools. Her tracheostomy tube was removed and the next day she was tried on room air. Her arterial blood gases on room air showed an arterial oxygen saturation of 85 percent. To combat hypoxemia we gave her continuous 40 percent nasal oxygen and continued to monitor her arterial blood gases to make sure that her oxygen saturation remained greater than 90 percent.

Ms. R. was transferred to a surgical ward on the eighteenth postoperative day. Her course was complicated by several pulmonary emboli, signaled by dyspnea and chest pain, and by a massive retroperitoneal hemorrhage from excessive anticoagulation. Nevertheless, with transfusions and protamine her condition became stable within several days.

Pleural effusions, which caused shortness of breath and chest discomfort, continued to be a problem. These were treated with thoracentesis when necessary. Often a pleural tap caused symptomatic hypovolemia due to rapid fluid transfer. As her cardiac and pulmonary status improved her capacity to tolerate room air without developing hypoxemia increased gradually, even with increased bodily activity. The effusion gradually subsided. She returned home six weeks after leaving the surgical intensive therapy unit.

Ms. R. was a remarkable patient, not only because of the complications she experienced, but because of her personal strengths in coping with her situation throughout her many physiological crises. Her daughter was not able to visit often, but Ms. R. was not alone. She received emotional support from the physicians and nurses who were actively involved in her care. We talked with her, encouraged her, and informed her of her progress and treatment plans. She was very aware of many of her complications both because of the way she felt and the procedures

272

that were done. She needed and received the most support during the initial postoperative bleed, the cardiopulmonary arrest, the tracheostomy, and the retroperitoneal bleed.

Close cooperation between the medical and nursing staffs of our unit was responsible for Ms. R.'s recovery after a postoperative course beset by almost every imaginable complication. In this unit the classical and, we believe, largely artificial and outmoded distinctions between what constitute medical and nursing assessment and intervention blurred, to the evident benefit of the patient.

From the *American Journal of Nursing* 72:2021-2025, Nov. 1972.

Unusual Sensory and Thought Disturbances After Cardiac Surgery

ROSEMARY ELLIS

Sensory deprivation only partially explains the sensory and thought disturbances patients experience postoperatively.

Since 1954, when Fox, Rizzo, and Gifford published their report of a study of patients undergoing mitral surgery, there have been numerous reports of unusual sensory and cognitive disturbances experienced by cardiac surgery patients during the postoperative period(1-14). The disturbances have been variously called "postoperative delirium," "cardiac psychoses," "cardiac delirium," or "postcardiotomy delirium."

In a small percentage of cases, psychiatric hospitalization or shock therapy has been deemed necessary. But, the vast majority of patients who suffer psychotic-like disturbances recover completely in a relatively short time. Though these experiences appear to be generally transient, they are very frightening for some patients. A nurse reporting her own postoperative experience following surgical repair of a congenital atrial-septal defect describes it as follows:

One part of my mind knew that the symptoms which distressed me

DR. ELLIS *is a professor of nursing at Case Western Reserve University, Cleveland, Ohio. She received an A.B. degree from the Univ. of Calif. at Berkeley, a B.S. degree in nursing from the Univ. of Calif. at San Francisco, and M.A. and Ph.D. from the Univ. of Chicago.*

[hallucinations of a bared-fang menacing black bear, and of two copper rods that exuded a vile smell] *were not actual, though the periods of awful nameless fear which I suffered were quite beyond my control*(6).

Patients may experience such recurring sensory hallucinations or illusions with or without disorientation to time, place or person during the experience(1,8).

Interest in unusual sensory experiences, or what are termed indeterminate stimulus experiences (shortened to ISEs), at Case Western Reserve University School of Nursing and in thought disturbances of postoperative patients started with interest in clinical sensory deprivation.

In 1963, a research project, titled "Sensory Deprivation and Effective Nurse Intervention," supported by a grant from the USPHS Division of Nursing (NU-00068), was initiated by nurse investigators at the school of nursing.[1] The research was originally designed to study the sensory and thought disturbances of hospitalized patients who were experiencing reduced sensory input as a result of eye or ear surgery.

While these studies were in progress, graduate students in nursing and some nursing school faculty members noticed the similarity between the unusual sensory and thought disturbances of some eye surgery patients and those of some cardiac surgery patients. At this time, the investigators also were beginning to recognize the inadequacy of sensory deprivation as a total explanation for the phenomena observed in about 50 percent of the postoperative eye surgery patients interviewed.

Similarly, it did not seem logical to argue that sensory deprivation could adequately account for all the unusual experiences of postoperative cardiac surgery patients. Some of these experiences occurred after discharge from an intensive care unit.

Also, although a patient in the intensive care facility may experience some perceptual deprivation and may be exposed to monotonous stimulation, he also may be overstimulated by pain, by frequent interruptions for vital observations or care, and by alterations in his usual pattern and environment for sleep. To gather more information on the type, frequency, and possible causes of unusual sensory and cognitive indeterminate stimulus experiences of cardiac surgery patients, a study of postoperative cardiac surgery patients was initiated under the sensory deprivation research project.

Indeterminate stimulus experiences, or ISEs, are experiences of a patient for which there is no apparent appropriate stimulus within the

---

[1] The project director for the study was C. Wesley Jackson, Jr., Ph.D.

patient's environment. A patient may misperceive or misinterpret something he sees, hears, or feels. If there is some stimulus for his experience which an objective observer can recognize as a possible source for the patient's experience, this is *not* an ISE. If, however, the patient sees something, like a menacing black bear, for which there is no *appropriate* stimulus in the environment, this is considered an ISE.

THE ISE STUDY

Partial data were collected on a total of 74 patients. However, data collection could not be completed on 31 patients, so the sample for the study consisted of 43 patients who had had cardiac surgery.

The 43 patients in the final study sample were all adults, ranging in age from 21 years to 66 years. Twenty-one of the patients were female, and 22 were male. All were English speaking, had sufficient hearing to easily communicate verbally, and were willing and able to participate in the study. The patients had had either open or closed heart surgery for valvular disease or congenital defects, or surgery to improve coronary circulation for coronary artery disease.

Data were collected from the medical and nursing records of each patient and from a series of three interviews with him. The first interview was conducted preoperatively. In this session, the interviewer introduced himself and the study to the patient and obtained his consent to participate. Information from the patient about ISEs or thought disturbances were sought through two postoperative interviews, which were conducted after the patient had been transferred out of a surgical intensive care unit and returned to his hospital room. Typically, these interviews were conducted on the fifth and seventh postoperative days.

The postoperative interviews included a series of questions which were structured to obtain increasingly specific information. The first series included vague, general questions: "How have you been feeling?" "What have you been doing?" Questions in the second series were slightly more specific: "Has anything unusual happened?" The questions in the third series were very structured and were introduced with a explanatory phrase: "The reason I've been asking you these questions is that sometimes people who have had heart surgery see things and wonder if they are real. Has anything like this happened to you?" A similar question was used for each sense, including body touch.

THE FINDINGS

From the interview data and from the physicians' and nurses' notes, it was found that 29 of the 43 patients, 67 percent, had experienced one or more ISEs consisting of a thought disturbance or a change in some sensory function. Of the 43 patients, 35 percent had two or more such experiences. In determining whether a patient had had an ISE or thought disturbance, any experience which could reasonably be associated with a physical problem was not included in our count. Thus, the number of patients with ISEs or thought disturbances reported above does not include, for example, patients who had experiences which could be attributed to postoperative neurological changes as a result of cerebral emboli or other causes.

DEGREE OF STRESS A rating of patient stress associated with the experiences was made by the investigators based on the recorded and transcribed interview protocols and notes in patients' records. Twelve of the 29 patients who had some experience were judged to have moderate or high stress with the experience. A patient with no apparent stress reported an ISE as:

I have seen colors. I stared at the wall and I have seen purple spots . . . I'd blink my eyes and spots would just keep blinking all over the wall as if they were a bunch of neon lights blinking on and off.

After describing this experience, the patient commented, "I gave it no thought whatever."

Another patient had a cognitive disturbance on the second postoperative day which was judged highly stressful. In the patient's hospital record, the physician noted that the patient was "somewhat confused and verbalizing paranoid-like ideas." The nurses' notes contained the following:

Continues to talk of nurses outside her door talking about her. . . . States 'they are trying to put me out of my room. They are going to send me home before I can have a change to get well. . . . They thought I was going to report them.'

This 37-year-old woman, in an interview on the fifth postoperative day, answered the general question. "How have you been feeling?" as follows:

I'd hear voices when no one was there. . . . I probably made accusations about it to people . . . maybe I caused a lot of trouble which I didn't mean to. . . . If I, uh, hurt anyone, if I did say anything about anyone, uh, I didn't mean to. I feel awful sorry about a lot of things if it was done, but right now I don't know.

This patient was described as "apprehensive" at the time she was having the experience and on the fifth postoperative day, she was still concerned about what she might have said to the surgeon and to the nurses, though she said she was not quite sure exactly what had happened. During her lucid periods she did not discuss her experiences with the nurses either to find out exactly what had happened or the possible reasons for her experiences.

KIND OF ISES The types of experiences reported by patients or described in their records included visual, auditory, smell and taste ISEs, as feeling one's body was in cement, and disturbances in orientation or in other thought processes. Some experiences were termed "unusual dreams": these were dreams which the patient clearly distinguished from regular dreams and dreams which he volunteered in response to such nonspecific questions as, "How have you been feeling?"

POSSIBLE EXPLANATIONS The patient's explanation, if he had one, for what he thought might have caused the experience was sought along with information on whether he had told anyone about the ISE and what, if anything, he or anyone else had done about it; whether he had had any previous experiences; and what the patient was doing at the time, who was with him, and when the experience occurred. Also, information on the drugs the patient received, abnormal blood values, temperature elevations, and so forth was obtained.

From the analysis of all of these data, there is no evidence to account for the experiences by age, sex, type of surgery, or any other single factor commonly considered to be a cause in the occurrence of postoperative disturbances of this type. For example, the average age of the patients who had experiences was 43.6 years while that of the group who did not have experiences was 44.0 years. From the literature and from this investigation, one cannot rule out drugs, perceptual deprivation, overstimulation, sleep deprivation, or physiological imbalances as causal factors, but each of these is inadequate to explain *all* the phenomena.

It seems more useful at this stage of knowledge to consider that the unusual sensory, emotional, and thought experiences which occur postoperatively with some cardiac surgery patients (and with other surgery patients as well) are of multiple types and are probably caused by multiple factors. Perhaps patients' reality-orienting capacity is impaired by such psychological factors as a patient's premorbid personality, the press of current family or other life problems, and the meaning of his illness and of the surgery. It can also be impaired by such undesirable physiological states as electrolyte disturbances, pain, temperature elevations, and by drugs such as narcotics, analgesics, and hypnotics. Or, it may be impaired by unfamiliar, stressful environments with either monotonous or ambiguous stimuli, such as the recovery room, intensive care facility, and other hospital environments. The vulnerable patient, from whatever cause, then experiences some failure in his reality-orienting function and is prone to the sensory and thought disturbances observed.

NURSING IMPLICATIONS

The exact cause of ISEs is still a mystery, though more is known about the nature of the experiences and the conditions under which they occur than before the research was done. From the research findings, we can offer suggestions to nurses caring for patients who have disturbing postoperative sensory or thought experiences.

UNCONTROLLED PAIN First, a significant number of patients associated with occurrence of ISEs, unusual dreams or thoughts, to having pain which was not adequately controlled. Typical of this is the following experience related by a patient. The experience occurred on the fifth or sixth postoperative day following surgery for coronary artery disease:

I had discomfort . . . unpleasant sort of half dreams, sort of like a hazy unpleasantness. . . . I think it has to do with the fact that you have the pain that you can't control. . . . [In the dream] I was hooked up to a computer type of recovery and something went wrong . . . dreams that just didn't make sense . . . an unreal kind of dream nightmare.

The patient said he was afraid of being addicted and had not taken medication for pain as often as necessary. His feeling of living in what he called a "half-real world" and the "hazy unpleasantness" were relieved when he was given an injection for pain.

Another patient after a closed mitral commissurotomy reported that the whole operation went back through his mind on the evening of the first postoperative day:

It was just like I was back on the operating table again . . . step by step, only there seemed to be more pain . . . I don't know whether it was just nerves or what it was, but to me it was very vivid . . . it was real to me.

The patient reported that the experience was interrupted a short time after a nurse gave him a "pain shot" and told the patient what was wrong and what was happening.

In retrospect, it would appear that these patients, and several others with similar experiences, could be helped by a nurse's skillful management of their pain.

Several patients were sufficiently disturbed by nightmares, unusual dreams, or dreamlike unpleasant experiences to be afraid to go to sleep. The fear of "going off his rocker" was expressed by one such patient. Another patient who reported very disturbing dreams stated that he watched the late, late show and did other things to keep from going to sleep. Such patients may offer a challenge to a nurse, but an empathic, skillful nurse in whom the patient can develop trust ought to be able to mitigate the fears that accompany some experiences.

DISCHARGE FEARS Some patients were unusually disturbed by the anticipation of discharge. The patient who erroneously thought the nurses were trying to put her out on the second postoperative day manifested this fear in the immediate postoperative period. Another patient reported she "panicked" on the eighth postoperative day after her surgeon had told her she might go home in several days:

I had a thought last night when they told me I might go home Friday. I panicked. It scared me to think about going out . . . because I didn't feel like I felt well enough to go out. . . . I just don't feel like I can trust myself. If I get a pain or something, I'll probably panic.

This 27-year-old woman had had rheumatic fever at the age of nine months and had had a heart murmur since that time. She remained asymptomatic until five months before open heart surgery for repair of her mitral valve. Her preoperative symptoms were increasing fatiguability and a "swollen liver" for which she took diuretics as necessary. She had marked cardiac enlargement. This patient and others need a skillful nurse to assist them in working through discharge fears.

CLINICAL CONDITION Another kind of phenomenon of interest to nurses also was identified in the experiences of these patients. An appreciable number of experiences contained some element which could be associated by content with the patient's actual disease process or its symptoms. A clear example of this occurred in a 24-year-old woman during the postoperative period after mitral commissurotomy.

The patient had experienced shortness of breath attributed to mitral stenosis from rheumatic heart disease over a period of five years prior to surgery. She had had peripheral edema for a period of one year and took "water pills" as necessary at home. In talking about her past illness she remarked that during a pregnancy, one year prior to cardiac surgery, she had edema up to her knees. As she put it, "I started swelling and started worrying."

On the fifth postoperative day, she was asked in interview, "Have you been sleeping as you usually do?" She replied, "I slept fairly good, but I had troubles too." She then related the "troubles" she had had in the intensive care unit:

Like everyone else after surgery . . . I started seeing water blisters on myself and I was filled with water and it sprayed out all over my body and, if I looked at people, they had water blisters on them.

She also saw "wet wavy lines" on the blank wall on the third postoperative day. The evening of surgery she asked the nurse, "Do I breathe all right when I'm asleep?" She was very apprehensive when she had the hallucinations. She knew she was seeing things that were not really there. She later reported, "I was hysterical. I wondered why the doctor wasn't doing something about it (the water blisters and spraying water)." One can readily relate the content of her hallucinations to a concern about edema, "water pills," breathing, and the condition of her heart.

A clinical relationship was a component in the reported experiences of a number of other patients. For example, a male patient, obviously concerned about his cardiac condition, felt that some of his peculiar thoughts were emanating from his heart rather than from his mind.

MISPERCEPTIONS AND OTHER COMMUNICATION PROBLEMS Another sort of problem presents from the experiences of the 37-year-old woman who was concerned about whether she had said something offensive or had made unjust accusations. Her suspicions and concomitant visual and auditory hallucinations occurred over the first four postoperative days. In the interview on the fifth postoperative day, it was apparent the patient recognized that her hallucinations were not real, and that she had probably made unjust accusations during them for which she felt sorry. She seemed very troubled that she might have offended the surgeon or the nurses.

She reported she had told her husband and her surgeon about her hallucinations and her accusations, but she had not told the nurses on the convalescent unit. The intensive care unit nurses, who had observed the woman during her experiences, were the target of her accusations.

From this small beginning, it is possible to conjecture some of the problems which can ensue. Whether the intensive care unit nurses described this patient's experiences to the convalescent unit nurses or not the patient likely believed they did and could only imagine the possible details of their descriptions. The situation, of course, becomes even more complex if, indeed, the nurses know nothing of the patient's experiences. It is possible that this patient, wrought by feelings of guilt that she had "caused trouble" or offended someone, might then misperceive or exaggerate some unintentional lapse or chance remark of the nurse. If her bed inadvertently was not made or her breakfast was delayed, it is possible that such a guilty-feeling patient would feel the nurses were retaliating or punishing her.

To avoid such a possibility there should be adequate communication about any of the patient's experiences. What may seem inconsequential to a nurse in the intensive care unit can fester and be magnified by a patient, and result in the patient's subsequent misunderstandings with other nurses who may not know the source of the patient's feelings.

The patient who was preoccupied with her body filling up with water had a different type of communication problem. She related her experience to the doctors and nurses but received no information from them. She reported she overheard her doctor explaining to a nurse that the patient had experienced thoughts about her body filling up with water before. The patient recognized the rationality of the physician's explanation which she had overheard, but she reported she felt mad that the doctor explained it to the nurse instead of telling the patient herself. Though the patient was having hallucinations, she was also alert to her real environment and was resentful that an explanation had not been given to her directly.

It is easy to overlook the fact that a patient who is having ISEs can be keenly aware of reality at the same time and can talk rationally about the experiences even when they are going on. For this reason, such terms as "psychosis" or "delirium," which may connote more impairment than the patient is experiencing or have a negative connotation, might best be avoided. At best, they describe a multidetermined syndrome rather than an individual patient's exact state, which should be the nurse's focus.

CONCLUSIONS

It is difficult to offer any specific actions which will help all patients in all experiences. A useful orientation is offered by Weisman and Hackett from their work with cataract surgery patients. They stress a patient's need for a reliable, trustworthy, personal relationship (which might be supplied by a nurse) and actions specific to the individual patient to improve ego function and reality testing(15).

The husband of one of our patients was very helpful to his wife by constant explanation and clarification and by insisting that she try to focus on real-life activities, rather than drift into fantasy, which then led to frank hallucinations she could not control. Reality-orienting devices must be selected for specific patients and not be used indiscriminately without evaluation of their effectiveness with the individual patient.

An anecdote from the experience of a graduate student in nursing at Case Western Reserve University offers food for thought for those concerned with helping patients cope with disturbing postoperative hallucinations.

A patient in an intensive care unit was bothered by the hallucination of bugs crawling all over the wall. The nurses tried all one morning to relieve the patient's distress but were not successful. Finally, the ward secretary who had heard and observed what was going on could stand it no longer. She got up from her desk, picked up a book, and, without a word, walked over and slammed the book against the wall. She then turned to the patient and said. "Did I get it, Clem?" The patient replied, "Yeah, I'm okay now." Anything that works seems justified if it relieves the patient of disturbing experiences and fears!

REFERENCES

1. Fox, H. M., AND OTHERS. Psychological observations of patients undergoing mitral surgery. *Psychosom.Med.* 16:186-208, May-June 1954.
2. BLISS, E. L., AND OTHERS. Psychiatric complications of mitral surgery; report of death after electroshock therapy. *Arch.-Neurol.Psychiatry* 74:249-152, Sept. 1955.
3. ZAKS, M. S. Disturbances in psychologic functions and neuropsychiatric complications in heart surgery. IN *Cardiology: An Ency-*

clopedia of the Cardiovascular System, edited by A. A. Luisada. New York, McGraw-Hill Book Co., 1959, Vol. 3, pp. 167-171.

4. BLACHEY, P. H., AND STARR, A. Post-cardiotomy delirium. *Am.J.Psychiatry* 121:371-375, Oct. 1964.

5. EDGERTON, N., AND KAY, J. H. Psychological disturbances associated with open heart surgery. *Br.J.Psychiatry* 110:433-439, May 1964.

6. JOHN, C. A. Hallucinations after cardiac surgery. *Nurs.Times* 60:1347, Oct. 9, 1964.

7. ABRAM, H. S. Adaptation to open heart surgery: a psychiatric study of response to the threat of death. *Am.J.Psychiatry* 122:659-668, Dec. 1965.

8. KORNFELD, D. S., AND OTHERS. Psychiatric complications of open-heart surgery. *New Engl.J.Med.* 273:287-292, Aug. 5, 1965.

9. NAHUM, L. H. Madness in the recovery room from open-heart surgery or "they kept waking me up." *Conn.Med.* 29:771-772, Nov. 1965.

10. LAZARUS, H. R., AND HAGENS, J. H. Prevention of psychosis following open-heart surgery. *Am.J.Psychiatry* 124:1190-119. Mar. 1968.

11. MORSE, R. M., AND LITIN, E. M. Postoperative delirium: a study of etiologic factors. *AORN J.* 10:85-92, Nov. 1969.

12. BLACHER, R. S. Open-heart surgery patients. Part 3. Psychological aspects. *RN* 33:79-82, Apr. 1970.

13. ISLER, CHARLOTTE. Open-heart surgery patients. Part 2. Pre- and post-op nursing care. *RN* 33:44-50, Apr. 1970.

14. KIMBALL, C. P. Psychological responses to open heart surgery. *AORN J.* 11:73-84, Feb. 1970.

15. WEISMAN, A. D., AND HACKETT, T. P. Psychosis after eye surgery. *New Engl.J.Med.* 258:1284-1289, June 26, 1958.

From *Nursing Research* 23:341-348, July-Aug. 1974.

Effect of a Reorientation Technique on Postcardiotomy Delirium

SUZANNE BUDD • WILLA BROWN

Thirty-one patients—15 in a control group and 16 in an experimental group—took part in a study of a method of reducing incidence of delirium in postoperative open heart surgery patients in an intensive care unit. A specific reorientation procedure for orienting the patient to time, place, person, and physical status was administered postoperatively by intensive care unit nurses to experimental group patients. Experimental group patients subsequently demonstrated a significantly lower incidence of total symptoms of delirium, had significantly fewer postoperative complications, and were discharged from the hospital an average of four days earlier than control group patients.

Innumberable reports have appeared in the literature describing the phenomenon of postoperative psychosis, using such terms as "psychosis," "insanity," "states of excitement," and "delirium." With the advent of open heart surgery, clinical studies have validated that the highest percentage of postoperative delirium occurs in postcardiotomy patients. Among various groups of patients subjected to open heart surgery, the incidence of postoperative psychosis has been reported as ranging from none in some studies to 61 percent in others[1]. Ellis found that 29 of 43 patients studied (or 67 percent) had experienced thought or sensory disturbances following cardiac surgery[2].

Delirium can be defined as an acute brain syndrome characterized by an impairment of orientation, memory, intellectual functioning, judgment, and sensory discrimination(3). The usual process leading to a delirious state, as described by Lazarus and Hagens(4), includes a lucid period immediately after the postanesthetic recovery, followed by a subsequent period in which the patient becomes restless, apprehensive, and confused. The symptoms occur sequentially and progress to a state of delirium by the second or third postoperative day.

REVIEW OF LITERATURE

A higher incidence of delirium has been reported in postcardiotomy patients who have had psychiatric, organic, laboratory, or metabolic disorders. Psychiatric factors which have been found to lead to delirium include previous brain damage(5), family history of psychiatric disorders(6), overwhelming personal problems unrelated to surgery(6-8), verified history of alcoholism(5), significant degree of insomnia before surgery(9-10), a conscious fear of death(11), history of postoperative psychosis(6,7). Organic factors included: duration of procedure—if longer than four hours(12-14), presence of postoperative complications such as hemorrhage and cerebral anoxia(6, 14, 15), preoperative disorientation(4,5,16), sensory distortion(8), cerebral emboli(12,17,18), and valvotomy surgery(16). Laboratory and metabolic factors were found to be: abnormal electrocardiogram(5,7), blood irregularities such as albuminuria, alkalosis, anemia, azotemia, hypochloremia, hypokalemia, hyponatremia, and leukocytosis(6,13).

Several authors(4-6,10,12,15,19) stressed the significance of sensory distortion—which Norse and Litin labeled the deprivation syndrome(3). This syndrome includes a lack of sleep, both pre- and postoperatively, sensory distortion from extraneous noises such as the monitor beep and respirator sigh, and frequent wakening of the patient for monitoring vital signs.

Hebb, in his experimental work on perceptual isolation, suggested that monotonous sensory stimulation produces a disruption of the capacity to learn or even to think(20). Hebb's associate, Heron, found that with greatly reduced amounts and patterning of sensory input, his volunteers

SUZANNE PEARSALL BUDD (Micihigan State University School of Nursing, East Lansing; M.S., University of Michigan, Ann Arbor) is an instructor in medical surgical nursing, Michigan State University, East Lansing. WILLA BROWN (Tuskegee Institute School of Nursing, Tuskegee, Alabama; M.S., University of Michigan, Ann Arbor) is a clinical nurse at the Allen Park Veterans Administration Hospital, Allen Park, Michigan.

experienced inability to think or concentrate, anxiety, somatic complaints, temporal and spatial disorientation, visual phenomena, hallucinations, and deficits in task performance(21). Restrictions in physical mobility concurrent with deprivation in other modalities produced rapid and severe perceptual disturbances in many subjects. Danilowicz and Gabriel noted that non-English-speaking patients were more prone to develop postoperative psychosis following open heart surgery(22).

Nurses in an intensive care unit (ICU) who have long recognized innumerable symptoms of delirium that occur in the acutely ill concur that there is a higher incidence in postcardiotomy patients. Walker and Kasmarik found that "some patients who appear placid and stoic (in the preoperative phase) may become excitable, demonstrating erratic behavior" in the postcardiotomy phase, because of fear(23). They believed that fear could result from ignorance or false knowledge of postoperative procedures and ICU milieu. When Weiler interviewed open heart surgery patients postoperatively to ascertain what preoperative information would have been most helpful during the postoperative phase, patients' responses varied from information regarding disorientation and hallucinations, explanation of expected pain, explanation of coughing and deep breathing exercises, reasons for intravenous fluids and blood, to explanation of chest tubes and endotracheal tubes(24).

When McFadden and Giblin compared sleep patterns of patients in the pre- and postoperative ICU environment, 75 percent of the patients demonstrated behavioral changes; they related these changes to sleep deprivation during the postoperative phase(10). Worrell advocated that a "therapeutic nursing approach should be geared toward helping the patient understand the incoming stimuli", especially if the patient is experiencing sensory overload or distortion from the constant unpatterned sounds of the intensive care environment, or is deprived of meaningful communications with others(25). Lazarus and Hagens, Henrichs *et al.*, Danilowicz and Gabriel, and Worrell believed that the sensory distortion syndrome which leads to delirium could be lessened by reorienting the patient to time, place, person, and physical status in the ICU.

BACKGROUND OF THE STUDY

Purpose. Sensory deprivation is considered a major factor leading to disorientation which progresses to delirium. Because the clinical nurse practitioner has more control over sensory deprivation than any other possible etiologic factor, a nursing intervention tool, designed to minimize sensory deprivation and increase orientation of the patient to his surroundings, might be utilized by the nurse to decrease the incidence of delirium. The purpose of this study was, therefore, to determine if the nurse can reduce the incidence of postcardiotomy delirium in the ICU by the use of a specific reorientation procedure.

Significance of Study. The peak incidence of postcardiotomy delirium seems to occur in the ICU between the second and third postoperative days. During this critical period, many other problems are generated by the complication of delirium. These include danger of physical injury to the patient by his dislodging oxygen connections and/or intravenous or chest tubes, by chance of reopening incision and causing infection, or by disturbances in heart rhythm and rate; frightening experience for the patient and his family; prolonged hospital stay, with added expense and inconvenience to the patient. Theoretically, if the nurse can intervene to reduce the incidence of postcardiotomy delirium, a lessening of associated problems should result.

METHOD

Sample. The subjects for the study represented a presenting sample[1] of patients admitted to St. Joseph Mercy Hospital, Ann Arbor, Michigan, for planned open heart surgery. The patient population consisted of English-speaking and writing patients between the ages of 23 and 63. Patients were informed that participation was voluntary, all information would be confidential, and withdrawal of participation from the study would be granted at any time, upon request. The patients were told that the purpose of the study was to help nurses understand some of the feelings and experiences of patients who undergo open heart surgery in order to give comprehensive nursing care. They were also informed that patient participation would include completing a patient checklist preoperatively and a patient questionnaire postoperatively. Consent forms were signed. No one refused to participate in the study.

Permission for recruiting patients was granted, pending patients' consent, by all three thoracic surgeons who perform open heart surgery at St. Joseph Mercy Hospital.

A presenting sample of patients was assigned to the experimental and the control groups until a total of 31 patients was recruited. The first 15 patients were assigned to the control group; the second 16 patients, to the experimental group. The two groups were assigned and studied consecutively (first, control; second, experimental) rather than simultaneously to prevent accidental contamination of the control group by the

---

[1] Langley (1971) described a presenting sample as a consecutive series of patients who present themselves for treament of a certain complaint.

manipulative factor. Once the reorientation procedure (the manipulative factor) had been introduced, the ICU nurses might have found it extremely difficult *not* to use this procedure for patients in the control group. A preoperative orientation program was given by medical social workers at St. Joseph Mercy Hospital to both groups. The orientation consisted of: assessment of knowledge, coping abilities, financial difficulties, and any specific problems imposed by illness; offering information regarding visiting policies, family comforts, and an explanation of the usual sequence of going to the operating room, the recovery room, and awakening in the ICU on the day of surgery; and conducting a tour of the ICU to acquaint the patient and his family with environment, equipment, and personnel.

Zukerman's Multiple Affect Adjective Check List (MAACL) (26), was administered preoperatively to both groups to obtain a base-line reading of the patient's preoperative anxiety level. The checklist was administered by one of the nurse investigators one day prior to surgery.

Procedure. A nursing intervention tool, called the reorientation procedure, was designed for patients in the experimental group to decrease sensory distortion and increase orientation to surroundings during the postoperative period. The procedure included:

Orient the patient to time by informing him of the time of day and by placing a clock or wristwatch within easy access. Orient the patient to the day of the week by stating the month, the day, and the date and by placing a large "one-day" calendar within easy view. Orient the patient to place by stating that he is in the intensive care unit at St. Joseph's Mercy Hospital. Promote personal identity by addressing patients by name and by referring to significant others. Information obtained from nursing assessments and/or medical social worker reports will provide clues to persons and topics that are of interest to the patient. Keep the patient informed of his physical progress to promote a sense of accomplishment, allay fears, and eliminate misconceptions. For example, the nurse might converse with the patient as follows:

"Good morning, Mr. Breen. It is 9 o'clock, Wednesday morning, June the first. You are in the intensive care unit at St. Joseph Mercy Hospital. How are you feeling after yesterday's surgery? Your blood pressure, pulse, and temperature are all within normal limits. You are progressing very well. Your wife and daughter are waiting to see you. Do you feel up to seeing them now?"

The success of the reorientation technique depends on its implementation on a planned, organized, and consistent basis. Each time nursing care is given, the nurse should use this technique. The technique should be organized and administered on an individual basis, according to the patient's greatest need: that is, if the patient is aware of time and place but questions his physical progress, then greatest emphasis should be placed on orienting him to physical status. Patients who exhibit no signs of disorientation should still receive the reorientation technique on a consistent basis to prevent the occurrence of disorientation. Should signs of disorientation being to appear, the frequency of administering the reorientation technique should be accelerated to counteract the disorientation.

Following open heart surgery, patients were admitted to the recovery room and transferred to the ICU the same evening. Patients in the first group, the control group, were observed for only overt signs of delirium. Experimental group patients were observed for delirium signs, whereupon the reorientation technique was implemented by the ICU nurses and continued throughout their ICU stay. Overt signs of delirium were recorded on a prepared form (Figure 1).

Each time the patient verbalized that he was experiencing any unusual sensory experiences or confusion in thinking, one unit check was placed in the appropriate category. When the patient perceived objects or sensations with no reality or external cause as stimulus, he was considered in one of the "hallucinations" categories. An example would be if the patient stated, "Get that grizzly bear out of this room!" (And there was none present.)

When the patient demonstrated either by word or by action or by a combination of both that he had a misinterpretation or belief about what was really present in the environment, these experiences were recorded as "illusions." For example, a patient might say, "That machine is moni-

Figure 1. Example of Nurses' Form for Recording Incidence of Delirium for Each Patient in the Control and Experimental Groups

HALLUCINATIONS					ILLUSIONS	DELUSIONS	MENTAL CONFUSION				BEHAVIORAL MANIFESTATIONS OF CONFUSION
VISUAL	AUDITORY	SMELL	TOUCH	TASTE			TIME	PLACE	PERSON	PHYSICAL STATE	
Bear					Heart Monitor					Patient's perception of his physical state	Re: withdrawn hostile abusive marked restlessness inappropriate laughter

toring my thoughts." When the patient maintained a fixed, false belief, despite evidence to the contrary, the experience was recorded as a "delusion." For example, the patient might state, "I know they have taken my heart out and replaced it with someone else's heart."

Repetitions of the same communication were taken as an indication of unrelieved thought problems of sufficient intensity to be recorded as additional units of measure.

The final categories for guiding observations provided for tabulating confusion or disorientation as to person, time, place, or perception of physical status as verbalized by the patient.

The behavioral manifestations column was included under the mental confusion category so that the patient's behavior could be recorded. Any noncompliant behavior—such as overt hostility, depression, or withdrawal—was recorded. Reduced conscious awareness, such as that induced by drugs, and momentary confusion and drowsiness related to the manifestations of sleep were not recorded as an incidence of delirium. The ICU nurse used her judgment to decide whether the symptoms disappeared within moments of conversation. For example, upon awakening, the patient might say, "Oh, for a moment I thought I was at home in my own bed." Such an incident should not be considered evidence of disorientation but rather a natural occurrence.

If it was necessary to facilitate the data collection, the nurse precipitated a patient's verbalization by asking him about time, place, person, or physical status (if he had an endotracheal tube intact, he was asked to write the information on a tablet or respond by nodding to the correct choice).

Questions on the first day included: Do you know what time it is (day or night)? Do you know what month this is? What is your first name?

On the second day: Can you tell me how many children you have? Can you tell me what day this is (day of week)? What is your full name?

On the third day: Can you tell me where you are in the hospital? Can you tell me the name of your hometown? Can you tell me your wife's (or husband's) full name? Can you tell me what type of surgery you had?

Patients in both the control and experimental groups were observed for 30-minute intervals three times each day—morning (8:00 A.M.–12:00 NOON), afternoon (12:00 NOON–5:00 P.M.), and evening (5:00 P.M.–10:00 P.M.)—for the length of their ICU stay. Each patient's chart was reviewed for pertinent, ongoing descriptions of behavior during all three shifts.

Subjects in both groups were asked to fill out a simple 25-item patient questionnaire on the tenth postoperative day. In two cases, the patient questionnaire was given on the eighth postoperative day because of early recovery and discharge of the patients. In two other cases, the patients were still in the ICU on the tenth postoperative day. These two patients, one in the experimental group and one in the control group, received the questionnaire three days post-ICU discharge, on the twentieth and twenty-eighth postoperative day.

The questionnaire was designed to ascertain: the patient's view of his level of orientation or disorientation while in the ICU, the most helpful preoperative information for preparing the patient for ICU experiences, and, for the experimental group, the components of the reorientation procedure that were most helpful in keeping him oriented.

Sample questions are:

I. Were you aware of the time?
   1. All of the time
   2. Most of the time
   3. Some of the time
   4. Seldom
   5. None of the time
   6. Don't remember

VI. Were your lights dimmed at night?
   1. All of the time
   2. Most of the time
   3. Some of the time
   4. Seldom
   5. None of the time
   6. Don't remember

IX. Did the nurse inform you that you were in the Intensive Care Unit?
   1. All of the time
   2. Most of the time
   3. Some of the time
   4. Seldom
   5. None of the time
   6. Don't remember

XVIII. Were you informed of your progress and physical condition each day?
   1. Yes
   2. No
   3. All of the time
   4. Most of the time
   5. Some of the time
   6. None of the time
   7. Don't remember

In addition, nurses kept a record of how many times each day they used the reorientation procedure for each patient.

Data Collection. Base-line data which might correlate with some of the etiological factors and data compiled from empirical observation were collected for each patient.

FROM PATIENTS' CHART
Age
Sex
Medical diagnosis
Type of surgery
Minutes on heart-lung machine
Number and amount of pre- and postoperative tranquilizers and pain medications
Surgeon's name
Number of days in ICU
Abnormal pre- and postoperative physical findings
Incidences of delirium
Day discharged post-ICU
Shift with highest incidence of delirium

FROM THE PATIENT
Marital status
Education (years)
Number of children
Religion
Insomnia—presurgical sleep pattern (number of hours)
Occupation,
History of previous delirium
Alcohol—usual intake
Answers to postoperative patient questionnaire

FROM THE PHYSICIAN
Degree of cardiac impairment

FROM THE NURSE INVESTIGATOR
MAACL test score
Incidence of delirium
Day of onset of delirium
Nurse-patient ratio
Shift with highest incidence of delirium

RESULTS AND DISCUSSION

Demographic Variables. Analysis of demographic variables revealed no significant differences between control and experimental groups. The mean age of the patient population was 49 years (experimental mean age, 48; control, 50). There were 12 males and four females in the experimental group and 14 males and one female in the control group.

Twenty-seven of the patients were married. The mean level of education was 12 years for the experimental group, 11 years for the control group. The mean number of children for both groups was four. Occupational data classified both groups as equal, falling in the five occupational categories of professional, technical, clerical, semi-skilled, and laborer. A majority of the patients in both groups were Protestant (control group, nine; experimental group, 12). Four in each group were Catholic.

Organismic Variables. Thirteen patients in each group were diagnosed as having coronary artery disease. Preoperative physical and laboratory findings revealed no differences between the groups. Two patients in each group had elevated blood urea nitrogen (BUN) (normal 10–20 mgm. 100/ml.; control group, 22 and 50; experimental group, 28 and 40). Three patients in each group had elevated cholesterol values (normal 250 mgm./100 ml. or below; control group highest value, 350; experimental group highest value, 840).

The degree of cardiac impairment as graded on the four-point American Heart Association scale, showed a mean grade of three for both groups. The preoperative mean hours of sleep per night for both groups was 7.6 hours. Patients in both groups revealed average alcoholic intake to range from infrequent to light consumption (one to five ounces a week).

No patients in either group received pain medication preoperatively. One patient in the control group received a tranquilizer preoperatively (Thorazine 25 mgm. *per os ter in die*). No one in either group reported a history of previous delirium; MAACL anxiety scores revealed mean scores of 6.4 for the control group and 6.2 for the experimental group, both within the normal range of 6–8 for preoperative anxiety level. There was no statistical difference between the groups for time on the heart-lung machine (mean time—139 minutes).

Surgical procedures for control patients included: repair of ventricular aneurysm, one; mitral valve replacement, one; single bypass, three; double bypass, four; triple bypass, one; aortic valve replacement with mitral commissurotomy, one; single aortic bypass and valve replacement, one; double aortic bypass and ventricular aneurysm, one; double aortic bypass and aortic valve replacement, one; double aortic bypass, Vineberg procedure, and ventricular aneurysm, one. Experimental group patients had surgery as follows: repair of atrial-septal defect, one; mitral valve replacement, one; Vineberg procedure, one; single bypass, four; double bypass, three; triple bypass, four; quadruple bypass, two.

No statistical significance could be demonstrated on the basis of type of surgery performed. No relationship was noted among type of surgery, surgeon, and incidence of delirium, nor was there a relationship between nurse-patient ratio and incidence of delirium. The mean number of patients per nurse remained constant throughout the study: two patients per nurse.

The experimental group demonstrated a significantly lower incidence of postoperative complications when subjected to chi-square analysis ($X^2 = 4.034$, 1 df, $p = .04$). Among experimental group patients, 13 had no complications, three had primary complications, none had secondary complications. The primary complications were urinary tract infection, one; cholecystitis, one; low cardiac output syndrome, one. In the control group, eight had no complications and seven patients had primary complications of which four had secondary complications also.

Complications among control group patients were: urinary tract infection, three; pneumonia, one; cholecystitis, one; myocardial infarction, three; pericardial tamponade, one; low cardiac output syndrome, one. One patient died.

The two patients who were diagnosed as low cardiac output syndrome experienced severe symptoms of delirium, and the patient in the control group died. The reorientation procedure was administered to the patient in the experimental group 106 times during his 16-day ICU stay. This patient recovered. (See Table 1 for number and kind of postoperative complications.) There were no statistically significant differences between the groups for mean values of selected postoperative laboratory and vital signs. Mean values for the signs, for experimental and control patients, respectively, were: high BUN, 30 (control) and 31 (experi-

Table 1. Number of Postoperative Primary and Secondary Complications for Control and Experimental Patient Groups

COMPLICATIONS	PATIENT GROUPS			
	CONTROL		EXPERIMENTAL	
	PRIMARY COMPILATIONS	SECONDARY COMPILATIONS	PRIMARY COMPILATIONS	SECONDARY COMPILATIONS
No complications	8	11	13	16
Urinary tract infection	2	1	1	0
Pneumonia	0	1	0	0
Cholecystitis	1	0	1	0
Hemorrhage	0	0	0	0
Myocardial infarction	2	1	0	0
Pericardial tamponade	1	0	0	0
Low cardiac output syndrome	1	0	1	0
Death	0	1	0	0
Total	15	15	16	16

mental); low oxygen, 95.6 and 95.0; low hemoglobin, 12.2 and 12.5; low hematocrit, 37.2 and 37.5; high systolic blood pressure, 138 and 143; high diastolic blood pressure, 88 and 90; low systolic blood pressure, 81 and 88; low diastolic blood pressure, 50 and 55; low pulse, 71 and 75; high pulse, 133 and 115; high respiration, 27 and 23; low respiration, 11 and 11; low temperature, 99.1 and 98.8; high temperature, 103.36 and 102.46. We are unable to account for elevated postoperative BUN values in either group, although only the highest BUN value was recorded for each patient. No relationship could be detected between BUN and incidences of delirium. Patients in the experimental group demonstrated a lower mean value for high temperature postoperatively. These patients also demonstrated lower mean values for postoperative high pulse. The Student's t analysis for temperature resulted in $t = -2.42398$, 29df, $p < .02$; for pulse, $t = -2.5898$, 29 df, $p < .01$.

The mean length of ICU stay for control group patients was 6.0 days; for experimental patients, 4.1 days. The mean discharge day from the hospital after ICU was 11.2 days for the control group; 9.3 days, for the experimental group. This earlier discharge of 3.8 days for patients in the experimental group did not reach statistical significance.

Incidence of Delirium. Onset of delirium in the ICU was observed the second day in control group patients and the fourth day in experimental patients. When analyzed according to Student's t-test, statistics were $t = -3.2884$, 29 df, $p < .002$. Occurrence of hallucinations (visual, auditory, smell, touch, and taste) was rare. Only three incidences of hallucinations occurred in the control group, two auditory and one visual. No hallucinations were observed in the experimental group. Two incidences of illusions and three incidences of delusions were noted in the control group; none was observed in the experimental group. One patient with illusion interpreted the heart monitor as an airplane control panel; the other patient thought the continuous sighs of his respirator were guns being fired in the background. Delusions expressed were, "They are trying to kill me" or "I know that (intravenous infusion) is full of poison." One patient thought he was in Asia Minor and shouted, "The tanks are coming." Several incidences of mental confusion were noted. For control group patients, 50 incidents regarding time confusion were recorded; of place, 28; of person, 12; of physical status, one. In the experimental group, 14 incidents of confusion of time and 14 of place were experienced by one patient. Mental confusion of time and place was significantly lower in the experimental group ($t = -1.8869$, 29 df, $p = .06$).

Behavioral manifestations were more prevalent in control patients; marked restlessness, 38; hostility, 25; abusiveness, 10; inappropriate laughter, four; withdrawal, four. Only one experimental patient showed behavioral manifestations—four incidences of marked restlessness. Confused behavioral manifestations were exhibited by control group patients at a fignificantly more frequent rate ($t = -2.4029$, 29 df, $p < .003$).

The total incidences of delirium were 180 for control group patients, 32 for experimental group patients. Thirteen (83 percent) of the 15 control group patients demonstrated some symptoms of delirium. One (six percent) of the 16 experimental group patients demonstrated symptoms of delirium, in spite of consistent administration of the reorientation technique. When all variables were reanalyzed, no differences were found between this patient and others in the experimental group. The Mann Whitney U analysis of *total* symptoms of delirium reached a statistical significance between the two groups ($t = -2.0916$, 29 df, $p < .04$). There were equal occurrences of delirium among the three shifts.

Lazarus and Hagens (1968) suggested that symptoms of delirium may follow a progressive pattern, and symptoms of delirium in the patients observed in this study did, in fact, follow such a pattern. First, disorientation to time and then to place occurred. These events were followed by marked restlessness and then withdrawal, paranoid ideation, hostility, and abusiveness. In some cases these symptoms progressed to illusions and delusions, completing the pattern of delirium.

This raised the question, "At what point in the progression of symptoms is the reorientation technique most effective?" All patients in the experimental group, except one, remained oriented to time, place, person, and physical status; for them, the reorientation technique had been implemented immediately following postoperative return to consciousness in the ICU. Because the experimental group demonstrated a low (six percent) incidence of delirium, we believe that the reorientation procedure must be implemented upon admission to ICU to prevent disorientation to time and place, person, and physical status at an early point. The most crucial point in halting the progression of symptoms leading to delirium is prior to onset. Our findings supported those of Danilowicz and Gabriel (1971), Worrell (1971), Henrichs et. al. (1971), and Lazarus and Hagens (1968), that the sensory distortion syndrome which leads to delirium can, in fact, be diminished by reorienting the patient to time, place, person, and physical status.

Postoperative Patient Questionnaire. While in the ICU, control group patients may have received some type of orientation to time, place, person, and physical status from family, friends, or staff, on an *incidental* basis, whereas patients in the experimental group received a planned, organized reorientation technique *consistently*. This process of orienting the patient on an indepth and frequent basis was reflected by responses given to the patient questionnaire. Statistically significant differences between the groups were observed in many of the answers.

For example, to the question, "Were you aware of the time of day?" 13 experimental group patients and six control group patients answered affirmatively. The difference was significant, $X^2 = 10.128$, 5 df, $p < .07$). When asked, "Was a watch or clock helpful?," 11 experimental group patients thought so, but 11 control group patients answered in the negative. This reached statistical signifance ($X^2 = 14.297$, 5 df, $p < .01$). Experimental group patients found the calendar most helpful in keeping them oriented as to the day of the week, whereas patients in the control group answered that no calendar was available ($X^2 = 13.665$, 4 df, $p < .0084$).

Patients in the experimental group were more aware of ICU sleeping time and responded in the first three categories of short, moderate, and long periods of time slept. Patients in the control group demonstrated that they were less aware of sleeping time and responded equally in all six categories—short, moderate, long, all the time, none of the time, don't remember. Statistics were: ($X = .4563$, 5 df, $p < .0922$).

Twelve patients in the experimental group believed that their being informed on an organized and consistent basis while they were in the ICU was helpful in keeping them oriented to place. Only five control group patients who were informed inconsistently found this helpful. This was statistically significant ($X^2 = 7.4117$, 3 df, $p < .05$).

Although 13 patients in the experimental group and eight in the control group felt that the nurse's calling them by name helped keep them oriented as to personal identity, this did not reach statistical significance. Answers to the questions, "Did the nurse refer to your family members and events?" and "Was this helpful in enhancing personal identity?" illustrated a marked difference between the groups. Eleven experimental group patients and four control group patients recalled a nurse's reference to family; five experimental and ten control group patients did not. This was statistically significant ($X^2 = 11.393$, 5 df, $p < .04$). Ten in the experimental and three in the control group found it helpful, while six in the experimental and 11 in the control group did not. Again, the finding reached statistical significance ($X^2 = 11.688$, 5 df, $p < .04$). Most of the patients in both groups found the equipment in ICU familiar and reassuring. No one perceived the equipment as frightening.

A majority of the patients (13 experimental, 11 control) stated that an explanation of nursing procedures was given prior to performance and was valuable in helping them understand what to expect. Apparently, this was standard practice among ICU nurses prior to implementation of the reorientation procedure.

Most patients in both groups (14 experimental, 10 control) believed that they were informed daily of their physical progress and perceived this as helpful in promoting a feeling of physical progress or accomplishment. A majority of the patients in both groups (14 experimental, 11 control) answered that family members were also informed of the patient's daily progress and that this facilitated the family's understanding of their progress. We concluded that patients and their families in both groups were informed by their physicians of physical progress. This also was standard practice and no differences were demonstrated between the two groups.

Eight patients in the experimental group and two in the control group were visited by their minister. All expressed that these visits were very helpful. Ten patients in the experimental group answered that the nurse was the most helpful person in keeping them oriented in the ICU. The patients in the control group answered that the social worker, spouse, and nurse were equally helpful. No statistical significance was demonstrated.

The question, "What preoperative information would have been most helpful in preparing you for your ICU experience?" revealed a significant difference between the groups ($X^2 = 6.614$, 2 df, $p<.04$). The patients in the experimental group wanted more information regarding discomfort, pain, and pain medication. Although it was not within the scope of this study to determine the amount of pain experienced by either group, questionnaire responses indicated that the experimental patients were more concerned with pain.

Patients in both groups received nearly equal amount of morphine and Valium postoperatively in the ICU (morphine—22 doses to experimental patients, 19 doses to control patients; Valium—six doses or 33 mgm. to experimental patients; 6.7 doses or 38 mgm. to control patients). No other pain or tranquilizer medication was given.

Patients who experienced more incidences of delirium, the control group, wanted more information regarding possible states of disorientation in the ICU. These responses to the patient questionnaire add validity to the study by showing that the experimental group was more alert and aware of pain, and the control group was more concerned with disorientation. Both groups were equal in their desire for information regarding coughing and deep breathing, endotracheal tubes, and visiting hours.

Based on the analysis of the two groups, the reorientation procedure administered by the ICU nurses was most successful in keeping the patients in the experimental group oriented. Incidence of delirium by experimental patients in the ICU was significantly reduced. The following components of the reorientation procedure were judged most significant by the data compiled from the patients' subjective answers to the postoperative questionnaire: Access to a watch or clock, a calendar placed within easy view, and dimming the lights at night were most helpful in orienting the patient to time. Consistently informing the patient that he was in the ICU was valuable for his orientation to place. Personal identity was enhanced by the nurse's referring to family members and family events. For some patients, the minister's visit was also helpful. A sense of physical well-being and progress was facilitated by nurses, doctors, and family members emphasizing physical progress.

Based on patient responses, preoperative orientation programs should include information regarding expected discomfort and pain, availability of pain medication, possible states of disorientation, importance of coughing and deep breathing, presence of endotracheal tubes, visiting hours in the ICU, and chest tubes. Preoperative orientation should also include a tour of the ICU to acquaint patient and family with the equipment and environment. Time should be planned to provide opportunities for the patient and family to ask questions regarding information given and to discuss their concerns.

Nursing Implications. The increase in open heart surgery and the high incidence of postcardiotomy delirium indicate a preponderance of problems that ICU nurses face. To alleviate the problems associated with delirium, nursing intervention should be initiated immediately following surgery. As indicated in this study, nurses can reduce incidence of postcardiotomy delirium by orienting the patient to the intensive care milieu. An orientation program should encompass orientation to time, place, person, and physical status. Interactions between patient and nurse should be focused on things *meaningful* to the patient. Continual assessment of the patient's response to incoming stimuli is essential to prevent sensory distortion. Situations which tend to provoke disorientation for a particular patient require major emphasis for that patient's orientation plan. Evaluation of the patient's responses to orientation should be systematically made so that components judged most successful for a given patient are communicated and utilized by all who are involved in his care. The crucial factor in determining the success of an orientation program in this study was implementation on a planned, organized, and consistent basis. The practice of informing patients and their families of physical progress was helpful in promoting a feeling of well-being. This practice should be incorporated in every reorientation plan. The simplicity of the reorientation technique makes implementation easy. Not time-consuming, it can be carried out during routine nursing care. Nurses should not fear that conversing with patients disturbs them. As demonstrated, meaningful conversation contributes to the patient's state of orientation. Family members and other medical personnel can also administer the technique.

Educational systems, such as schools of medicine, nursing, and social work, should incorporate within their curriculums the concepts of orientation. Patients, entrusted to their care, may be subjected to situations which alter states of orientation. If doctors, nurses, and medical social workers develop an awareness of situations which may induce disorientation, they will become effective in preventing and/or in helping patients cope with disorientation. The concepts of orientation should be included in continuing education and in-service programs so that all paramedical personnel involved in the care of patients will become contributors to the orientation process for the benefit of the patients.

Suggestions for Future Study. Although data were not collected once the patient was transferred from the ICU to the general medical-surgical floor, we were informed by the nursing staff that some patients in both the experimental and control groups demonstrated symptoms of disorientation. Future nursing research should be conducted to study patient orientation-disorientation experiences post-ICU discharge. Specific preventive measures and techniques could then be designed and implemented.

Since the frequency of delirium is usually higher among postcardiotomy patients than among other surgical patients, further research should be conducted by physicians and nurses to discover the physiological and psychological etiology of postcardiotomy delirium. This investigation should be replicated, using a larger number of subjects. Subsequent studies would yield more information to provide more guidelines for nursing intervention which could then be incorporated into the reorientation technique.

REFERENCES
1. HAZEN, S. J. Psychiatric complications following cardiac surgery. Part 1. *J.Thorac.Cardiovasc.Surg.* 51:307-319, Mar. 1966.

2. ELLIS, ROSEMARY. Unusual sensory and thought disturbances after cardiac surgery. *Am.J.Nurs.* 72:2021-2025. Nov. 1972.
3. MORSE, R. M., AND LITIN, E. M. Postoperative delirium. *Am.J.Psychiatry* 126:388-395, Sept. 1969.
4. LAZARUS, H. R., AND HAGENS, J. H. Prevention of psychosis following open-heart surgery. *Am.J.Psychiatry* 124 1190, Mar. 1968.
5. ZISKIND, E. G. Hypnoid syndrome in sensory deprivation. *Recent Advances Biol.Psychiatry* 5:331-344, 1963.
6. EGERTON, N., AND KAY, J. H. Psychological disturbances associated with open-heart surgery. *Br.J.Psychiatry* 110:433-439, May 1964.
7. KNOX, S. J. Severe psychiatric disturbances in postoperative period —five year survey of Belfast hospitals. *J.Ment.Sci.* 107:1078-1079, Nov. 1961.
8. HENRICHS, T. E., AND OTHERS. Psychological adjustment and psychiatric complications following open heart surgery. *J.Nerv.-Ment.Disorders* 152:332-345, May 1971.
9. AIKEN, H. J., AND HENRICHS, T. F. Systematic relaxation as a nursing intervention technique with open heart surgery patients. *Nurs.Res.* 20:212-217, May-June 1971.
10. MC FADDEN, E. H., AND GIBLIN, E. C. Sleep deprivation in patients having open-heart surgery. *Nurs.Res.* 20:249-254, May-June 1971.
11. JANIS, I. L. *Psychological Stress.* New York, John Wiley and Sons, 1958.
12. GILMAN, SID. Cerebral disorder after open-heart operations. *N.Engl.J.Med.* 272:289-297, Mar. 11, 1965.
13. KORNFELD, D. S., AND OTHERS. Psychiatric complications of open-heart surgery. *N.Engl.J.Med.* 273:287-292, Aug. 5, 1965.
14. TUFO, H. M. Neurological abnormalities following open-heart surgery. *J.Thorac.Cardiovasc.Surg.* 58:502-507, Oct. 1969.
15. RIMON, RAMON, AND OTHERS. Psychiatric disturbances after cardio-vascular surgery. *ACTA Psychiatr.Scand. (Suppl.)* 203:125-130, 1968.
16. KNOX, S. J. Psychiatric aspects of mitral valvotomy. *Br.J.Psychiatry* 109:656-668, Sept. 1963.
17. HILL, J., AND OTHERS. Experience using a new Dacron wool filter during extracorporeal circulation. *Arch.Surg.* 101:649-652, Dec. 1970.
18. LEE, W. H. JR., AND OTHERS. Effects of extracorporeal circulation upon behavior, personality and brain function. Part 2. *Ann.Surg.* 173:1013-1023, June 1971.
19. JACKSON, C. W. JR., AND ELLIS, ROSEMARY. Sensory deprivation as a field of study. *Nurs.Res.* 20:46-53, Jan.-Feb. 1971.
20. HEBB, D. O. *Organization of Behavior.* New York, John Wiley and Sons, 1941.
21. HERON, WOODBURN. Cognitive and physiological effects of perceptual isolation. IN *Sensory Deprivation*, edited by Philip Solomon and others. Cambridge, Mass., Harvard University Press, 1961, pp. 6-33.
22. DANILOWICZ, D. A., AND GABRIEL, H. P. Postcardiotomy psychosis in non-English-speaking patients. *Psychiatry Med.* 2:314-320, Oct. 1971.
23. WALKER, M. L., AND KASMARIK, P. E. Continuity of care in cardiac surgery. *AORN J* 9:67, Feb. 1969.

24. WEILER, SR. M. CASHEL. Postoperative patients evaluate preoperative instructions. *Am.J.Nurs.* 68:1465, July 1968.
25. WORRELL, J. D. Nursing implications in the care of the patient experiencing sensory deprivation. IN *Advanced Concepts in Clinical Nursing*, ed. by K. C. Kintzel. Philadelphia, J. B. Lippincott Co., 1971, pp. 130-143.
26. ZUKERMAN, MARVIN. *Multiple Affect Adjective Check List.* San Diego, Calif., Educational and Testing Services, 1965.

Section VI   Hypertension and Peripheral Vascular Disease

Hypertension is a major health problem in the United States. As Dr. Aagaard points out in the first article in this section, 20 to 30 percent of adults have elevated blood pressures, and many of these people are unaware of it or are untreated. Nurses have a major role to play in hypertension detection and treatment, particularly in the important area of patient counseling.

A second chronic cardiovascular problem—peripheral vascular disease—affects mostly older people, and is associated with activity limitation, pain, and potential infection. While drug therapy, dietary restrictions, careful hygienic practices, and, occasionally, surgery can slow the disease's progress, many patients need continuous nursing management to prevent complications. The articles related to this subject identify assessment factors, describe the treatment of chronic arterial and venous occlusion, and give some clues for the long-term management of these patients.

From the *American Journal of Nursing* 73:620-623, Apr. 1973.

Treatment of Hypertension

GEORGE N. AAGAARD

Hypertension is one of our nation's most important health problems. From 20 to 30 percent of adults in the United States have blood pressures equal to or greater than 160 mm. Hg systolic and 95 mm. Hg diastolic. In a recent study, 75 percent of the persons with elevated blood pressure were either unaware of it or were untreated(1). This number of undiagnosed and untreated people is tremendously significant because insurance company statistics and epidemiological studies show that morbidity and mortality increase with increases in either systolic or diastolic pressure.

The most important causes of complications and death from hypertension are cardiovascular disease, such as congestive heart failure and myocardial infarction; cerebrovascular disease, chiefly stroke; and progressive renal failure. Modern treatment can prevent much of the disability and many of the deaths now caused by hypertension.

The Veterans Administration Cooperative Study demonstrated a significant decrease in morbidity and mortality in male patients who received drug treatment(2,3). Among those men with initial diastolic pressures above 105 mm. Hg, significantly fewer complications, such as stroke and episodes of congestive heart failure, and a decreased number of deaths occurred in the treated patients as compared with the untreated control group. For men with diastolic pressures below that level, the differences were not statistically significant but did suggest that drug treatment was beneficial.

DR. AAGAARD (*M.D., University of Minnesota, Minneapolis*) is chairman of the subcommittee on Hospital-Based Education in Therapeutics of the American Society for Clinical Pharmacology and Therapeutics. He is also professor of medicine, University of Washington School of Medicine, Seattle.

Before embarking on a treatment program, it is important to determine if there is any specific cause of the hypertension. Pheochromocytoma, aldosterone-producing adenoma, renal artery stenosis, and coarctation of the aorta are some of the specific and curable causes of elevated blood pressure. However, the hypertension of 90 to 95 percent of new patients with elevated blood pressures has no demonstrable cause and is classified as essential hypertension.

NONPHARMACOLOGIC CONTROL MEASURES

Certain general treatment measures should be initiated in all patients with hypertension, even those with very mild blood pressure elevations. These modalities carry no risk and are sufficient to reduce some patients' blood pressure to satisfactory levels. For other patients, drug therapy may be required but dosage may be lower.

Weight control should be strict enough to keep the patient on the lean side of the standard weight for a given height. Since many charts of average weights are too generous, it may be helpful to estimate the thickness of the patient's subcutaneous fat layer and to keep this close to the lower limits of normal.

The diet ought to be restricted in sodium content. All grossly salty foods should be eliminated, and no salt should be used in preparing food at mealtime.

Daily exercise should be initiated and increased until the patient is walking briskly for 30 minutes per day, unless there is some specific contraindication. Other more vigorous sports are recommended for patients who are physically fit—tennis, handball, basketball, baseball, swimming, and skiing.

Relaxation techniques are particularly useful to those patients who are obviously nervous, tense, hyperactive, and restless. Progressive muscular relaxation, autogenic therapy, various yogic exercises, and transcendental meditation may help the patient to obtain more profound relaxation.

The patient should be urged to carefully consider his life style. Hurry is to be avoided. Work and play and mealtime should be leisurely and enjoyable. People who work on a schedule ought to space their appointments or work activities so that they can work and concentrate on the task presently at hand without having to hurry for the next appointment.

Probably the most important aspect in the general management of hypertension is to teach the patient that hypertension is a chronic condition that tends to persist and, in fact, to get worse unless treatment is carefully and persistently followed. Even patients whose blood pressure returns to normal without drug therapy should have periodic checks of blood pressure. Patients must be motivated to continue their therapeutic program, which may last a lifetime. Unfortunately, too many patients follow a treatment program only until their symptoms are relieved or blood pressures return to normal.

DRUG THERAPY

I advocate drug treatment if diastolic pressure remains at 100 mm. Hg in males and 105 mm. Hg in females despite the general treatment measures. Epidemiological studies show that women tolerate elevated blood pressure better than men.

We are fortunate today in having several groups of drugs which can lower blood pressure significantly. Although none of these drugs is uniformly effective nor free of side effects, they can, when properly used, control blood pressure in almost all hypertensive patients. For many patients, it may be necessary to try different medications, alone and in combination, and at different dosage levels, to find the treatment which is effective and tolerable.

The individual patient and his family may have to learn to monitor blood pressure. Blood pressure can be a guide to drug dosage and may help to reassure the patient that it can be controlled.

Drugs available at present for the treatment of hypertension may be classified as diuretics, adrenergic inhibitors, and vascular smooth muscle dilators.

DIURETICS Mild oral diuretics include thiazides and chlorthalidone, which are closely related to the sulfonamide chemotherapeutic agents. How they lower blood pressure is not entirely clear. Initially, there is a decrease in plasma volume, but some studies have suggested that the hypotensive effect of the diuretic persists even after the plasma volume returns to normal, as it does after several weeks. Opinion is divided on this matter.

Other studies suggest that the diuretics cause a decrease in the sodium content of vascular smooth muscle and thus make it less responsive to the effects of sympathetic nerve stimulation and the release of norepinephrine at the sympathetic terminal. At any rate, diuretics appear to decrease peripheral vascular resistance without producing significant postural hypotension. The maximum effect of the diuretics on blood pressure does not usually appear for two or three weeks. Often in mild or moderate hypertension, a diuretic alone may lower pressure to an acceptable level.

Patients with significant impairment of kidney function may need a more potent oral diuretic, furosemide. This drug can be given in increasing doses until diuresis takes place. Continuing administration of furosemide will control extracellular-fluid volume in patients with impaired renal function and make the other drugs which are available for treatment more effective.

The oral diuretics are relatively safe drugs. Mild gastrointestinal symptoms, such as nausea and anorexia and even vomiting, may occur but can be prevented or minimized if the drug is given initially in small doses and gradually increased. Perhaps the most important side effect of the diuretics is excess potassium excretion that can lead to hypokalemia. This may cause muscular weakness and cardiac arrhythmias. Hypokalemia is of particular concern in patients with hypertensive heart disease requiring digitalis, since it increases the hazard of digitalis-induced disturbances in cardiac rhythm.

Patients taking oral diuretics should be encouraged to eat potassium-rich foods, like bananas and citrus fruits. If serum potassium falls below the normal range, potassium chloride should be prescribed. If serum potassium still cannot be maintained at a satisfactory level, it may be necessary to reduce the dose of the thiazide diuretic or chlorthalidone and supplement this reduced dose with a potassium-sparing diuretic, such as spironolactone or triamterene.

Increased serum uric acid is another biochemical effect of oral diuretic therapy and sometimes precipitates gouty attacks. Allopurinol may be used to reduce the serum uric acid level.

Hyperglycemia is another adverse effect of the oral diuretics; it usually does not require therapy. If significant glycosuria or other symptoms of diabetes occur, antidiabetic measures should be taken.

Skin rash and photosensitivity are other side effects. Jaundice, vasculitis, and hematologic complications are rare adverse effects.

ADRENERGIC INHIBITORS The adrenergic inhibitor drugs include several that act through slightly different mechanisms to reduce sympathetic nervous system effects on the cardiovascular system. These drugs will be briefly considered in ascending order of potency.

Reserpine, an alkaloid of rauwolfia, decreases the sympathetic tone, primarily by depleting the postganglionic nerve terminals of their stores of catecholamines. Reserpine action ordinarily develops slowly and usually requires two or three weeks to reach its full effect when the drug is given by mouth. It is a mild hypotensive agent and may reduce blood pressure only slightly when given alone. When reserpine is taken with an oral diuretic, its blood pressure-lowering effect may be accentuated.

The most serious adverse effect of reserpine is depression. Fortunately, this is not common, but the drug should probably not be prescribed for patients who have a history of depression or who tend to be depressed without any medication. Change in the sleeping pattern, such as early awakening and inability to go back to sleep, may be the first sign of depression related to the use of reserpine. This should be regarded as an

HIGH SOURCES OF POTASSIUM[1]

	mg./100 Gm.
All-Bran cereal	1,200
Almonds, raw	690
Apricots, dried	1,700
Beans	
Dry, Navy	1,300
Fresh, Lima	680
Beef—lean, raw	360
Beets—fresh greens	570
Brussels sprouts, fresh	450
Chocolate—milk, candy	420
Chicken—raw, breast meat	320
Coca-Cola	52
(Pepsi-Cola, by contrast, has 3 mg./100 Gm.)	
Coconut—dry shredded	770
Cod—frozen fillets	400
Coffee	
Instant, Nescafe, dry	3,100
Roasted, decaffeinated, Sanka, dry	2,000
Crackers, rye	600
Dates—semidry, California	790
Flour, buckwheat	680
Lentils, dry	1,200
Liver—raw, calf	380
Lonalac, dry	1,000
Oranges—Temple, pulp and juice	220
Peaches, dried	1,100
Peanut butter	820
Peas—dry, split	830
Pettijohn's cereal, dry	380
Tea—India-Ceylon-Java blend, dry	1,800

* Reproduced from: Sodium and potassium in foods and waters, determination by flame photometer, C. E. Bills, F. G. McDonald, W. Niedermeier, and M. C. Schwartz, J. Amer. Dietet. A. 25:304, 1949 by permission of the copyright owners. The table used here is excerpted from WAYLER, T. J., AND KLEIN, R. S. Applied Nutrition. New York, Macmillan Co., 1965, pp. 152-157.

indication for reducing the dose or stopping the drug. Many patients complain of general weakness or lack of pep; they may find the drug intolerable. Nasal congestion may make breathing difficult and cause sleeplessness at night.

Methyldopa is a more potent adrenergic inhibitor; its mechanism of action is not yet entirely clear. It appears to reduce the amount of norepinephrine at the sympathetic nerve terminal by substituting a less potent catecholamine derivative. Methyldopa has a greater hypotensive effect than reserpine and may be used as a single drug for the treatment of mild hypertension.

Adverse effects of methyldopa include lassitude, weakness, and depression, although these occur less frequently than with reserpine. Skin rash may also occur. Sexual impotence is a distressing side effect for male patients who are taking fairly large doses of methyldopa. Many patients develop positive Coombs tests after a year of large-dose therapy with methyldopa, but significant hematological complications are rare.

Guanethidine is the most potent adrenergic inhibitor now available. It decreases sympathetic tone by blocking the transmission of the sympathetic nerve impulse and causes depletion of norepinephrine at the nerve terminal. Guanethidine, too, is potent enough to lower blood pressure satisfactorily in many patients with mild hypertension. Its potency is markedly increased when it is used with an oral diuretic.

Guanethidine, like the other adrenergic inhibitors, may cause lassitude, fatigue, and general weakness and may be intolerable for some patients unless dosage is carefully controlled. Diarrhea is not uncommon and the urgency associated with it is very distressing to the patient. Large doses of guanethidine may impair sexual function in the male, usually by producing an inability for normal ejaculation.

Perhaps the most dangerous adverse effect of guanethidine is postural hypotension. At the extreme, syncope may occur. Patients must be warned to sit or squat at the first feeling of light headedness or dizziness to avoid serious injury from falling. They should be taught to assume an erect position slowly and to pause before walking.

Propranolol is a beta adrenergic receptor blocker not presently approved by the Food and Drug Administration for treating hypertension. Propranolol has been used with other drugs in severe hypertension and may act by decreasing renin release. The place of propranolol in the treatment of hypertension is still to be established.

Propranolol should not be given to persons with asthma or heart failure. Lassitude may be a side effect. Diarrhea or abdominal cramps or both may be a factor in determining dosage level.

VASODILATORS Hydralazine probably acts as a vasodilator through its direct action on vascular smooth muscle. In uncomplicated hypertension, it is usually given with a diuretic and an adrenergic inhibitor. A three-drug treatment program with hydrochlorothiazide, reserpine, and hydralazine was very effective in severe hypertension in the Veterans Administration Cooperative Study(4). Adverse effects of hydralazine include headache, nausea, and fatigue. Tachycardia, palpitation, and anginal-type distress are important side effects. These are minimized if the patient is receiving an adrenergic inhibitor before hydralazine is started.

PATIENTS AND DRUGS

When a satisfactory drug treatment program has been worked out, it is important that the patient understand it and follow it. Many patients simply forget to take their medications on schedule. Some people find it helpful to put out all their day's medications in a convenient but obvious place in the morning. They know that those medications must be taken before the day is over.

Although all drugs currently available for treating hypertension have notable shortcomings, they will reduce the toll of disability and death when properly used. Our goal at present is to see that they are used when indicated. Further improvement in our ability to control hypertension should improve as patients come under treatment earlier and as new and more effective drugs become available.

REFERENCES

1. SCHOENBERGER, J. A., AND OTHERS. Current status of hypertension control in an industrial population. *JAMA* 222:559-562, Oct. 30, 1972.
2. U.S. VETERANS ADMINISTRATION, COOPERATIVE STUDY GROUP ON ANTIHYPERTENSIVE AGENTS. Effects of treatment on morbidity in hypertension: Part 2. Results in patients with diatolic blood pressure averaging 90 through 114 mm. Hg. *JAMA* 213:1143-1152, Aug. 17, 1970.
3. ———. Effects of treatment on morbidity in hypertension; Part 3. Influence of age, diastolic pressure, and prior cardiovascular disease; further analysis of side effects. *Circulation* 45:991-1004, May 1972.
4. ———. Effects of treatment on morbidity in hypertension; results in patients with diastolic blood pressures averaging 115 through 129 mm. Hg. *JAMA* 202:1028-1034, Dec. 11, 1967.

From the *American Journal of Nursing* 73:624-627, Apr. 1973.

Primary Hypertension Patients' Learning Needs

ELIZABETH WELK GRIFFITH • BLANCHE MADERO

Controlling blood pressure requires patients' understanding of hypertension and their responsible involvement in their own care. Patients' misunderstandings constitute an obstacle that they themselves, their families, nurses, and physicians need to be aware of. Since both case finding and teaching are part of nursing practice, perhaps nurses can intensify their efforts to help patients start and then continue in treatment.

During the past five years we have been involved, as nurse instructors, in an experimental hypertension clinic emphasizing patient education and motivation. We have treated and monitored approximately 500 hypertensive patients according to a formal protocol, under the supervision of a physician-consultant. The patients have been members of a prepaid health plan which is fairly representative of the socioeconomic profile of the general population in the area. We have become aware, in our continuing care of these patients, of differing interpretations, misconceptions, and certain patterns of reasoning which indicate common learning needs.

Caldwell and others investigated the reasons that patients discontinued antihypertensive therapy[1]. Among the reasons patients gave were that

MS. GRIFFITH and MS. MADERO *are nurse instructors in the Hypertension Clinic, Health Education Center, Division of Preventive Medicine, Kaiser-Permanente Research Medical Center, Oakland, Calif. Ms. Griffith was graduated from Deaconess Hospital School of Nursing, Milwaukee, Wis. She has a B.S.N., Western Reserve University; and an M.S., University of Michigan. Ms. Madero was graduated from St. Joseph's Hospital School of Nursing, San Francisco, Calif. and holds a B.S. from the College of the Holy Names, Oakland, Calif.* Research activities of this project were supported by the Kaiser Foundation Research Institute.

they felt well, received poor instruction, were in financial need, were dissatisfied and discouraged, lacked family support, and experienced drug side effects.

Inferred reasons for continuing treatment were good knowledge of the disease, the harmful effects of inadequate hypertensive treatment on family members, emotional satisfaction, physical comfort, and family support. The researchers concluded that patient and spouse education offers one approach to help patients continue treatment.

Rosenberg and others studied the relationship of patient information to the frequency and length of hospital readmission(2). They theorized that persons who know the why, what, and when of their care would be more likely to cooperate with prescribed regimens than persons who are simply prescribed for; and that hospital readmissions and hospital days would be reduced. The investigators' data led them to conclude that planned education is effective.

From these studies and our experience, it is evident that several factors must be considered to help patients carry out control measures which, in present circumstances, are expected to be lifelong. Ongoing assessment of each person provides the basis for action and interaction. Not every patient needs to know everything about hypertension to adapt well. Sufficient knowledge for some to participate and feel confident in their care is insufficient for others. Here, we discuss content that is generally useful to most patients.

The following descriptions illustrate a spectrum of patients' interpretations of and approaches to primary hypertension.

A YOUNG COLLEGE GRADUATE Mr. J., a college graduate, was denied employment when a physical exam revealed he had hypertension. He has since found a job, but is anxious about his blood pressure. "Here I am only 24 years old, in the prime of my life, and I'm worse off than some men of 40. And it's obvious I'm getting worse because I've gone from taking phenobarbital to thiazide and now reserpine is being added."

Mr. J. has not been able to eat foods high in potassium for the past three weeks because he has been short of money. He has been eating mostly pork and beans, and he feels guilty because he's heard that pork makes hypertension worse. His present weakness and difficulty in concentrating worry him; he is afraid he might make serious errors at work.

Mr. J. wonders why he has hypertension and what is happening to his body. He doesn't feel any different. Is he aging faster than someone who does not have hypertension? Are his arteries older than those of other people his age? Why has his medicine been increased? Why must he take the potassium solution? How will the medicine bring his pressure down? What is a normal blood pressure anyway? How long will all of this go on?

A MIDDLE-AGED ENGINEER Mr. C., a 45-year-old engineer, is thin and soft spoken, and appears relaxed. He follows directions accurately and feels highly honored that people take such interest in his good health. He appreciates all suggestions and information and keeps his appointments. Occasionally, he asks questions about his diet or the articles on exercise, blood pressure, and heart disease, which he has read.

AN EMBARRASSED WOMAN Ms. B. has had hypertension for 13 years. In the past, her blood pressure has been under poor control. She was not aware of the importance of taking her medicine as directed. Ms. B. was embarrassed to seek medical care, since her obesity had been implicated in the cause of her hypertension. She was afraid that her blood pressure readings were incorrect because sometimes a wide cuff was used and other times a regular-size cuff was used. She thought that she should not work because of her hypertension, and yet her family was poor.

Ms. B. attends a weight-control program. Her blood pressure is controlled and she hopes to be employed.

A PROFESSOR Mr. P., a 49-year-old university professor, has been followed 11 years for labile hypertension. Recently, his blood pressure has been consistently elevated. Mr. P. feared that he would not be given any information about his condition simply because he is well educated and might be expected to understand hypertension. He was relieved to hear that this assumption would not be made and he expressed a desire to learn about hypertension and how to take better care of himself.

A THREATENED MAN At age 36, Mr. F. became quite upset when he needed antihypertensive medication for his consistently elevated blood pressure. For the last seven years he has been having his blood pressure checked routinely, but he has never really been concerned about having hypertension. His father and mother have hypertension and "seem to be doing all right."

Why did his blood pressure suddenly go up when all these years he's been doing so well? Because of something he did? Maybe his jogging, which he recently started? Or perhaps something he ate? What would happen if he didn't take any medicine? If he did take medicine, how would he feel? How long will he need medicine?

Mr. F. is disheartened since he thinks that "Once I start taking medicine I'll never get rid of the high blood pressure." Friends who have hypertension and who felt well are having "all kinds of problems" now that they have begun taking medicine. Mr. F. doesn't want this to happen to him.

A TRUSTING WOMAN Ms. S. recently learned during her annual physical examination that she has hypertension. She does not ask questions about hypertension; readily replies, "anything you say," to suggestions; and seems perfectly satisfied with her care. Anticipating what Ms. S. must know becomes especially important. She is highly motivated to do anything to stay in good health and trusts that what doctors or nurses tell her is the best advice.

HYPERTENSION AT 22 At 22 years of age, Mr. W. cannot believe he has high blood pressure. During his first visit he asked to have his blood pressure taken several times to be sure it was elevated. He is much concerned about hypertension and how it will affect his coming marriage. He does not know his family history because he was adopted, and he frequently mentions the possibility that other problems he is not aware of could develop.

He worries about the "bad things" drugs can do to the body, about taking a sedative because it is habit forming. He dislikes "popping pills." He acknowledges being nervous and tense, especially when he comes for checkups because he is afraid that his pressure will be very high. He often asks if something he is doing causes his hypertension. Why can't he "just have a drink" to calm him instead of medicine?

AN ANXIOUS YOUNG MAN Mr. J. is 25 years old. He and his wife have just had their first child. He came to have his blood pressure checked the day his wife was in labor. After missing several previous appointments and not responding to letters and telephone calls, he finally came because he was having severe headaches and thought his blood pressure might be high. He was anxious, spoke rapidly, fidgeted, and asked many questions, repeating some two or three times. Moderate hypertension was recorded and he was started on medication.

For the next several days, Mr. J. called almost daily. Why did he still have headaches? Would his blood pressure go down right away? Would he be all right? Would he have a stroke? What could he eat? So many people had said not to eat certain foods that he had eaten almost nothing in the last three days. He had lost five pounds. He pleaded to have his blood pressure checked again to see if it was lower.

His pressure was somewhat lower on his next visit, but he remained extremely anxious. More medication was added, his blood pressure was controlled, headaches infrequent.

Mr. J. has not completed his laboratory tests to exclude secondary hypertension because other family members have hypertension and he thinks he has inherited the disease. Now Mr. J. misses regular appointments. If he has headaches, he calls to have his blood pressure checked right away; subsequently, he skips the next scheduled appointment.

Adjusting to primary hypertension often begins with developing an awareness of the condition, a phase common to nearly all patients in their adjustment to chronic illness. The realization that one is hypertensive may not come easily. Difficulty may arise because patients frequently feel well; they cannot associate their sense of well-being with their usual concept of the presence of illness.

Most patients are amazed that they are asymptomatic or that their symptoms are not necessarily related to elevated blood pressure. For example, patients commonly attribute headaches to high blood pressure and think that when they do not have headaches their pressure is normal. Headaches and high blood pressure may or may not be associated.

Patients with labile pressures may think that medical personnel err in measurement and are unreliable, or that the fluctuations are not significant because medication is not prescribed. Lacking tangible evidence of their disease—evidence they can feel—some persons cannot incorporate its presence in their self-concept or follow through with therapy.

Other patients become apprehensive as they remember relatives who had high blood pressure and strokes that were followed by invalidism or death. They fear that hypertension requires withdrawal from their usual life-styles and that the disease or its therapy will damage their bodies. Dealing with conflicting advice from several well-meaning friends may cause apprehension. The asymptomatic characteristic of the disease bothers the patient who wants to know by the way he feels whether his blood pressure is controlled.

Patients search past or present behavior for cause-and-effect relationships. For example, some attribute their hypertension to physical overexertion, fatigue, unusual or continued emotional stress, overweight, overeating of pork, salt, and sweet or spicy foods, exposure to noxious substances, and heredity. Many patients actually believe that the diagnosis of hypertension means nervousness and emotional tension, not high blood pressure.

If patients continue to have this misconception, they are likely to assume that the hypertension will disappear when their emotional stress is relieved. Or, if they foresee no relief of emotional tension, they may think nothing can be done to control the blood pressure, or that nothing need be done. Some feel the added stress of guilt if they regard nervousness as a character flaw, something they should but cannot overcome. Exploring these thoughts in a relaxed environment helps the person get in touch with a relatively intangible situation. Discussing experiences he has in common with others makes his hypertension more real to him. Talking helps him become aware of the change in his body and alerts us to his special needs. His expression of fears and search for a cause reveal his view of his problem, his knowledge and misconceptions, his attitudes and motivation, and aspects of his personality.

As the details emerge, teaching content appropriate to the patient's and family's understanding and attitudes is selected. Specific learning experiences are arranged recognizing that information-giving is not equivalent to the ongoing process of learning.

FOCUSING ON THERAPY

Nearly all patients who require treatment for primary hypertension receive medication. The use of medication is clearly a source of concerns and problems.

Many patients find it difficult to take medicine accurately and routinely. Some simply forget. Some are embarrassed by having to take medicine and by the inappropriate remarks of friends and co-workers. Sometimes, patients strongly fear psychological and physiological drug dependency or the potentially damaging effects of any drug.

Some think that taking medicine wastes time and money if it does not make them feel different; they equate taking medicine with feeling ill and relieving symptoms. The patient who feels well initially, then takes a drug and feels worse, may discontinue all treatment because "The cure is worse than the disease."

The belief that medicine will be needed only for a while, like antibiotics, is more common among patients who are symptomatic at the start of antihypertensive treatment. As they begin feeling better with medication, they are apt to equate their improvement with cure and discontinue the drug.

Sometimes patients will not admit to emotional stress or will feel guilty about taking medicine to relieve emotional tension. Some think they should be able to relax without medicine. Some do not understand that medicines may contain more than one substance, an ingredient to help them relax, another to open the lumen of blood vessels. Therefore they take their medicine only when they recognize the need for the relaxing component.

Many patients expect that one drug is right for all people with primary hypertension and do not appreciate individual differences in disease patterns and responses to medication. Some patients think that, once their blood pressure has been controlled with a medication, they will take the drug at that dosage the rest of their lives. Believing that "if a little is good, more must be better," some increase dosage. Others do the opposite—try to get by on less than prescribed—often to simplify the dosage schedule or save money. Understanding the potentiating interactions between some drugs and alcohol, some patients change their medicine schedule or omit their medicines so they can drink.

Some patients are perplexed by the array of drugs available, while others are encouraged. Among all the drugs, surely something will be right for them! Of course, many worry about drug costs, especially the patients who take several drugs, and all who face lifelong usage.

To encourage treatment, we have found the following approaches helpful. We stress that patients need to take their medicines correctly and tell us how they are feeling in order to select the most effective and acceptable therapy. We emphasize that medicine controls blood pressure only during the time it is taken regularly. It is not useful to scold a patient for not taking his medicine. Rather, one explores his reasons and attempts to modify the circumstances or the medication.

We do not think it is advisable to say, "Your blood pressure is normal." Add or substitute, "Your blood pressure is being well controlled by your medicine at this time." The patient could interpret the first statement to mean that his disease has been cured and assume that more medicine is unnecessary. The second statement reinforces his need to continue treatment and follow-up.

Use of home remedies like vinegar and honey, garlic solution, or other foods is a sensitive point. Here, it seems best to say that the remedy will not harm him (if true), but that additional treatment is still necessary.

We try to gain a patient's acceptance of alternative methods of contraception when birth control pills are not advisable or possibly are implicated in causing the hypertension. An alternative method to relieve menopausal symptoms may be needed when estrogens must be discontinued for some reason.

We help patients understand facts and modify behavior related to specific drug actions, diet, weight and blood lipid control, relaxation, exercise, and smoking cessation.

Discussing the conflicting or interesting ideas a patient has encountered in reading or talking with friends can also promote learning. It is essential to repeatedly reinforce the patient behavior favorable to continued care with facts about the risks of uncontrolled hypertension; that is, that the goal of therapy is to prevent cardiovascular complications.

REFERENCES

1. CALDWELL, J. R., AND OTHERS. The dropout problem in antihypertensive treatment. *J.Chronic.Dis.* 22:579-592, Feb. 1970.
2. ROSENBERG, S. C. Case for patient education. *Hosp.Formulary Manage.* 6:14-17, June 1971.

BIBLIOGRAPHY

CRATE, M. A. Nursing functions in adaptation to chronic illness. *Am.J.Nurs.* 65:72-76, Oct. 1965.

FREIS, E. D. The chemotherapy of hypertension. *JAMA* 218:1009-1015, Nov. 15, 1971.

INTER-SOCIETY COMMISSION ON HEART DISEASE RESOURCES. Part 1. Cardiovascular disease—primary prevention. Primary prevention of hypertension. *Circulation* 42(Suppl.): A39-A41, July 1970.

MOYER, J. H., III. Optimum therapy for essential hypertension. *Am.Fam.Physican* 5:103-114, June 1972.

REDMAN, B. K. Patient education as a function of nursing practice. *Nurs.Clin.North Am.* 6:753-580, Dec. 1971.

WILBER, J. A., AND BARROW, J. G. Reducing elevated blood pressure. Experience found in a community. *Minn.Med.* 52:1303-1306, Aug. 1969.

From the *American Journal of Nursing* 74:910-912, May 1974.

Group Work with Hypertensive Patients

ANDREA CONTE • MERLE BRANDZEL • SUSAN WHITEHEAD

The person with hypertension may face a life-long regimen of medications, dietary restrictions, and—if there is organ involvement—curtailment of activity. Since the onset of hypertension is likely to be silent and progressive, rather than dramatic and sudden, a disparity between how a patient feels and an existing serious condition, as reflected by his medical regimen, often prompts denial. Emotional factors such as denial may play a role in the hypertensive patient's lack of adherence to prescribed regimen, especially if he has little knowledge of the condition.

At the Boston City Hospital Hypertension Clinic, which is primarily a consultation clinic for evaluation and treatment of hypertensive patients, we observed that many patients did not adhere strictly to their prescribed regimens. The patients had many concerns and questions regarding their illness and seemed anxious to discuss their problems. We postulated that a person with hypertension who understood and accepted his condition and treatment would be more likely to carry out the physician's advice and would have less anxiety about his hypertension.

With physician support, we worked closely with small groups of patients to achieve an understanding of their concerns, questions, and thoughts about hypertension, and to gain insight about the possible rela-

MS. CONTE *is a graduate of Mercy Hospital School of Nursing, Springfield, Mass., and holds a B.S. degree from the University of Washington, Seattle. She is a professional instructor for Searle Medidata, Inc., Lexington, Mass.* MS. BRANDZEL *holds a B.A. degree from Washington University, St. Louis, Missouri, and a master's degree in social work from Western Reserve University, Cleveland, Ohio. She is a medical social worker at Beth Israel Hospital, Boston, Mass.* MS. WHITEHEAD *is a graduate of Rice University, Houston, Texas. She is a medical systems analyst with Bolt Beranek and Newman, Inc., Cambridge, Mass. This project was supported in part by Regional Medical Program Grant #1-G03-RM-00062-01.*

tionship of these factors to adherence to a regimen. Our intent was to demonstrate an effective and efficient method of patient education through collaborative efforts of nursing and social service. The group meetings were intended as a complement to, not a substitute for, the roles of the clinic and the physicians.

The objectives of our patient groups were to discuss the nature and treatment of high blood pressure and to explore patients' emotional responses to a chronic, though not necessarily debilitating condition. Group sessions were described to the participants as an opportunity for them to learn more about hypertension and its treatment, and to share with others the experience of having it.

Organizing and planning the group in terms of content and dynamics required a major commitment of time and effort. Another demanding activity was learning to function as co-leaders in a group situation. Learning to anticipate each other's behavior and to function harmoniously in the group was a slow, sometimes painful, always meaningful process.

THE GROUPS

Two consecutive groups were organized with eight participants in the first group and six in the second. Participants' ages ranged from 28 to 61 years. Meetings, conducted in a building adjacent to the outpatient department, were held for one hour and fifteen minutes each week. The first group met for six weeks, the second for eight weeks. The meetings were taped with the consent of the patients and each week the recording was listened to and discussed by the co-leaders and a group work consultant, who helped us to interpret the group process.

The criteria for selection of patients were an established diagnosis of hypertension, ability to communicate, interest, and willingness to invest the specified time. We attempted to screen out persons with known psychiatric problems which would have been beyond the scope and focus of the group.

Prospective group participants were identified in clinic by the community health nurse, social worker, physicians, or self-referral. After the initial screening process, each of the eventual participants was approached in clinic by either a nurse or social worker who explained the proposed group to the patient.

To gather baseline information and to measure change in level of knowledge about hypertension, a questionnaire was devised by the clinic physicians, the community health nurse, the social worker, and the cardiovascular biometrician. Both multiple-choice and open-ended questions were used, as well as statements requiring only "yes" or "no" answers. The questionnaire was administered to each prospective group member as a pre-test. Within a week after termination of the group, a subset of the pre-group questions was administered as a post-test.

To counteract the literacy factor and the possibility of "leading" a patient's responses, an objective third party, the cardiovascular biometrician, administered the questionnaires orally. To minimize anxiety and to encourage honest and thorough responses, the questionnaire was kept anonymous, being letter-coded for matching pre- and post-group questionnaires.

Some test questions were revised for the second patient group as a result of difficulties encountered in the first group. For example, patients in the first group were given a list of about 20 foods and asked to indicate whether or not they could eat a food if they were on a low-salt diet. The patients consistently had difficulty responding to this question and tended to answer in terms of whether or not they usually ate the food mentioned. Therefore, patients in the second group were presented with a series of colored pictures of different foods and were asked to separate the pictures into two groups, those high in salt and those low in salt. With this approach, patients were better able to identify foods they should restrict.

The nurse or the social worker interviewed each group member at home prior to the group meetings for orientation purposes. These interviews provided valuable information about the medical, educational, and emotional status of the group participants. More important, this individual contact facilitated their transition into the group. Motivation to attend was a crucial element. Many of the participants were inner city residents who led relatively isolated lives, and who had had little or no previous experience with group or "talk" therapies.

In preparation for the group meeting, clinic physicians outlined the topics they considered important for discussion. We hoped to involve the participants in the learning process by pooling their experiences and then exploring, discussing, and clarifying those experiences. For example, in the first group meeting each patient was asked to relate when and how he learned he had high blood pressure. Each participant's contribution illustrated in a direct and meaningful way the various symptoms of hypertension—or lack of them. This particular exchange also led to discussion of the cause and chronicity of hypertension. To augment group discussion on other topics, we made use of such visual aids as pictures of commercial foods allowed or restricted on a low-sodium diet and diagrams of the circulatory system.

The group belonged to the members in attendance and they determined, within defined limits, the topics of discussion. It was imperative that the group deal not only with what clinicians believed to be important, but what the participants believed important.

RESULTS

Medications and their side effects was the most frequently discussed topic and the one which was of most concern to our patients. Antihypertensive medications taken by group members included thiazide diuretics, spironolactone, rauwolfia, methyldopa, hydralazine, and guanethidine. While no single individual was taking all of these medications, each patient was taking at least two of these drugs. Side effects mentioned by the patients ranged from drowsiness and easy fatigability to decreased libido and failure to ejaculate. Often when a troublesome side effect was mentioned by one group member some other person in the group reported experiencing the same reaction. Sharing concerns about medications and side effects stimulated discussion not only about hypertension and its treatment, but also about emotional responses.

The nature of blood pressure and of high blood pressure, diet (both weight-reduction and low-sodium), hypertensive complications, and problems causing emotional stress also were discussed. With each successive meeting, the participants became more familiar with each other and expressed themselves more openly.

Many of our patients expressed sadness ("I get so tired of taking my pills . . . sometimes I feel like sitting down and crying"), anger ("Why? Why me? Why did this have to happen to me?"), guilt ("If I had only gone to the doctor sooner, maybe it wouldn't be so bad today"), and denial ("If they don't know what causes it and they can't cure it, how do they know I have it?").

Some of our patients revealed that when they were first advised to take anti-hypertensive medications, they had doubts as to the accuracy of the diagnosis. Some said they had taken their hypertension seriously only after an unusual or frightening event had occurred as a result of their hypertension or after they learned of its dangers. This suggests that early patient education regarding hypertension could prevent many unnecessary complications.

The post-group questionnaire was administered to all but two of the participants; one was involved with a family crisis and the other had moved. Comparison of the results of pre- and post-group questionnaires revealed that changes in response tended to be more qualitative then quantitative. For example, most pre-test responses to the question "Why is it important for an overweight person with hypertension to lose weight?" were in terms of it being "hard to carry a lot of weight." On the post-test, the majority of patients were able to answer in terms of "lowering blood pressure" and "decreasing the strain on the heart."

The participants had a new understanding and acceptance of the fact that they would need to take medications for the remainder of their lives. In addition, after the group experience all patients were able to give some response to the question on "possible causes" of hypertension, with half of them recognizing the cause as usually unknown.

Post-group interviews were conducted within one week after the last meeting to determine each participant's reaction to, and evaluation of, the group experience. Each interview lasted from 30 to 60 minutes.

The interviews revealed that the patients felt they were now better informed. Many said they were no longer as concerned about having hypertension because they knew much more about it. As one man said, "I know now that just because you have hypertension doesn't mean you have to die from it . . . you can control it with the medicines." Several persons indicated that they weren't as likely to skip their medications and realized the importance of taking them regularly. This suggests that a stricter adherence to regimen in the future might be an outcome of the group experience. A number of people were able to verbalize specific things they had learned concerning diet and symptomatology. During one group meeting, the patients agreed that they were the lucky ones, because they knew they had hypertension and could control it.

The participants expressed positive feelings about having the opportunity to share their thoughts, concerns, and ideas about hypertension with others. Each of the participants seemed to feel a sense of community in being part of a group where having high blood pressure was the norm. During the group sessions we found that patients teaching patients was most effective. The groups permitted patients to be active participants on the health care team, and resulted in greater personalization of the clinic and hospital. The mutually supportive atmosphere permitted and encouraged patients to share with and understand each other, reducing the isolation and loneliness many of them felt.

The use of patient groups as an adjunct to the ongoing treatment of persons with hypertension merits further exploration and refinement. Ideally, there should be long-term follow-up to determine whether such group experience and increase in the level of knowledge about hypertension having a lasting effect on behavior.

BIBLIOGRAPHY

BREST, A. N., AND MOYER, J. H. Treatment of the ambulatory patient with diastolic hypertension. In *Hypertension-Recent Advances*, ed. by Albert N. Brest and John H. Moyer. Philadelphia, Lea and Febiger, 1961, pp. 485-492.

CHOBANIAN, A. V., AND LANZONI, VINCENT. Current concepts of the drug therapy of hypertension. *Med.Counterpoint* 3:18-40, Mar. 1971.

GARLAND, J. A., AND OTHERS. A model for stages of development in social work groups. IN *Explorations in Group Work: Essays in Theory and Practice*, ed. by Saul Berstein, Boston, Boston University School of Social Work, 1965 pp. 12-53.

HARPER, D. A. Take my work—patient follow-up of medical advice: a literature review. *J.Kans.Med.Soc.* 72:265-271ff. June 1971.

U.S. PRESIDENT'S COMMISION ON HEART DISEASE, CANCER AND STROKE. *Report to the President—A National Program to Conquer Heart Disease, Cancer* and Stroke, Volume 2, Washington, D.C., U.S. Government Printing Office, 1965.

U.S. VETERANS ADMINISTRATION, COOPERATIVE STUDY GROUP ON ANTIHYPERTENSIVE AGENTS. Effects of treatment on morbidity in hypertension, Part 1. *JAMA* 202:1028-1034, Dec. 11, 1967.

———. Effects of treatment on morbidity in hypertension. Part 2. *JAMA* 213:1143-1152, Aug. 17, 1970.

WOOD, J. E., AND OTHERS. Primary prevention of hypertension. *Circulation* 42:A39-A41, July 1970.

From the *American Journal of Nursing* 74:1450-1452, Aug. 1974.

A Rural Hypertension-Control Program

GRETRUDE M. LEE

Is it feasible for rural health departments to undertake a massive screening and treatment program for hypertension? It seemed worthwhile to find out in three rural counties in northwestern Florida, where cardiovascular death rates were higher than for the state as a whole.

Half the families in the tricounty area were medically indigent, and the number of private physicians was low, one physician to just over 4,000 people. A rural hypertension program, conceived by the county health director of the Tricounty Unit of Holmes, Washington, Walton Counties, and the administrator of the Heart Disease Control Program of the Florida Division of Health, was launched in the spring of 1969.

The stated purpose was to demonstrate the feasibility and practicality of controlling arterial hypertension in a rural population, 50 percent of whom were medically indigent. More specifically, the program was designed to find an efficient means of early detection of hypertension and a practical means of using the limited number of local physicians and health department staff as a team to diagnose and treat persons with hypertension.

The program was designed to take as little physician time as possible

MS. LEE *is a public health supervisor, Holmes County Health Department, Bonifay, Fla., and was program coordinator for the project described in this article. She is a graduate of the Sacred Heart Hospital School of Nursing, Pensacola, Fla. The project was under the overall supervision of James E. Fulghum, M.D., chief, Bureau of Adult Health and Chronic Disease; and M. E. Groover, Jr., M.D., administrator, Heart Disease Control Program, Division of Health, Jacksonville, Fla., and the local administrative supervision of William G. Simpson, M.D., director of Holmes, Walton, and Washington County Health Departments, Bonifay, Fla.*

and still provide quality health care. This was originally planned as a five-year demonstration with an application for a National Institutes of Health grant. Plans changed, however, and the Florida Regional Medical Program, Inc., of Gainesville, funded a three-year rather than a five-year project. Time lost with funding notification, establishing positions, and recruiting personnel resulted in 27 months of actual operation, from December 1968 to March of 1971. Today, a hypertension program continues as an integral part of our overall health department program.

Early in the project the public health nurse supervisor from the Holmes County Unit was designated project coordinator and given great latitude to develop the program and coordinate it with the ongoing services in the three county health departments.

Personnel recruitment posed something of a problem. Registered nurses were in short supply, and the medical society, in approving the program, stipulated that nurses employed in hospitals were not to be recruited. We found and hired three inactive registered nurses. None had any experience in public health nursing. Because all nurses in the health departments provide generalized public health nursing service, we had to orient the newcomers to a generalized public health program. Staff had to have a refresher orientation to hypertension control. Three community health workers (a new class of nonprofessional worker in our three departments) and a clerk-typist were employed.

Procedural guidelines were established to (a) identify early asymptomatic cases (b) recheck patients with positive findings on initial screening and refer them to their own doctors or indigent clinic, and (c) do follow-up on suspected cases.

CASE FINDING

Our hope was to screen all residents aged 14 years or older. This gave us a target population of 29,650. The referral level was 150/90 for people over 20 years old, and 120/80 for younger people. These levels were determined at a meeting of cardiologists with the physicians who originated the program.

We tried many methods of reaching people to do the screening. Nurses and health department community health workers did all the screening. We began by contacting the local civic, church, and professional groups. At program meetings of many organizations, we spoke, handed out information on hypertensive disease, and screened members who were present. We held walk-in blood pressure screening clinics in various sections of the counties. The grocery stores all over the cities and counties allowed us to use space on Fridays or Saturdays.

We also had "blood pressure parties." A popular neighborhood woman would invite friends and relatives to her home during evening hours, usually 7:00 to 9:00 P.M., for blood pressure screening. The community health workers did some house-to-house visitation to take blood pressure readings. This last turned out to be the least effective method for reaching people to screen.

We did a total of 17,601 screenings. For original screenings, we took a reading in the left arm, with the person sitting in a comfortable position with his arm at approximately heart level. If blood pressure was elevated, it was rechecked at an early date with the patient standing, sitting, and reclining.

If these recheck readings were elevated, the person was scheduled for fasting blood specimens for sugar, cholesterol, uric acid, triglycerides, hemoglobin, and uric nitrogen. If the triglyceride level was high, the laboratory determined lipoprotein levels. We also did a cardiovascular, hypertensive-disease history and an electrocardiogram on this visit.

After test results were reported, we referred the person to his private doctor or the medical clinic of the health department. Some people on the borderline of indigency were under private medical care, but obtained antihypertensive drugs through medical clinic.

Persons whose blood pressure was extremely high were referred for immediate medical care, before test results could be received. The original guidelines were to schedule each person with a reading above 150/90 within a month, but we learned early that such cases were too numerous. Therefore, we established a higher level, 170/100, for immediate recheck. We scheduled people with readings between 150/90 and 170/100 within three months.

A record system was devised for computer tabulation at specified intervals. Manual tabulation could be done daily, monthly, or quarterly to determine progress. The record system was cross-indexed so that the same people would not be screened again and again.

Once a private doctor, consultant cardiologist, or the medical clinic started a patient on a regimen of antihypertensive drugs and dietary control, the public health nurses assisted patients in medication adjustment and gave dietary instructions and supportive care.

DRUGS AND DIET

Diet recommendations included advice to avoid red meats and saturated fats and to restrict amounts of unsaturated fats and salt. Patients were advised to restrict eggs and dairy products until their blood pressure was well controlled and to use them in moderation afterward. They were advised to eat fish and fowl, but not duck, to eat fruits and vegetables, particularly those high in potassium, and, unless they were grossly overweight, they were allowed at least three servings of bread.

Two drugs were used in the program. One was a combination of reserpine, hydralazine chloride, and hydrochlorothiazide, and the other was guanethidine sulfate. These were given alone or in combination.

Public health nurses were informed regarding levels of blood pressure desired for individuals and the limitations on antihypertensive drugs. One week after a patient started on medication, he returned to the public health nurse clinic. The nurse took blood pressure readings while the patient sat, stood, and reclined. She collected a urine specimen for albumin, glucose, and blood.

If the patient showed no evidence of response to the medication after a time in therapy, the nurse increased the dose. If the blood pressure dropped below the desired level, she decreased the dose. On each visit, the nurse questioned the patient closely about problems and, if warranted, referred the patient back to the medical clinic for reevaluation. The nurse made home visits when patients failed to keep appointments. Patients on medication were seen at least once each week, or more frequently if indicated, until their blood pressure was fairly well stabilized. Then the nurse saw them once a month.

Many people, especially those who had had extremely high blood pressure for several years without medication, complained of feeling unwell and of general malaise as their blood pressure began to decrease. We encouraged them to continue on the medication until their bodies adjusted to a lower blood pressure and suggested eating foods daily that were high in potassium. Many had previously taken antihypertensive drugs, but had stopped because drugs made them "feel so awful." Counseling these patients, many of whom were elderly, was time-consuming.

HOW 100 FARED

This program ended prematurely, and we have not tabulated indisputable evidence that shows conclusively that controlling hypertension in a rural population is possible. We did conduct a survey of 100 people who took medication for one year; 99 reported that after the initial few weeks of medication they felt much better than they had in years, were more alert, and could do much more work.* Most reported they were improved to such an extent that they were sacrificing other needed items

---

* GROOVER, M. E., JR. Early detection and treatment of hypertension—the Northwest Florida hypertension program. Scientific Exhibit, 99th Annual Convention, Florida Medical Association, May 9-13, 1973.

in order to obtain their medication.

The program really evolved into a multiphasic screening program. We discovered numerous cases of diabetes and brought the diabetes under control before complications began. Many young people with high uric acid levels and joint pains were placed on drug therapy and given dietary counsel. Many overweight people were persuaded to lose some of their excess weight.

We believe that the program was effective in discovering early hypertensive disease and getting those affected under treatment. We believe that it demonstrated that medical coverage can be materially extended by registered nurses, if guidelines of function are clearly defined and each profession feels mutual trust. We also think that most of the people in our communities are much better informed in many areas of health maintenance than they were before this program.

We encountered many problems and objections along the way. It took almost a year to orient our new nurses and community workers. Some physicians were resistant to the health departments' involvement in treatment. Some nurses were resistant, too. Some nurses voiced resentment at being expected to do "the work of a physician" and did not want the added responsibility of making decisions about medication.

Part of this attitude was probably due to the fact that nurses were already overloaded, and there was no one to whom they could delegate some of their tasks. Sheer number of cases were overwhelming.

We found that nurses who had previously adjusted medications, for example, in diabetic clinics functioned well in the hypertension clinics, but nurses without such experience were very reluctant to adjust antihypertensive medications at first.

The public health nurses' case-finding skills have been sharpened by their work in the hypertension-control program. Our interest is still so keen that whenever an adult seeks any service in our county health departments, his blood pressure is read before he leaves. If indicated, a cardiovascular profile including the electrocardiogram is made available. Hypertension case finding and control have been adopted as a high-priority, ongoing, public health program in these three Florida counties.

From the American Journal of Nursing 74:2178-2179, Dec. 1974.

Hypertensive Emergencies

ANDREA B. O'CONNOR

The progressive changes of chronic hypertension can be fatal. In response to elevated pressure, artery walls slowly thicken, vessel lumens narrow, and blood supply to the various organs diminishes gradually. These changes cause kidney failure, heart failure, stroke, and aneurysm. But when arterial blood pressure rises dramatically, as it does in accelerated-phase hypertension (malignant hypertension) or in other acute hypertensive states, its damage is pronounced and severe, and organ failure is abrupt.

Accelerated hypertension is manifested by the sudden, severe onset of a markedly elevated diastolic pressure, usually above 120 mm. Hg, and the development of acute central nervous system signs and symptoms; renal failure and azotemia, proteinuria, cylindruria, and hematuria; and retinopathy, with or without papilledema(1). Untreated, accelerated hypertension can cause death in four years—or a few hours(2).

Accelerated hypertension is characterized by acute vascular changes, mostly in the arterioles. The arteriole lumen narrows and thickens. A necrotizing arteriolitis develops and fibrinoid changes occur. The afferent arterioles no longer can supply blood to the organs, most notably the kidney and brain, so tissues die. Necrotic arterioles may rupture, causing small hemorrhages into organs(3).

The precise mechanisms involved in the pathogenesis and course of accelerated hypertension are unknown. The vascular lesions may be caused by the mechanical effects of the severe arterial pressure elevation, but this conjecture has not been supported by research. Another hypothesis suggests that subtle changes in the vessel walls alter renal hemody-

MS. O'CONNOR, R.N., M.A., *was an associate editor of the* American Journal of Nursing *at the time this article was written. Her past experience includes nursing in a 15-bed coronary care unit.*

namics. This alteration stimulates renin release, which, in turn, stimulates the production and release of angiotensin. Angiotensin stimulates excessive secretion of aldosterone. This may cause the pronounced vascular changes that accompany accelerated hypertension and may immediately affect organ function and survival(2).

Persons with essential hypertension can develop a sudden exacerbation of their disease. Accelerated hypertension can be triggered by a severe emotional experience, increased salt consumption, the abrupt discontinuation of antihypertensive medications, or general poor management of the person with hypertension(4). A previously normotensive person can develop accelerated hypertension abruptly, but sudden onset usually suggests a secondary cause(2).

Most people with hypertension have chronic, essential hypertension, and so most accelerated hypertension is of unknown etiology. However, several secondary disease states can lead to, or present as, hypertensive crises.

Adrenal medullary tumors (pheochromocytomas) produce and release large amounts of norepinephrine and epinephrine, both powerful pressors. Most kidney diseases, for example, chronic glomerulonephritis, pyelonephritis, renal artery stenosis, and unilateral renal infarct, can cause accelerated hypertension, possibly by activating the renin-angiotensin system. Periarteritis nodosa often results in accelerated hypertension because the disease produces fibroid and necrotic changes in arteries.

Hypertensive crises can be caused by the combined action of monoamine oxidase (MAO) inhibitors with certain drugs and foods. The antidepressant drugs isocarboxazid (Marplan), nialamide (Niamid), and tranylcypromine (Parnate), and the antihypertensive drug pargyline (Eutonyl) are all MAO inhibitors. These drugs potentiate the action of sympathomimetic agents, such as levarterenol (Levophed), adrenalin, amphetamine (Benzedrine), methyldopa (Aldomet), dopamine, and tyramine. The pressor actions of sympathomimetic drugs are greatly potentiated when MAO inhibitors are administered simultaneously. The natural pressor effects of norepinephrine and epinephrine also are increased when a person taking MAO inhibitors eats foods that contain tyramine, such as beer, wine, pickled herring, chicken liver, yeast, coffee, broadbean pods, canned figs, and the natural and aged cheeses, particularly cheddar, Camembert, and Stilton(5).

Although rare, hypertensive emergencies can also develop during the course of acute glomerulonephritis, eclampsia, or collagen vascular disease; or hypertensive crises may occur secondary to drug ingestion, head injury, or coarctation of the aorta.

HYPERTENSIVE ENCEPHALOPATHY is the most serious complication of accelerated hypertension. Widespread cerebral arteriolar constriction and arteriospasm lead to vascular insufficiency and cerebral edema. Multiple small thrombi and petechial hemorrhages pepper the brain tissue. The elevation in arterial pressure usually is preceded by severe headache. Transitory cerebral phenomena, seizures, and coma follow. The patient may complain of nausea and dizziness in addition to headache. He may vomit. Personality changes, confusion, and lethargy are noted. Focal neurological signs, notably nystagmus and other visual disturbances, reflex asymmetries, localized paraplegia, and positive Babinski, wax and wane because of the sudden alterations in cerebral blood flow. Fatal intracranial hemorrhage may develop(1,6).

Aggressive drug therapy is the treatment of choice for patients with hypertensive encephalopathy. Death can ensue in hours if the patient is not treated. During parenteral hypertensive therapy, the patient's blood pressure must be monitored carefully to prevent a too rapid drop in blood pressure to too low levels. For the same reason, intravenous medications given by drip must be regulated precisely. A vasopressor drug should be readily available to combat excessive hypotensive reactions. Blocks under the head of the bed enhance the actions of some antihypertensives(2).

As with any patient subject to seizures, bed siderails should be padded and kept up at all times. A tongue blade should be at hand. Pupil response, level of consciousness, reflexes, and handgrips should be tested at regular intervals to detect increasing intracranial pressure and progressive cerebral damage.

HYPERTENSIVE RETINOPATHY is associated with the cerebral vascular changes. Cotton-wool exudates, striated hemorrhages, and papilledema are noted on ophthalmoscopic examination. The patient may complain of blurred vision(1). Blindness occurs when spastic constriction completely obliterates the retinal arteries. Vision returns when the hypertension is controlled and the arteries again become patent(6).

HYPERTENSIVE NEPHROPATHY is manifested by progressive renal impairment, may develop with accelerated hypertension, and is often present terminally. The degree of renal failure depends on the degree of renal arterial and arteriolar pathology(7). Fibrinoid necrosis of the afferent glomerular arterioles and endarteritis fibrosa of the interlobular arteries of the kidney cause renal ischemia and hemorrhage(8). Proteinuria, occasionally heavy, is the first sign of impairment. Microscopic or gross hematuria, cylindruria, and azotemia also are noted.

Parenteral antihypertensive therapy may worsen renal function initially, but this is usually reversed as arterial pressure is controlled. Frequent measurements of urinary output should be recorded, and fluid and sodium intake restricted.

CARDIAC DECOMPENSATION develops as the left ventricular workload increases. Coronary insufficiency and myocardial infarction may complicate both accelerated hypertension and its treatment. Left ventricular hypertrophy may lead to pulmonary edema. If pulmonary edema develops, the patient should be treated with morphine, digitalis, diuretics, and rotating tourniquets before aggressive parenteral antihypertensive therapy is begun. If the blood pressure is not controlled by diuresis, antihypertensive drugs should be given, preferably those that do not increase cardiac work(6).

STROKE is always possible with accelerated hypertension, because of the significant cerebrovascular changes which accompany the elevated arterial pressure. Stroke can be distinguished from hypertensive encephalopathy by the persistence of lateralizing neurological signs.

DISSECTING AORTIC ANEURYSM is actually a dissecting hematoma within the aortic wall. The bleeding splits the tunica media of the vessel, separating the intima from the wall. In the presence of accelerated hypertension, increased hemodynamic stresses on the aorta may prompt pathological changes that cause hematoma.

The weakened aortic wall may rupture, causing exsanguination, or it may leak. Or the dissection may proceed upward to the heart and cut off coronary blood flow (MI) or cause cardiac tamponade. Because any vessel that branches from the aorta can be occluded by the dissection, the aneurysm can mimic cerebral vascular accident, acute abdominal crisis, or peripheral vascular occlusion. Prompt lowering of the blood pressure can postpone the need for surgery, or, sometimes, obviate it altogether(6).

Most patients with dissecting aneurysm complain of chest pain similar to the pain that accompanies myocardial infarction. The patient may appear to be in shock, with anxiety, sweating, pallor, tachypnea, and tachycardia, but his blood pressure is elevated. Because differentiating between aneurysm and Ml is often difficult, the blood pressure of any patient suspected of having had an Ml should be checked in both arms. A great difference in the readings may indicate a dissecting aneurysm.

While antihypertensive therapy is being given, the nurse must check closely for signs of organ ischemia. The peripheral pulses on both sides of the body are evaluated and compared. Urinary output is monitored.

Once the crisis has passed and the patient's blood pressure is under control, he must learn the specific dietary and drug regimen that will control his hypertension and prevent future life-threatening crises.

REFERENCES

1. KOCH-WESER, JAN. Hypertensive emergencies. *N.Engl.J.Med.* 290:211-214, Jan. 24, 1974.
2. DELGRECO, FRANCESCO, AND KRUMLOVSKY, F. A. Malignant hypertension. *Hosp.Med.* 9:8-26, July 1973.
3. WINTROBE, M. M. AND OTHERS, EDS. *Harrison's Principles of Internal Medicine.* 6th ed. New York, McGraw-Hill Book Co., 1970, pp. 225-228.
4. BURRELL, L. O., AND BURRELL, Z. L. *Intensive Nursing Care.* 2d ed. St. Louis, C. V. Mosby Co., 1973, pp. 95-97.
5. GOODMAN, L. S., AND GILMAN, ALFRED. *Pharmacological Basis of Therapeutics.* 4th ed. New York, Macmillan Co., 1970, pp. 181-186.
6. FINNERTY, F. A., JR. Hypertensives in crisis. *Emerg.Med.* 8:59-66, Feb. 1974.
7. BREST, A. N., AND OTHERS. *Hypertension and its complications.* Philadelphia, Jefferson Medical College, 1970. (Pamphlet)
8. BEESON, P. B., AND MCDERMOTT, WALSH, EDS. *Cecil-Loeb Textbook of Medicine.* 13th ed. Philadelphia, W. B. Saunders Co., 1971, pp. 1194-1195.

From the *American Journal of Nursing* 75:1132-1133, July 1975.

Peripheral Pulses

COLLEEN SPARKS

Palpation and evaluation of peripheral pulses are significant steps in a thorough vascular assessment. Most peripheral pulses are difficult to locate, so practice is needed to develop this skill.

A pulse is felt when the arterial wall expands in response to the increase in aortic pressure when the left ventricle contracts and ejects blood into the filled aorta. Peripheral pulses are located over vessels in parts of the body other than the trunk—the head, neck, and extremities.

When a pulse cannot be palpated, the problem may be faulty heart function, as in congestive heart failure or cardiac arrest; decreased blood volume, as in hemorrhage; or some obstruction to blood flow, such as a thrombus or embolus proximal to the point where the pulse should be palpable.

When a patient is not being monitored electronically, the presence or absence of the femoral or carotid pulse quickly establishes whether cardiac arrest has occurred. These pulses also are used to evaluate the adequacy of perfusion during resuscitation.

After major vascular surgery, such as repair of an aortic aneurysm or iliac-femoral bypass graft, absence or decrease in the quality of a peripheral pulse may be the first indication of vessel blockage due to a thrombus or embolus.

Arteriovascular disease predisposes to obstruction of circulation to the

MS. SPARKS, R.N., M.S., *is an assistant professor of nursing at the University of California, Los Angeles.*

lower extremities or head. This can be due to spasm and constriction of the arteries, as in Raynaud's disease, but more frequently the obstruction is due to an atheromatous plaque, a thrombus, or an embolus. Occlusion can occur following a decrease in blood pressure or blood volume or when there are such predisposing factors as atherosclerosis.

Atherosclerosis usually affects the larger arteries, such as the aorta, carotid, iliac, and femoral arteries. Plaque formation in these vessels is spotty rather than continuous. These plaques narrow the lumen of the artery and so impair circulation, or the rough edges of the plaques can disrupt the smooth flow of blood, facilitating thrombus formation. These thrombi can break off and become emboli to smaller vessels, such as the cerebral or pedal arteries.

In any of these arteriovascular conditions peripheral pulses taken over a period of time, during several clinic or office visits or over the course of hospitalization, for example, can be helpful in establishing the severity and progress of a vascular condition. Occlusions usually occur one segment higher than the site of overt symptoms—pain, numbness, or gangrene.

SITES

Pulses are usually palpated over arteries which lie close to the body surface and over a bone or other firm surface that supports the artery when pressure is exerted. The most commonly used sites for peripheral pulse palpation are over the temporal, carotid, brachial, radial, femoral, popliteal, dorsalis pedis, and posterior tibialis arteries. Because the radial and brachial sites are used so frequently, identification of these sites will not be discussed.

The *temporal* pulse can be felt just anterior to the middle of the ear, at the mandibular joint. It can also be felt lateral to the eyebrow and anterior to the hairline, at the temple.

The *carotid* artery runs between the larynx and the sternocleidomastoid muscle in the neck. To palpate the carotid pulse, approach the patient from the front, push the sternocleidomastoid muscle to the side, and palpate the pulse against the lateral wall of the larynx. Or, because palpation against the trachea could occlude the airway, find larynx, run fingers to groove of muscle, and palpate there.

Locate the *femoral* pulse where this artery passes through the groin in the femoral triangle. This triangle is bordered superiorly by the inguinal ligament, laterally by the sartorius muscle, and medially by the adductor longus. The right and left common iliac arteries lead directly from the abdominal aorta, then split into the external and internal iliac. The exter-

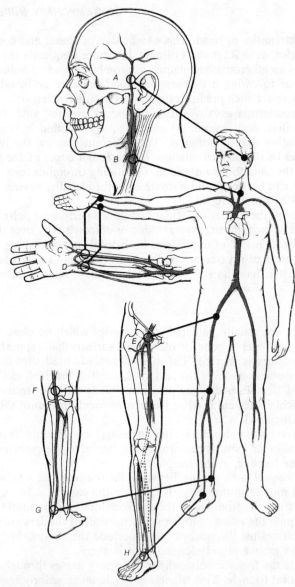

Peripheral pulses *give important clues to the patient's cardiovascular status.*
Some are more difficult to locate than others, so practice is necesary.
The most commonly used pulses include the temporal (A), carotid (B), radial
(C), ulnar (D), femoral (E), popliteal (F), posterior tibial (G), and dorsalis pedis (H).

nal iliac artery becomes the femoral artery as it passes under the inguinal ligament and enters the leg.

The femoral artery becomes the *popliteal* artery as it enters the knee. At the indentation in the back of the knee, the popliteal fossa, the popliteal artery is close to the surface and can be palpated. It is most easily felt if the patient can lie on his abdomen and flex his knee approximately 45 degrees.

The *dorsalis pedis* pulse is felt on the top of the foot, usually between the first and second metatarsal bones just above the longitudinal arch. However, in eight to 10 percent of the normal population, this pulse is either congenitally absent or so anomalously placed as to be undetectable. Therefore, absence of this pulse without other symptomatology is not indicative of arteriovascular disease.

The *posterior tibialis* pulse can be felt just posterior to the internal malleolus (ankle bone) on the inner aspect of the ankle.

HOW TO DO IT

Using the first three fingers, select the palpation site and place the fingers along the length of the artery. If the person's pulses are normal, the pulse usually can be felt immediately. Press the artery gently against the bone or underlying firm surface to occlude the vessel. Gently and gradually release the pressure. The pulse will be palpable as the blood again starts through the artery. If the carotid pulse is being palpated, be certain not to exert too much pressure, as stimulation of the carotid sinus can precipitate atrio-ventricular block, particularly in patients with MI.

The pulse rate and rhythm should be noted, and when evaluating peripheral pulses, it is important to assess the strength of the beat: full, bounding, weak, or faint. Another way of describing pulse quality is by numbers: 4+ is normal; 3+ is just slightly weaker or fainter; 2+, weak or faint; 1+, very weak; 0, no pulse palpable. The strength of the pulse also should be compared to the same pulse in the other extremity and to the next proximal pulse.

When pulses are difficult to locate and palpate, mark their location with a pen to facilitate locating them the next time. If a pulse is undetectable, vary the site slightly, and change the amount of finger pressure because pressure can obliterate a pulse.

In the absence of other symptoms, a weak or absent pulse should not be considered indicative of vascular problems. Again, comparisons should be made between the two limbs being assessed.

Color, skin condition, and temperature indicate the degree of circulatory insufficiency. These vary with the severity and cause of disease. The patient may experience numbness and tingling caused by poor oxygenation and ischemic neuropathy. Pain occurs and increases as circulation and oxygenation to an extremity are compromised.

Palpation of peripheral pulses, correlation of these data with other significant signs and symptoms, and correct interpretation of these parameters are important aspects of vascular assessment. This assessment is always important, but it is particularly vital in emergency situations, after major vascular surgery, or in patients with arteriovascular disease.

From the *American Journal of Nursing* 72:928-934, May 1972.

Chronic Peripheral Arterial Disease

BETTIE SPRINGER JACKSON

If you have ever been a "people watcher," you probably have noticed elderly persons walking very slowly and after a short distance, casually stopping, perhaps to window shop, and then continuing on. As they walk, this pattern is repeated. They may limp or have a guarded gait. They may stroke their limbs in the direction of arterial flow. You may well have been watching how people with chronic obstructive peripheral arterial disease or arteriosclerosis manage walking. (Here, the terms arteriosclerosis and atherosclerosis will be used interchangeably, for though they are different pathologically, long-term management is the same.)

Pathologically, the arteries of these people are either completely occluded by plaques or the elastica has broken down in such a way that there are minute sacculations. After a period of exercise, such as walking, tissue hypoxia and the build up of lactic acid, blood flow through saccular overstretched arterioles (the same mechanism as migraine headaches), or a combination of these produce weakness and pain, intermittent claudication, which is relieved by rest.

A patient may not know the physiology of his problem, but he has discovered that the only way to relieve calf pain while walking is to rest. Over a period of time, he may have found that he used to be able to walk four blocks without pain, then three, and so on until he may only be able to take a few paces without resting. Depending on the level of the

MS. JACKSON *received her B.S. in nursing from Columbia University, New York City. She worked with patients before and after arterial surgery and, as a graduate student at Columbia University Teachers College, she became interested in the medical management of the majority of patients who are ineligible for surgery. She has since received her M.Ed. from Teachers College.*

occlusion, he may complain of calf pain, calf and thigh pain, or deep pain in the buttocks extending down the legs. The disease may be unilateral or bilateral. With older persons, bilateral disease with leg muscle wasting and weakness is likely. Rubbing limbs to mechanically pump blood has no effect; the rest period is the critical factor.

Because arterial disease is a generalized process, coronary arteries may also be compromised. On one-half block exertion, a patient may have to stop because he is short of breath or is having an angina attack.

Reflex peripheral arterial constriction due to a cold environment further compromises arterial flow. Because of the poor circulation, sufferers of peripheral artery disease often complain of being cold all the time and usually seem to be overdressed for the weather.

CLINICAL DIAGNOSIS

Clinical diagnosis of obstructive peripheral arterial disease is not difficult. But, often this disease is left undiagnosed and untreated as sufferers attribute such subtle changes as hearing loss, failing memory, sight changes, and decreased exercise tolerance to "old age" and never report them.

In a history, a patient may report claudication, shortness of breath, hearing and sight failure, impotence, poor memory, and perhaps some expressive or receptive aphasia or both, or other neurologic symptoms. He may have leg pain when resting and find that sitting up is the only way to relieve the ache. Gravity may assist arterial flow. Limb positioning may be a problem if he has venous stasis as well. Dependent edema may occlude already precariously patent arterioles. In this situation, the patient may spend a great deal of time in bed with legs horizontal.

Classic appearance of affected limbs may include absence of hair, bluish pallor, blanching or paradoxic rubor, many degrees of ulcers or gangrene, coldness, thickened discolored nails, and absence of the dorsalis pedis, posterior tibial, and popliteal pulses depending on the level of the blockage. When his leg is raised and then lowered to a dependent position, arterial filling will be retarded or absent (indicated by failure of skin to return to its normal pink hue). His toes may be extremely tender and he can barely allow anyone to touch them. He may feel as though he is always walking on gravel. Neuropathy secondary to ischemia is commonly seen in this condition.

Arteriography is a useful diagnostic procedure if isolated occlusions are suspected. But, for patients with diffuse chronic arterial disease, arteriography is an involved procedure which requires hospitalization and only documents what can be seen on physical examination.

The pathophysiology of arteriosclerosis is slowly being elucidated as more is discovered about cholesterol and, more specifically, triglyceride metabolism, but we are a long way from using this knowledge in cither a first line of defense or an offense against this disease. Once the arteriosclerotic process begins, there are no definitive weapons that can be prescribed to reverse it. There are only measures which may retard it.

EPIDEMIOLOGIC APPROACH

Using an epidemiologic framework, we can examine what is known about chronic occlusive arterial disease.

AGENT FACTORS Beta-lipoproteins have been identified as the key agent in chronic arterial disease. Cholesterol has long been implicated as the primary causative agent whether due to dietary intake or the body's own synthesis. In the 1960's researchers found that serum cholesterol is independent of dietary control and the body has its own feedback-regulating system to maintain a fairly constant level. However, dietary intake of saturated fats increases circulating serum triglycerides which have been identified as primary causative agents in atherosclerosis.

Whether dietary management has any effect on already existing arterial disease is controversial. Some physicians say it does and prescribe low fat diets while others see diet therapy as a futile effort once the disease process has begun. But, because controversy does exist at this point, dietary management should be included in the treatment.

HOST FACTOR Striking pathologic findings on autopsy reveal atherosclerotic changes in the most apparently healthy teenagers. This is more evident in boys than in girls because of the differences in circulating estrogen levels which affect fat metabolism. Women are apparently protected by estrogen until about the fifth decade. Then, after menopause, women's arteries become sclerotic at a rapid rate which soon brings their level of disease up to that experienced by men.

International studies have been done on classes and occupations of people and their psychosocial milieu. Coronary occlusions and occupations with associated emotional tensions have high correlations. Fight, fright, and flight evoke specific physiologic responses including arterial spasm, occlusion, and shunting of blood, which can produce hypoxia in both the periphery and the myocardium.

ENVIRONMENTAL FACTORS Nationality differences in prevalence of atherosclerosis are quite remarkable, but they are not static. Dietary variances, changes in food preparation, physical activity, and emotional milieu are all contributing to changing international population statistics.

There is evidence that the incidence of atherosclerosis is increasing in Americans, who, as a population, are living longer. Generally, incipient signs and symptoms of arterial disease appear in the fifth decade and become more obvious with age.

Also, Americans continue to consume the largest amounts of saturated fats. Despite the fact that they are generally a weight-conscious people, they are overweight. Arterial circulation in fat tissue is minimal and main arteries, especially when they are plaqued with disease, are unable to supply excess tissue with oxygenated blood.

Exercise stimulates the formation of collateral circulation because of tissue oxygen demands under hypoxic conditions. This is a healthy process. However, among many Americans, physical exercise is not a pleasurable pastime, but a burdensome strain. Thus, a vicious cycle is established: people who do not exercise or practice dietary discretion do not develop substantial collaterals while they do slowly develop arterial occlusions, which in turn limit their ability to exercise.

TREATMENT

The majority of patients with peripheral arterial occlusive disease can only be treated medically because of the diffuse nature of the disease. The regimen usually includes a vasodilator drug, orders to stop smoking, exercise, meticulous foot care, and fat controlled diet.

SMOKING Nicotine is a potent vasoconstrictor-vasospastic agent. Smoking severely jeopardizes a patient's already impaired circulation. No battery of medicines and physical exercises can be effective if a patient continues to smoke. On the other hand, there have been improvements in oscillometrics (measurement of arterial pulsation through a limb) and foot temperature in patients whose only therapy has been to stop smoking.

MEDICATIONS Statistics on the effectiveness of various vasodilators, arterial antispasmodics, and hypocholesteremic drugs vary from study to study. There are wide discrepancies in what a drug company calls effective, what the physician sees clinically, and how a patient feels.

So often when patients first seek treatment, they are encouraged when the doctor prescribes a few drugs. They anticipate dramatic results when they really should be advised against great expectations. Foot temperature and oscillometrics may improve, but this is hardly convincing evidence of improvement to the patient who feels no better.

344

It isn't easy, but the nurse can help a patient to understand that although he may not feel any different, the tests show there is improved circulation due to a combination of drugs, diet, exercise, and not smoking. She can explain that this means blood is flowing better to areas that were being nourished very poorly or not at all, and she can point out that leg ulcers are healing or at least not worsening. Patients' symptoms may not change, but the treatment is preventing or minimizing chances of complications such as gangrene. The nurse must be extremely understanding, patient, and persistent in helping patients to adhere to the regimen despite their impulse to quit.

Some patients are not candidates for vasodilators because of coronary artery disease and borderline cardiac function and could be harmed by vasodilators which cause reflex tachycardia. Also, some physicians feel that some claudication is a sort of safety valve against more vigorous activity which might precipitate angina or a myocardial infarction.

A patient who does not get a prescription for "the special pill my friend is on to open up his arteries" needs to know that they would not benefit him and, in his individual situation, might do him more harm. Other aspects of care should be emphasized as best suited for him.

Antihypertensive drugs are being used but with some caution. If a patient has long-standing hypertension secondary to arteriosclerosis, his whole body has adjusted its function to that setting. When his blood pressure is lowered, there is a risk of decreased renal circulation, cerebral hypoxia, and generalized decreased peripheral perfusion.

Antilipemic drugs offer some hope presently. Sodium dextrothyroxine (Choloxin), other thyroid drugs, and the female estrogens have lowered serum cholesterol levels but they are not without inherent unpleasant and sometimes intolerable side effects, particularly in men. Clofibrate (Atromid S) offers new hope in reducing triglycerides and cholesterol. While it will not reverse already existing disease, it is proving to be effective in retarding the progress of atherosclerosis by decreasing serum lipids.

A B-complex vitamin may be prescribed, but its effect in reducing symptoms of ischemic neuropathy is questionable.

Drug expense may be a problem. If so, the physician may decide not to prescribe certain medications which have an unproved effect. Also, the nurse can suggest resources available to help the patient pay for necessary medications.

Often, patients medicate themselves for pain. Knowing what, when, and the amount of drugs a patient is already taking and whether these drugs are effective will give some hints as to how severely he is affected.

DRUGS USED IN TREATING PERIPHERAL ARTERIAL DISEASE

nonproprietary name	proprietary name	single oral dose	effects	remarks
VASODILATORS VASCULAR ANTISPASMODICS			Act at various sites to relax smooth muscle of blood vessel walls to increase the diameter of constricted vessels and increase blood flow to hypoxic tissues. Their effect on blood vessels made rigid by atherosclerotic plaques is questionable.	
adrenergic blocking agents: azapetine phosphate phenoxybenzamine HCl pentolamine HCl tolazoline HCl	Ilidar Dibenzyline Regitine Priscoline	50-75 mg. 20-60 mg. 50-100 mg. 50-75 mg.	Decreases vasospasm by interfering with ability of adrenergic receptors in vascular smooth muscle to receive vasoconstrictor impulses from sympathetic nerve endings.	High doses cause systemic vasodilatation which decreases BP and produces dizziness, weakness, faintness, fatigue, postural hypotension, reflex tachycardia. Contraindicated for cardiac patients; may precipitate angina attacks.
ganglionic blocking agents: chlorisondamine chloride mecamylamine HCl pentolinium tartrate trimethidinum methosulfate	Ecolid Inversine Ansolysen Ostensin	10-50 mg. 25-25 mg. 20-60 mg. 20-40 mg.	Decreases transmission of vasoconstrictor impulses from sympathetic ganglionic relay stations in brain.	High doses cause same side effects of systemic vasodilatation as above. If vessels are too sclerotic to dilate, blood may be shunted away from areas where it is needed most.
sympathetic amines: isoxsuprine HCl nylidrin HCl	Vasodilan Arlidin	10-20 mg. 6 mg.	Structural resemblance to epinephrine. Increases blood flow through ischemic vessels in skeletal muscles in limbs by stimulating adrenergic receptors, which in skeletal muscle vessels are inhibitory and respond to sympathetic impulse by vasodilatation. Questionably effective for intermittent claudication.	Few side effects, no tachycardia. Contraindicated in coronary artery disease.
parasympathomimetic (cholinergic) agents: methacholine Br methacholine Cl	Mecholyl Br Mecholyl Cl	200 mg. (20 mg. S.C. and 0.2-0.5% sol. for iontophoresis)	Long acting choline ester causes peripheral superficial vasodilatation. Questionably effective for leg ulcers in arterial and venous disease.	Side effects similar to food poisoning, i.e. diarrhea, cramps. To avoid systemic action, drug often given directly into skin with an electric current (iontophoresis).
direct-acting vascular antispasmodics: cyclandelate nicotinyl tartrate	Cyclospasmol Roniacol	200 mg. 50-150 mg.	Acts directly to relax smooth muscles of peripheral vascular beds, increases local circulation. Effective for leg ulcers; not been proven effective for obstructive disease.	Dizziness, flushing as with nitroglycerine and papaverine for coronary artery disease.
ALCOHOL	brandy	½-1 oz. BID or TID	Peripheral vasodilatation, sense of well-being, euphoria.	Moral aversion, addiction, intoxication.
HYPOCHOLESTEROLEMICS ANTILIPEMICS			These drugs must always be used in conjunction with a controlled low fat diet. They do not improve the condition of already disease-damaged vessels. They may act by interfering with cholesterol metabolism, inhibiting biosynthesis of cholesterol in the liver, or speeding breakdown of cholesterol to bile acids. Initial cholesterol decrease is often negated by the body's response and production of cholesterol.	
beta-sitosterols cholestyramine colestipol	Cytellin Cuemid, Questran	½-1 oz. a.c.	Believed to interfere with absorption and increase fecal excretion of dietary cholesterol.	Must be used in conjunction with dietary regimen. Large doses may cause gastrointestinal upset.
neomycin and other antibiotics			Lowers cholesterol available for lipoprotein synthesis in liver by diverting cholesterol and bile acids from the gut into the feces which increases rate of excretion. (Surgical bypass of the ileum has similar effects.)	Any antibiotic (especially one effective against gram negative bacilli) may be used. Suppresses normal intestinal flora and may cause development of resistant bacteria.

The nurse can help the patient discuss pain and analgesics with the doctor, explore the reasons for pain, and suggest measures to relieve it.

None of the drugs listed here are free of side effects. These side effects may be compounded by other drugs the patient is taking. He may need

nonproprietary name	proprietary name	single oral dose	effects	remarks
aliphatic fatty acids	Triparanol (MER 29) AY 9944		Inhibits cholesterol synthesis in liver and other tissues.	Experimental. Not used on human subjects because of toxic effect in liver and adrenal glands.
clofibrate	Atromid S	500 mg. QID	Decreases elevated serum triglycerides and cholesterol possibly by interfering with cholesterol synthesis in liver. Also, brings about desirable reduction in coagulability of blood, It will not reverse already existing disease but may retard further atherosclerosis by decreasing serum lipids.	Fairly new. Because of experience with Triparanol (also hepatic biosynthesis inhibitor) liver and adrenal toxicity, drug used cautiously; to date only minor side effects noted: nausea, flatulence, diarrhea.
niacin aluminum nicotinate	Nicotinic acid Nicalex		In massive doses (as much as 50 times the daily requirement) may decrease cholesterol and other serum lipids.	Side effects include flushing, itching of face and neck, gastrointestinal upset.
dextrothyroxine sodium (thyroid hormone)	Choloxin	60-120 mg. BID or TID	In large doses may reduce cholesterol, by stimulating liver to increase breakdown and excretion of cholesterol.	Large doses may cause hyperthyroidism and hypermetabolism which may aggravate coronary artery disease. Should only be given to patients with normal thyroid function.
heparin		given I.V.	I.V. dose given after a meal known to clear plasma made cloudy by absorbed fats.	Antilipemic effect is not observed when given orally. The drug will not effect chronic arterial occlusion because of short term lipemia-clearing effect.
diethylstilbesterol (estrogens)	Stilbetin Stilbesterol	0.1-2.5 mg.	May reduce circulating serum lipids, based on clinical evidence of rare coronary artery disease in premenopausal women. Effectiveness in prophylaxis still to be established.	Large doses cause feminizing effects in men, uterine bleeding in post-menopausal women, and anorexia, nausea, and vomiting in both.
vitamin B_{12}			Questionably effective in reducing symptoms of diabetic peripheral neuropathy.	
ANTIHYPERTENSIVES	Lower arterial pressure by reducing peripheral resistance through vasodilatation.			
hydralazine HCl	Apresoline	40-400 mg.	Acts at vasomotor center and directly on smooth muscles of blood vessels to decrease peripheral resistance.	May be too stimulating for patients with coronary artery disease (combined with Rauwolfia may prevent tachycardia). Headache, fever, general malaise, gastrointestinal irritation may occur.
methyldopa	Aldomet	375-750 mg.	Close chemical relative of catecholamines. Reduces biosynthesis of sympathetic neurotransmitter, norepinephrine, to cause vasodilatation and decreased BP.	May cause moderate postural hypotension and shunting of blood from areas relying on higher blood pressure for perfusion. Drug tolerance may develop.

Information adapted from "Treatment of hyperlipidemia" by R. S. Lees and D. E. Wilson, New England Journal of Medicine, January 28, 1971 and Pharmacology and Drug Therapy in Nursing by M. J. Rodman and Dorothy W. Smith, J. B. Lippincott Co., 1968.

instruction on how to take and what to expect from other drugs as well as the vasodilators. The drug regimen can become quite involved, and the patient may benefit from a written schedule for reference.

It is important for a nurse to be with the patient when the physician is talking with him. Then, if he has no questions or is hesitant to ask about his therapy the nurse can ask for him. Afterward, she can sit down with him and review drugs and other aspects of treatment that have just been prescribed. Group classes may also be a consideration as an opportunity for a number of patients to get together to share their feelings and exchange helpful hints. Whenever possible, another family member should be included in any instruction sessions.

EXERCISE Exercise for a healthy 20-year-old and a 70-year-old with chronic occlusive peripheral artery disease mean very different things. But, often an elderly patient is told, without any specifications, that despite the pain in his legs he must exercise. Exercise, here, refers specifically to exercise for the patient over 50 years old with clinically diagnosed peripheral artery disease.

Flat-surface walking is the best form of exercise. Evaluate how far the patient is able to walk before he develops claudication and what kind of pace he sets. Acknowledge that he may be discouraged if he can only walk one-half block at a slow pace. Walk with him at a very slow pace and help him set short and realistic goals for himself: one block this week, a little farther next week, and so forth. Over a period of time, there should be some improvement. No matter how slight this improvement is, encourage him continually by comparing his current tolerance to his past: "Mr. Jones, I know it is difficult and frustrating, but remember six months ago you couldn't walk half a block without stopping because of the pain in your legs. Now you can even go to the grocery three blocks from your home."

Stairs can be monumental to maneuver. Climb stairs with the patient if he must do so at home. Evaluate what he can and cannot manage by himself. Perhaps a cane, a walker, or some other assistive device is necessary.

Different activities require different amounts of energy. Advise patients to rest when they develop pain. Their pain usually indicates that the arteries are inadequate to supply blood to meet the metabolic demands of that tissue.

Patients may benefit from exercises that they can do for a few minutes a day at home to stimulate collateral arterial formation.

However, even home exercises are difficult for a patient to do if the chilliness in his home causes vasoconstriction. Patients who live in poorly heated apartments may need help in contacting superintendents or landlords and in notifying the local department of housing to remedy the situation.

Home exercises, such as Buerger or Buerger-Allen exercises, use positioning and gravity to improve blood flow(1). Gravity is used to alternately fill and empty the arteries. One rule states that the legs should be in the down position three times as long as in the up position. Other phy-

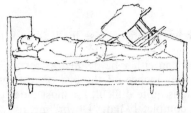

To Start: Straightback chair with a pillow or some other padding is placed on a bed. Patient lies flat on his back in bed.

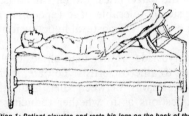

Position 1: Patient elevates and rests his legs on the back of the padded chair for about two minutes or until his legs become pale.

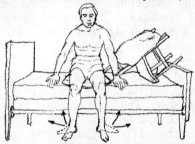

Position 2: Patient lowers his legs, sits up, and dangles for about three minutes or until his legs become pink. While dangling, he moves his feet through six positions: he points his toes down, up, in, out, spreads them, returns to neutral position, and repeats.

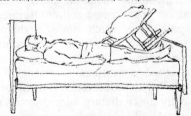

Position 3: Patient returns to flat starting position for about five minutes and then repeats the exercise.

Adapted from *Bed Exercises for Convalescent Patients* by Nila K. Coralt, Springfield, Ill., Charles C Thomas publisher, 1968, pp. 136-137.

sicians prefer to have a patient raise his legs until they blanch and then lower them until they become pink.

The up position can either be defined as resting flat as on a bed and raising the legs a few inches off the bed or just resting completely flat. Because leg raising is quite difficult for most older people, "up" is better defined as resting completely flat. "Down" means to dangle the legs over the edge of the bed.

Between 5 and 10 Buerger exercises, done 2 to 3 times a day, should help blood flow to the extremities. Patients need help at first in order to set a slow and physically tolerable pace (speed is not the objective) and to assure stability, especially if postural hypotension is a problem.

DIET THERAPY Triglycerides rather than cholesterol have been identified as the agent leading to atherosclerosis. To date, there is enough evidence to draw some correlations between diet and atherosclerosis; but, a number of such questions as to whether reducing serum cholesterol to normal will prevent development of further atherosclerosis or reverse the disease process and whether diet can prevent the formation of atherosclerosis in persons predisposed by familial prevalence, remain unanswered(2). Still, dietary management should be employed as a first line of preventing disease starting with infants and as a method of treating existing disease.

The American Medical Association, the American Heart Association, and the Department of Health, Education, and Welfare recommend various fat controlled diets. The basic objective of these diets is to reduce the triglycerides and, by using unsaturated fats, bring the ratio of saturated and polyunsaturated fat calories down from the usual 2:1, found in most diets, to 1:1(3).

An individualized diet is based on a comprehensive dietary history. What does the patient know about balanced nutrition? Does he know what foods are sources of saturated and unsaturated fats? Who does the cooking and shopping? How much money is there for groceries? What are his particular tastes based on cultural background, likes, dislikes, and allergies? What constitutes a typical meal for him? How is food prepared? How much food constitutes a serving? Is he used to having between meal snacks? This information should be used in helping the patient and his family make dietary adaptations so that their entire life style need not be drastically changed.

Dietary habits are considered by many people to be very personal and they are quite sensitive about their tastes and budget. Set aside at least one-half hour for your first contact with the patient about his diet and make the purpose of the interview crystal clear. Because your patient may or may not be hard of hearing or easily confused, depending on the extent of his disease, provide a quiet atmosphere for the session. Anticipate questions. Write things down and make adjustments in printed guidelines you may be using.

Older persons who require diet teaching may already be on one or more special diets, such as low salt, diabetic, low purine, and so forth. This makes diet teaching much more complex and, for the patient, much more confining. For instance, the Giovanetti diet used widely for renal failure is low in protein and high in fat in order to supply calories. The high fat component of this diet is incompatible with the low fat diet for patients with atherosclerosis.

Where more than one diet prescription must be combined, the nurse can either refer these complex dietary situations to the nutritionist or, before having a teaching session with the patient, obtain a dietary history from the patient and work out lists of compatible foods.

Follow-up instruction must be done and should be specifically scheduled rather than squeezed into time set aside for another purpose.

Again, anticipate that patients will probably not notice any changes in their circulation on the fat controlled diet. If they have lost considerable weight, they may feel generally better. But, as previously mentioned, it is not known if atherosclerosis can be reversed, and patients must be reassured that the diet is really aimed at reducing the progression of the disease and for that reason it is a necessity.

Finally, the federal government and local organizations around the country support a number of hot lunch programs for senior citizens. These are a wonderful means of supplying senior citizens with at least one well-balanced meal a day and they can often be individualized for people on special diets. But, often funds run short and these programs have to be discontinued. Part of the nursing intervention may be to let the appropriate people know of the vital need for such projects.

FOOT CARE The feet are at the body's periphery and are the last to be supplied by any blood that can be pumped through occluded arteries and arterioles. Take a careful look at the patient's feet. Is he a bathroom surgeon? Is there anything to suggest that he has been whittling his calluses? Are his feet dirty, dry, cracked, ulcerated? Are his socks clean and do his shoes fit properly?

Feet must be washed daily with soap and warm water. Cold water constricts vessels and, depending on his neurologic status, water too hot may burn or cause extreme pain. The patient should dry his feet thoroughly by gently patting rather than rubbing abrasively and then cream them with lanolin or petroleum jelly to prevent cracking. Lamb's wool may be placed between the toes to prevent irritation.

Toenails grow very slowly and need trimming infrequently. This is best done after the bath. Toenails should be trimmed straight across. If they are too thick to cut, they may be filed, or better, cut by a chiropodist. When the patient inspects his feet, he should look for any signs of blisters, ingrown toenails, or infection. Small breaks in the skin may never heal because of the patient's diminished circulation. If discovered, they should be bandaged, left alone, and reported immediately to the physician or nurse.

It is not unusual for a patient to wash his feet and put on clean socks because he is coming to see the doctor. The nurse ought to stress the importance of wearing clean socks or stockings every day. The fabric should be wool or cotton, not nylon. Nylon is not as absorbent and feet remain soggy and macerate.

Sometimes, patients with arterial and venous disease wear support stockings or socks which are tight enough to occlude arterioles. Check with the physician regarding the patient's use of such support hose. In any case, the patient must be instructed not to wear constricting garters, foundation garments, or hosiery. If the patient's feet get cold during the night, he should be told to wear bed socks instead of using hot water bottles or electric heating pads to keep his feet warm.

Sitting with crossed legs, sitting or standing in one position for prolonged periods, and sleeping under tightly drawn bed linen should be discouraged because these retard arterial and venous circulation.

Shoes, of course, should be comfortable and non-constrictive. New shoes should be broken in gradually to prevent initial irritation. Leather soles are preferable to rubber soles because rubber interferes with proper ventilation. Wet or damp shoes should be dried slowly on shoe trees or stuffed with paper to help them retain their shape(4). And, patients ought never to go barefooted.

NO GUARANTEES

At best, medical management of arteriosclerosis is palliative and maintaining. At worst, it is utterly discouraging, expensive, ineffective, and cannot guarantee against complications.

The effectiveness of the various therapies prescribed are often directly related to the patient's willingness and determination to follow each aspect of the regimen. The nurse can have a direct effect on this. However, it is only realistic to acknowledge that the highest level of nursing care does not guarantee patient enthusiasm and participation. Nor do all the nurse's efforts and patient response guarantee success in disease treatment. What docs the nurse say to a patient who has been encouraged and supported and then develops gangrene and other circulatory problems anyway? No combination of therapy offers a guarantee of success, but it may offer more time without complications and may help to minimize the gravity of complications that do occur.

REFERENCES

1. BELAND, IRENE I. *Clinical Nursing: Pathophysiological and Psychosocial Aspects.* 2d ed. New York, The Macmillan Co., 1970, p. 422.
2. WILLIAMS, SUE R. *Nutrition and Diet Therapy.* St. Louis, C. V. Mosby Co., 1969, p. 524.
3. *Ibid.*, p. 528.
4. BRUNNER, LILLIAN S., AND OTHERS. *Textbook of Medical-Surgical Nursing.* 2d ed. New York, J. B. Lippincott Co., 1970, p. 330.

BIBLIOGRAPHY

CECIL, R. L., AND LOEB, R. F. *Textbook of Medicine.* 12th edition edited by Paul B. Beeson and Walsh McDermott. Philadelphia, W. B. Saunders Co., 1963.
DIET AND VASCULAR DISEASE. *Lancet* 1:183, Jan. 24, 1970.
ELIZABETH, SISTER MARY. Occlusion of the peripheral arteries: nursing observations and symptomatic care. *Am.J.Nurs.* 67:562-564, Mar. 1967.
LEES, R. S., AND WILSON, D. T. Treatment of hyperlipidemia. *N.Engl.J.Med.* 284:186-193, Jan. 28, 1971.
MAVOR, G. E. Advances in the treatment of peripheral vascular disease. *Practitioner* 203: 468-482. Oct. 1969.
RODMAN, M. J., AND SMITH, DOROTHY W. *Pharmacology and Drug Therapy in Nursing.* Philadelphia, J. B. Lippincott Co., 1968.
SHANNON, J. A. Medical reseach: some aspects that warrant public understanding. *N.Engl.J.Med.* 284-80. Jan. 14, 1971.
TESTS *of Fat-Controlled Diets for Prevention of Coronary Heart Disease.* (An annotated bibliograph) Englewood, N.J., Best Foods Research Center, CPP International, June 1970.

From the American Journal of Nursing 74:258-259, Feb. 1974.

Chronic Leg Ulcers

JAMES C. COBEY • JANET H. COBEY

Different physiological mechanisms are responsible for the development of arterial and venous ulcers, and they require different treatment.

Nurses practicing in outpatient clinics and in community settings are often the primary professionals responsible for the ongoing treatment of patients with chronic leg ulcers. Most patients with leg ulcers are over 40 years old, and many have other chronic diseases as well as social and economic problems that may affect the treatment of these diseases. Success in treating these patients requires that the nurse assume responsibility for the day-to-day evaluation of illness and treatment.

Patients are referred to nurses after an initial examination by a physician. Frequently these patients are referred without a clear diagnosis of the type of ulcer and without a treatment regimen.

Proper diagnosis is essential because treatment results depend on an understanding of the pathophysiology of leg ulcers. Arterial diseases must be differentiated from venous insufficiency since the mode of treatment for each is quite different.

Arterial ulcers are caused by occlusion of large or small vessels. The usual manifestations of large vessel disease are sudden pain, pallor, pulselessness, coolness, or chronically progressive intermittent claudication. To diagnose large vessel occlusions, femoral, popliteal, anterior

DR. COBEY *received his M.D. and M.P.H. degrees from Johns Hopkins Schools of Medicine and Hygiene, Baltimore, Md. He is affiliated with the Department of Orthopedic Surgery, Yale University Medical School, New Haven, Conn. MS. COBEY received her B.S.N. degree from the University of Michigan, Ann Arbor, Mich. and her M.P.H. from Johns Hopkins School of Hygiene.*

tibial, and posterior tibial pulses in both legs must be palpated. An absent or diminished pulse may indicate a proximal obstruction that can be corrected surgically. Acute large vessel arterial disease alone usually does not produce chronic ulcers.

Small vessel arterial disease is caused by chronic occlusion of small arteries or arterioles, usually in patients with diabetes or atherosclerosis. The leg is cold and pale, with loss of hair and atrophy of the skin. Ulceration, infection, and gangrene can complicate small artery disease.

In treating small vessel disease one must be certain that there are no localized infections in the extremity and that there are no localized pressure areas from poorly fitted shoes. The patient must be taught to protect his feet from any form of trauma.

If arterial ulcers do occur, they must be kept clean and dry to prevent secondary infection. Pressure can be avoided by using sponge rubber or polyurethane boots to distribute weight evenly over the foot.

Venous ulcer disease is a consequence of one or more episodes of thrombophlebitis. There are two venous systems in the lower leg, the deep system and the superficial saphenous system. Blood is returned to the heart in the deep system by muscular action of the legs supported by the tight fibrous fascia of the leg. The superficial saphenous system has no surrounding heavy fascia to give it support. Between the two systems, small perforating veins with valves allow blood to flow from the external saphenous system into the internal system, then back up to the heart. After thrombophlebitis, the affected veins often recanalize and are patent again, but without valves. Therefore, the hydrostatic weight of a column of blood from the heart to the lower extremity tends to cause peripheral edema which can cause ulcerations.

Patients with peripheral edema complain of an aching discomfort, tenderness, or heaviness in the lower leg. Physical findings include edema, brawny induration, brownish discoloration, dryness, and scaling.

Patients with long standing peripheral edema may develop stasis ulcers. These venous ulcers are almost always found in the distal third of the lower leg and are particularly common posterior and superior to the medical and lateral malleoli where there is little subcutaneous tissue. The ulcers usually form over the perforating vessels that connect the deep venous system to the superficial.

Venous disease is treated with elevation and support of the saphenous system to promote venous return. The patient must keep his legs elevated as much as possible and wear support stockings or elastic bandages from the toes to just below the knees to give support to the superficial venous system and minimize peripheral edema. The upper part of the bandage must not be as tight as the lower part or a tourniquet effect will occur. Preferably, the bandage should not extend to the popliteal area; if it must, it should not be wrapped tightly. If the bandages are to extend above the knee, adhesive tape strips applied on each side will keep the bandage from rolling up behind the knee.

A venous ulcer can be treated by collapsing the perforating vein and venules in the tissue under the ulcer. This prevents transmission of hydrostatic pressure to this tissue across the perforating venules. Some physicians advocate surgery to tie off perforating veins; however, surgery can be dangerous and may lead to many complications unless the ulcer is completely healed and epithelialized first. The most efficient method for collapsing perforating venules is to apply local pressure over the ulcer, using 4x4 all-gauge pads that are cut to the exact size of the granulating ulcer. Three to four layers are applied over the ulcer and the leg is wrapped with an elastic bandage. No cotton should be placed on the ulcer since the cotton fibers tend to stick to the wound. This dressing localizes the edematous tissue under the ulcer. As the ulcer heals, the dressings are cut to a smaller size.

Topical antibiotics, steroids, creams, petroleum jelly, or antibiotic gauzes are not indicated. All open sores, including leg ulcers, have bacterial flora which cannot be eradicated until epithelialization is complete. Systemic antibiotics may be given, however, if there is cellulitis in the legs. The leg should be washed daily with soap and carefully rinsed to remove all traces of soap. If soap is left on, it may macerate the skin. After the leg is dry, the dry dressing is applied. This is actually a wet-to-dry dressing since venous ulcers are wet to begin with. This often heals ulcers dramatically.

After the ulcer is healed, the patient should still wear elastic bandages to keep the veins from dilating again and ulcer from recurring. It is important to remember that, if the legs are washed, all the soap must be removed to prevent skin irritation. For older people with dry skin, mineral oil or lanolin oil helps keep the skin moist. After complete epithelialization of the ulcer, surgery may be indicated to correct the disease.

To summarize: chronic arterial ulcers are caused by small vessel disease, recognized by loss of hair and cool dry skin, and treated by keeping them clean, dry, and free from pressure; venous ulcers are caused by hydrostatic pressure secondary to poor venous return, recognized by indurated, discolored, edematous skin with ulceration over the malleoli, and treated by elevation, support of venous return, and local pressure to collapse perforating venules.

From the *American Journal of Nursing* 74:260-262, Feb. 1974.

Home Care After Peripheral Vascular Surgery

MARY ANN ROSE

The diabetic patient who enters an acute care facility for peripheral vascular surgery has particular needs requiring nurse assistance. But what happens to this patient and his family once he leaves the hospital?

For the past year I have been making home visits to these postoperative patients and their families on the referral of a vascular surgeon. The patients referred for home nursing care are usually elderly, diabetic, and may have other medical problems such as congestive heart failure. In addition, they frequently have ulcers on the heel or lower leg because of poor peripheral circulation.

People expect different things from me. The physician believes the nurse is an extension of himself and will keep an eye on the arterial reconstruction and watch for early warning signs of complications. The patients and families usually have some concerns about assuming total care themselves and express relief that "doctor is sending someone out." While these expectations are more narrow and limited than my own, they are not inconsistent with my aim of promoting optimal health.

To ensure continuity of care, I visit the patients in the hospital before they are discharged. This gives me an opportunity to talk with the nurses about any problems that have arisen, and the solutions they use. Also, I can help the family make realistic plans for home equipment. Usually, very little equipment is required for home care, but families are often

MS. ROSE *has a B.S.N. degree from Georgetown University School of Nursing, Washington, D.C. She has worked as a public health nurse and is now a graduate student at Case Western Reserve University, Cleveland, Ohio. She is coordinator of nursing for the Cancer Center of Northeast Ohio.*

eager to help and spend much money unnecessarily. I suggest to the patient and family that I visit soon after discharge and this seems to provide some reassurance. After the first visit, we work out together how often I will come. I prefer to see families at least every two weeks and to keep in touch by telephone between visits. Some patients, of course, require more frequent visits.

Once home, the patient and family take a good look at the incision. Usually it is partially healed, but it may be draining slightly, and some patients come home with sutures still in place. These are removed during the first office visit with the physician. Often, a patient's first question is "Who's going to take those out?" Most don't seem to care who does this as long as someone does.

The incision is washed daily with tap water and Dial soap and rinsed. I help the patient and family feel at ease doing this. A shaving brush is soft and easy to use in cleaning the incision. Unless there are orders for a dressing, I encourage the patient to leave the area open to air.

Most patients are concerned about the ulcers. Frequently these are rather large craters on the heel which may be covered with a black crust. The physician I work with has tried various treatments, but he prefers a wash with soap and water followed by an application of Betadine dressings. Betadine is a nontoxic disinfectant which patients describe as soothing. Since the dressing dries out in a few hours, it should be remoistened with Betadine in an Asepto syringe or redressed periodically during the day. Redressing is impractical for many elderly patients because the contortions required to dress one's own heel are difficult.

We generally use unsterile, four-by-four gauze pads and circular gauze. The pads are not expensive, but circular gauze is, and it is not readily obtainable in this community. Some patients buy cheesecloth, cut it in wide strips to use in place of circular gauze, wash it after use, and then reuse it. The Betadine does stain linen and dressings orange, but the stain washes out.

Crusted ulcers can heal. The crust gradually chips off as the circumference of the involved tissue shrinks. Sometimes the dry, scaly skin at the ulcer's periphery comes off in strips. If this happens, I urge the patient and family to keep "hands off." They are tempted to cut away the peeling tissue, but I fear they might inadvertently traumatize healed tissue.

Sometimes healing is delayed by fluid trapped under the crust. This fluid can be felt by tapping the crust very gently with a tongue blade. The fluid portion feels soft. The crust over this area must be cut off. This is a simple but painful procedure, and I prefer the physician to do it.

The unaffected skin on the foot or leg is often extremely dry. I suggest that the family spread a little Crisco on this skin. Crisco is cheap and it works very well. The family may need a reminder to put it around, not on, the ulcer.

Besides ulcers, a patient may have one or more black toes. If they can be kept clean and dry, the toes will fall off by themselves. The patient can clean his toes by sloshing his foot in a basin of water to which a little mild dishwashing soap has been added. After this he should gently dry the foot and then, with a medicine dropper, drop 90-percent alcohol on the toes to keep them dry. Alcohol drops should be used at least four times a day. Ninety-percent alcohol is readily available in drug stores and is inexpensive.

Dry, necrotic toes are blackish-gray, brittle, and painless. Many patients are singularly unconcerned about losing them. Should wet necrosis develop, the black area looks the same, but a rather foul exudate comes from the base of the toe or nail. The alcohol drops should be continued if this problem develops. Lamb's wool between the toes keeps them dry as long as there is not a great deal of exudate. With profuse drainage, lamb's wool quickly becomes soggy and can macerate adjacent healthy tissue. In this situation, it is best to wash the foot and apply alcohol more frequently.

When the patient is soaking his foot, the loose toes tend to float at a right angle to the foot. This is a bizarre sight and can cause alarm. When the toes do fall off, the patient does not have pain—one man never even noticed! The alcohol treatment should be continued to keep the stump dry while it is healing.

One patient developed maggots at the stump site. Maggots eat dead tissue and his physician felt that this was advantageous. However, the family found the situation intolerable. The patient associated the maggots with death and his family thought they implied filth. Ether dropped on the site kills maggots.

Patients worry about their ability to walk. Although none of ours has been bedridden, a few have been asked to limit walking as much as possible. I reinforce these restrictions and suggest using a walker or wheelchair. When there are no specific activity limitations, I usually discuss ambulation with the patient and have him increase his activity gradually, using pain, healing progress, and swelling as indicators for increasing or decreasing his activity.

When a patient is not walking, his foot and leg should be elevated to prevent dependent edema. Edema will slow healing. Most patients have some swelling of the foot and lower leg during convalesence, but because many of the patients are elderly, I check carefully for signs of congestive heart failure, such as increased pulse rate, shortness of breath, or rales, when swelling occurs.

Other observations during a home visit should include a check on the peripheral pulses. If a patient has progressive arterial disease and has had an endarterectomy, the popliteal and pedal pulses may not be palpable. It is important to find out about the pulses before a patient leaves the hospital. If he had a bypass graft, the pulse underlying the incision should be full and the pedal pulse should be present.

Ulcers may be painful but this pain usually is not severe and can be relieved with a mild analgesic like Darvon or aspirin. More severe pain may be a symptom of arterial insufficiency. Besides feeling the pulses, I look at and feel the extremity itself. If an artery is blocked, the patient will have severe pain and that part of the leg will be pale and cold. The pulse above the affected area may not be palpable and the patient may not be able to move the extremity.

Nutrition is also important to the patient's recovery. He may have dietary restrictions because of his diabetes or other diseases, and may need help in this area. I also encourage an increased protein intake to promote healing. Many diabetic patients with vascular problems express guilt about their condition and its relation to diet. They may say, "If only I had stuck to my diet . . .," or a relative may say accusingly, "If he'd eaten what I cooked for him, this problem wouldn't have happened." While some authorities maintain that careful medical management can slow the development of diabetic vascular complications, others, including the physician I work with, maintain that even a well-controlled patient develops vascular problems. Keeping this in mind, I listen to the patient and then try to convey to him and his family that the diet business surely must be difficult and tiresome. I point out that diet is important to the patient's well-being but that the doctor says even the most careful diabetics can develop vascular problems. Most patients are surprised, but they still seem angry so I again comment that the whole vascular problem is certainly a difficult one for everyone.

Safety is another important consideration. Patients should wear some kind of foot covering when walking to protect intact skin from trauma. This can be improvised from something larger than the usual foot covering to accommodate the heel dressing, such as a large sock or a slipper or shoe with a portion cut out of it. The patient and family also must be careful when preparing the foot wash. The water temperature should be checked with the wrist, before the foot is put in. One of our patients was transferred to the hospital from another facility where she had received second-degree burns of the foot. She had been soaking her foot and complained about the water being too cool. Someone added "warm" water to the basin while her foot was in it. The "warm" water was hot.

We hope to avoid trauma from knives and scissors, which patients and their families use to cut off dressings or trim toenails. The kinds of appliances people use on their feet and legs are amazing. One diabetic patient told me she used a little electric sander to smooth her toenails. Another woman with a partially healed incision scratched her itchy skin with a knitting needle and inadvertently poked the needle right into the unhealed part of the incision.

Rehabilitation goals are achieved slowly. An elderly patient who can now sit at home with his foot up may have achieved his goals. The 60-year-old woman who has been active with her family and community may be anxious and depressed because of her temporary role change. Many people become quite distressed about the time it takes for the ulcers to heal. By talking about their distress, pointing out gains as they occur, and helping these patients to achieve the maximum activity they can while convalescing, the nurse can guide these patients to behave constructively.

Another source of anxiety for many patients is the knowledge that, if the vascular surgery proves unsuccessful, amputation is a possibility. The nurse's reassurance must be tempered by the fact that this is a realistic fear.

A number of diabetic patients with vascular problems also have diabetic retinopathy. The nurse must help them cope with the prospect of diminished or lost vision. She may encourage them to see an ophthalmologist and follow his suggestions. She may also suggest a low vision clinic, if one is available, to help patients learn to lead full lives despite their visual losses.

Finally, a word about availability. All the patients are given my telephone number and told that they can call me or the doctor at any time. Both he and I have been impressed with the volume of calls—his has been going down and mine has been going up. We feel that this is partly due to the fact that patients are calling for simple reassurance that things are going nicely and a professional person is indeed interested. I am easier to reach than the physician, and some patients found that when they called the doctor with a problem he frequently referred them to me. Now they call me first. Usually I can screen problems for nursing or medical intervention and, in addition, am able to spend more time exploring with the patient the nature of his problem. Sometimes this is enough.